Cardiac Pacing: New Advances

Frontiers in Cardiology

Series Advisors

JOHN CAMM
DESMOND JULIAN
NORMAN KAPLAN
SPENCER KING III
ULRICH SIGWART

Published

Management of Acute Myocardial Infarction
Edited by Desmond G. Julian and Eugene Braunwald

Noninvasive Electrocardiology: Clinical Aspects of Holter Monitoring
Edited by Arthur J. Moss and Shlomo Stern

Molecular Interventions and Local Drug Delivery
Edited by Elazer R. Edelman

Endoluminal Stenting
Edited by Ulrich Sigwart

Clinical Trials in Cardiology
Edited by Bertram Pitt, Desmond G. Julian and Stuart Pocock

Cardiac Pacing: New Advances

Edited by

Mårten Rosenqvist

Associate Professor of Cardiology
Karolinska Hospital, Stockholm, Sweden

W. B. Saunders Company Ltd
London • Philadelphia • Toronto • Sydney • Tokyo

W. B. Saunders Company Ltd 24–28 Oval Road
London NW1 7DX, UK

The Curtis Center
Independence Square West
Philadelphia, PA 19106-3399, USA

Harcourt Brace & Company
55 Horner Avenue
Toronto, Ontario M8Z 4X6, Canada

Harcourt Brace & Company, Australia
30–52 Smidmore Street
Marrickville, NSW 2204, Australia

Harcourt Brace & Company, Japan
Ichibancho Central Building, 22-1 Ichibancho
Chiyoda-ku, Tokyo 102, Japan

A catalogue record for this book is available from the British Library

ISBN 0-7020-2215-2

Typeset by Paston Press Ltd, Loddon, Norfolk
Printed in Great Britain by The University Press, Cambridge

Contents

Contributors

Henning Rud Andersen
Department of Cardiology, Skejby University Hospital, Århus, Denmark

Gerardo Ansalone
Dipartimento delle Malattie Cuore, Ospedale San Filippo Neri, Rome, Italy

Antonio Auriti
Dipartimento delle Malattie Cuore, Ospedale San Filippo Neri, Rome, Italy

David G. Benditt
Cardiac Arrhythmia Center, University of Minnesota Medical School, Minneapolis, Minnesota, USA

Johan Brandt
Department of Cardiothoracic Surgery, Lund University Hospital, Lund, Sweden

Rosemary S. Bubien
Division of Cardiovascular Disease, University of Alabama at Birmingham, Birmingham, Alabama, USA

Charles L. Byrd
University of Miami School of Medicine; and Broward General Medical Center, Fort Lauderdale, Florida, USA

A. John Camm
Department of Cardiological Sciences, St George's Hospital Medical School, London, England

Serge Cazeau
Department of Cardiac Pacing and Electrophysiology, Centre Chirurgical Val d'Or, Saint-Cloud, France

J. Claude Daubert
Centre Hospitalier Regional and Université de Rennes, Rennes, France

Philippe Delfaut
Arrhythmia and Pacemaker Service, Eastern Heart Institute, Passaic, New Jersey, USA

Kenneth A. Ellenbogen
Medical College of Virginia and the McGuire Medical Center, Richmond, Virginia,
USA

Anders Englund
Department of Cardiology, Karolinska Hospital, Stockholm, Sweden

Martin Fromer
Division of Cardiology, Department of Internal Medicine, Centre Hospitalier
Universitaire Vaudois, Lausanne, Switzerland

Fredrik Gadler
Department of Cardiology, Karolinska Hospital, Stockholm, Sweden

David M. Gilligan
Division of Cardiology and Department of Medicine, Medical College of Virginia and
the McGuire Medical Center, Richmond, Virginia, USA

Irakli Giorgberidze
Arrhythmia and Pacemaker Service, Eastern Heart Institute, Passaic, New Jersey,
USA

Demosthenes Katritsis
Department of Cardiology, Onassis Cardiac Surgery Center, Athens, Greece; and
Honorary Consultant Cardiologist, St Thomas's Hospital, London, England

G. Neal Kay
Division of Cardiovascular Disease, University of Alabama at Birmingham,
Birmingham, Alabama, USA

Ryszard B. Krol
Arrhythmia and Pacemaker Service, Eastern Heart Institute, Passaic, New Jersey,
USA

Chu-Pak Lau
Department of Medicine, Queen Mary Hospital, University of Hong Kong

Sum-Kin Leung
Department of Medicine, Kwong Wah Hospital, Kowloon, Hong Kong

Cecilia Linde
Department of Cardiology, Karolinska Hospital, Stockholm, Sweden

Keith G. Lurie
Cardiac Arrhythmia Center, University of Minnesota Medical School, Minneapolis,
Minnesota, USA

Philippe Mabo
Université de Rennes, Rennes, France

B. Magris
Dipartimento delle Malattie Cuore, Ospedale San Filippo Neri, Rome, Italy

Carlos A. Morillo
Division of Cardiology and Department of Medicine, Medical College of Virginia and the McGuire Medical Center, Richmond, Virginia, USA

Arthur J. Moss
Heart Research Follow-Up Program, University of Rochester Medical Center, Rochester, New York, USA

Anand N. Munsif
Arrhythmia and Pacemaker Service, Eastern Heart Institute, Passaic, New Jersey, USA

Atul Prakash
Arrhythmia and Pacemaker Service, Eastern Heart Institute, Passaic, New Jersey, USA

Philippe Ritter
Department of Cardiac Pacing and Electrophysiology, Centre Chirurgical Val d'Or, Saint-Cloud, France

Mårten Rosenqvist
Karolinska Hospital, Stockholm, Sweden

Lars Rydén
Department of Cardiology, Karolinska Hospital, Stockholm, Sweden

Sanjeev Saksena
Arrhythmia and Pacemaker Service, Eastern Heart Institute, Passaic; UMD–NJ Medical School, Newark, New Jersey, USA

Massimo Santini
Dipartimento delle Malattie Cuore, Ospedale San Filippo Neri, Rome, Italy

Hans Schüller
Department of Cardiothoracic Surgery, Lund University Hospital, Lund, Sweden

Richard Sutton
Royal Brompton Hospital, London, England

Mark A. Wood
Division of Cardiology and Department of Medicine, Medical College of Virginia and the McGuire Medical Center, Richmond, Virginia, USA

Wojciech Zareba
Heart Research Follow-Up Program, University of Rochester Medical Center, Rochester, New York, USA

Preface

When permanent cardiac pacing was introduced into clinical practice some 40 years ago, it was fixed-rate ventricular pacing, reserved for patients with complete heart block and syncopal spells. Although no prospective randomized studies had been published, this treatment soon became accepted as a life-saving remedy for this severely disabled group of patients.

The development of pacemaker technology and arrhythmia management was quite slow during the 1960s and 70s, except that the devices became longer-lasting and smaller.

With the development of programmable pacemakers and reliable dual-chamber devices, new interest was shown in providing optimal treatment for individual patients as well as in expanding the indications for permanent cardiac pacing. It has now become evident that cardiac pacing might be beneficial not only for patients with primary bradycardias but also for other conditions like tachycardias and various types of cardiomyopathies.

In this volume, well-known scientists in the field of cardiac pacing, from Europe and from the United States, provide an up-to-date picture, covering new indications, optimal programming and advanced trouble-shooting. This volume offers an exciting journey in a very rapidly developing area of cardiology. Intentionally, some of the chapters overlap in their contents. However, it is my belief that certain areas in the field are so exciting that they benefit from being covered from different viewpoints and by different personalities.

MÅRTEN ROSENQVIST, MD
Stockholm

SECTION I

Applications

Pacing in Congestive Heart Failure

J. C. Daubert, P. Ritter, S. Cazeau and P. Mabo

Advances in pharmacological therapy, and the key contribution of ACE-inhibitors in particular, have significantly improved the survival and quality of life of patients with chronic congestive heart failure (CHF). Nevertheless, patients in NYHA classes III or IV still have a poor prognosis and limited exercise tolerance. Various nonpharmacological methods have been proposed in the last two decades to treat these patients, who are refractory to drug therapy. *Orthotopic heart transplant* is unquestionably the gold standard, but many problems continue to limit its development, especially the persistent and worrying lack of grafts. Chronically implanted *artificial heart* remains at the planning stage. Long-term results of *cardiomyoplasty* are questionable. In this context of relative disillusion, *cardiac pacing* has been proposed as a new primary treatment for patients with drug-refractory CHF. The aim of this chapter is to reassess the data currently available on the subject, and to propose new perspectives based on our own experience.

Dual-Chamber Pacing

Some years after the first report of a possible benefit from short-AV-delay DDD pacing in patients with end-stage dilated cardiomyopathy (and drug-refractory CHF), many investigations are continuing and the issue is still highly controversial.

In 1990, Hochleitner et al.[1] reported a series of 16 patients with idiopathic dilated cardiomyopathy (mean $LVEF = 16 \pm 8\%$), all in NYHA classes III or IV, with symptoms refractory to maximal drug therapy, including 7 patients referred for heart transplantation. No patient had any classic indication for permanent pacing. All patients were in stable sinus rhythm with a PR interval ranging from 140 to 320 ms (mean $= 198 \pm 43$ ms). Seven patients had a left bundle branch block. After implantation, the DDD pacemaker was programmed at a short and fixed AV delay value of 100 ms. The authors did not give any clear explanation for this deliberate choice. During the short-term follow-up study (2–14 days), the mean functional (NYHA) class decreased significantly from 3.6 ± 0.4 to 2.1 ± 0.5 ($p < 0.001$) while the LVEF increased from $16 \pm 8\%$ to $26 \pm 9\%$ ($p < 0.001$). Concurrently the echocardiographic study showed a significant decrease in left ventricular and left atrial (LA) dimensions.

LVEDD was reduced from 74 ± 11 to 72 ± 10 mm ($p < 0.05$), LVESD from 62 ± 10 to 60 ± 10 mm ($p < 0.05$), and LA diameter from 48 ± 5 to 45 ± 5 mm ($p < 0.01$). Furthermore the authors observed a significant increase in systolic and diastolic blood pressure, especially in the patients who were severely hypotensive and needed inotropic support before pacemaker implantation. The conclusions from this disturbing study were that 'DDD pacing could represent an alternative approach to the management of chronic heart failure related to dilated cardiomyopathy, especially for heart transplant candidates and patients who are not accepted for cardiac transplantation, but no longer respond to maximal drug therapy'.

Unfortunately these optimistic (and premature) conclusions were largely refuted by the long-term follow-up study published 2 years later by the same group.[2] Of the 17 patients included, 10 died after 2–32 months, 9 from sudden death (without any defined cause) and 1 from a non-cardiac cause. Four patients were transplanted after 5–11 months, and finally only 3 patients survived more than 3 years without heart transplant. So the cumulative survival rate without transplant was only 18% at 3 years (see Figure 1.1). Furthermore, it can be noted that the three long-term survivors had the highest LVEF values (more than 30%) at the time of inclusion, and that those patients demonstrated a dramatic increase in LVEF during follow-up (41%, 45% and 63% at 2 years, respectively). These observations lead to a questioning of the validity of the initial diagnosis (dilated cardiomyopathy)! However, and despite the disappointing survival results, two data are worth emphasizing from this study. First, most

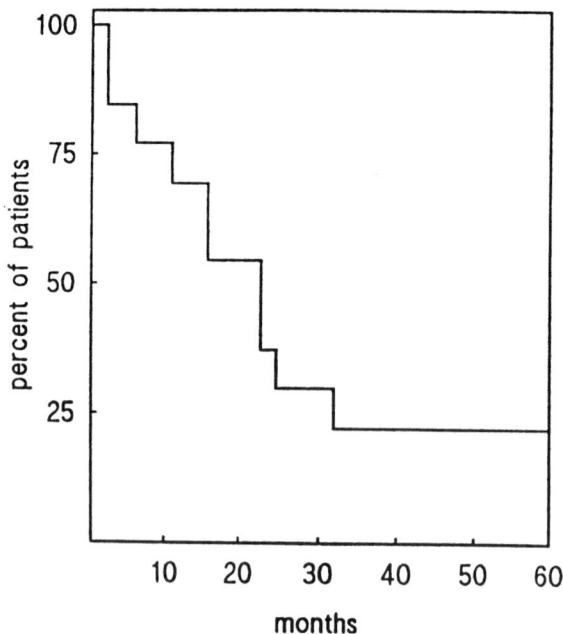

Figure 1.1 Cumulative survival rate in 17 patients with idiopathic dilated cardiomyopathy and end-stage congestive heart failure, treated by short-AV-delay DDD pacing. (Reproduced from reference 2 with the authors' permission)

deaths were sudden and did not result from refractory CHF. Secondly, most patients enjoyed a sustained and stable functional improvement until their death.

The initial enthusiasm produced by Hochleitner's report decreased considerably after the publication of subsequent studies of permanent DDD pacing.[3–5] These results, albeit contradictory, were generally unfavourable. Brecker *et al.*[3] studied the effects of programming different AV delays during temporary or permanent DDD pacing in 12 patients with dilated cardiomyopathy and short left ventricular filling time. With the individually optimal AV delay, the left and right ventricular filling times increased by an average of 65 and 90 ms, respectively ($p < 0.001$). It was estimated that left ventricular filling time increased by a mean of 35 ms for each 50 ms reduction in AV delay up to the optimal value. After implantation, exercise time duration and $\dot{V}O_2{}^{max}$ were significantly higher than baseline (no pacing).

Linde *et al.*[4] prospectively studied 10 patients in NYHA classes III or IV, with dilated cardiomyopathy (ischaemic in 7, idiopathic in 3). The mean LVEF was $21 \pm 9\%$. All patients had a stable sinus rhythm, and the PR interval was normal in most cases (mean value = 180 ± 40 ms). One day after DDD pacemaker implantation, the AV delay was individually optimized by Doppler echocardiographic measurements. The optimal AV delay ranged from 50 to 220 ms with an average value of 88 ± 26 ms, close to that empirically used by Hochleitner.[2] Patients were evaluated with regard to NYHA class, quality-of-life (questionnaire), cardiac output and LVEF (echocardiographic measurements) at 1, 3 and 6 months after pacemaker implantation. The AV delay optimization procedure on day 1 resulted in a significant increase in stroke volume (28 ± 12 *vs* 22 ± 7 mL at baseline; $p = 0.03$). But the mean stroke volume, cardiac output, NYHA class and LVEF values did not change significantly after 1, 3 and 6 months of permanent DDD pacing, in relation to the pre-implant values measured in spontaneous sinus rhythm. However, long-term response varied greatly from one patient to another. At 6 months, 1 patient deteriorated, 6 patients were unchanged, but the other 3 improved in functional NYHA class with a concomitant increase in overall quality-of-life score ranging from 30% to 55%. Nevertheless, consistent improvement of symptoms, cardiac output and LVEF was only observed in one of those three 'responder' patients.

Gold *et al.*[5] reported the results of a 'double-blind', randomized, crossover trial designed to assess the initial haemodynamic effects and the long-term clinical benefits of short-AV-delay DDD pacing in patients with chronic and drug-refractory CHF who presented with no classical indication for pacemaker implantation. Twelve NYHA class III or IV patients with a mean LVEF of $20 \pm 6\%$ were included in the study. Patients were required to be in stable sinus rhythm. The mean PR interval was 214 ± 45 ms and the mean QRS-complex duration was rather short at 130 ± 41 ms. On the day after implantation of a conventional DDD pacemaker, invasive haemodynamic measurements were done at varying AV delays up to 200 ms. Within these AV interval limits, no significant effect could be demonstrated on the different haemodynamic parameters: cardiac index, arterial pressure, right atrial pressure, pulmonary artery pressure and pulmonary capillary wedge pressure. At the optimal AV delay for each patient, neither cardiac output (4.7 ± 1.6 *vs* 4.5 ± 1.5 L/min) nor wedge pressure (17 ± 8 *vs* 16 ± 10 mmHg) improved significantly from baseline measurements with intrinsic conduction. After completing the acute haemodynamic study, 9 patients entered the 'long-term' protocol. Patients were randomized between either VDD pacing with a standard 100 ms AV delay or backup mode (VVI pacing at 40 bpm). After 4–6 weeks, a crossover to the alternative pacing mode was programmed. Follow-up was only based on the evaluation of functional status (NYHA class), drug regimen and LVEF as measured by radionuclide ventriculography. During the VDD pacing period, no patient improved with regard to their functional class and none had any increase in LVEF by >5%. The mean LVEF was $16 \pm 6\%$ with VDD pacing and $18 \pm 4\%$ in backup mode ($p =$ NS). The authors concluded that 'routine use of pacemaker therapy with a short AV delay as a primary treatment of heart failure without standard arrhythmic indications is *unwarranted'*. This very definitive conclusion, however, is to be considered cautiously. Although it was controlled, this study had important methodological and technical limitations: very small population (only 9 patients completed the 'long-term' protocol); very short follow-up; fixed-AV-delay programming at 100 ms; and finally, the use of conventional pacemaker technology, with a ventricular lead placement at the RV apex.

Considering the results of all these preliminary studies, either controlled or uncontrolled, we can conclude that *conventional short-AV-delay* DDD pacing provides variable, but on average nonsignificant, effects in patients with chronic CHF due to dilated (primary or ischaemic) cardiomyopathy. There is, however, a strong presumption of short- and long-term efficacy in some subgroups of patients. The problem is therefore to identify 'responder' patients before implantation and to define the technical prerequisites that need to be met to achieve optimal benefit. This implies that the mechanisms by which pacing therapy may produce a beneficial effect have to be understood first.

Possible Mechanisms of a Beneficial Effect from Pacing in CHF

We can assume that pacing therapy works primarily by correcting the electromechanical asynchrony in the left heart, which is a constant feature in dilated cardiomyopathies, either primary or of ischaemic origin. Asynchrony results, at least partially, from the nearly constant and often severe conduction disturbances that impair the atrium, the atrioventricular conduction system, and the ventricle to variable extents.

Conduction Blocks in Dilated Cardiomyopathy: Electromechanical Consequences

P-wave abnormalities

Atrial conduction disturbances are frequently observed in DCM patients and may severely alter AV synchrony in the left heart by delaying the timing of LA activation and contraction. In 12 consecutive patients (LVEF = $18 \pm 6\%$) referred to our institution for electrophysiological and haemodynamic evaluation before pacing therapy as a primary treatment for drug-refractory CHF, the mean interatrial conduction time (IACT) measured during spontaneous sinus rhythm was 102 ± 25 ms (range: 75–130). In DDD-paced patients, the deleterious haemodynamic effects of long IACT are well known and may result in the so-called 'DDD(R) pacemaker syndrome' owing to (1) the late occurrence of LA kick striking against the closed mitral valve, with a complete loss of LA contribution to LV filling; (2) a major LA wall stretching with neuro-humoral activation; and (3) LA-pulmonary venous regurgitation.[6,7]

PR interval

Serial electrocardiographic changes in necropsy-proven idiopathic DCM were eval-uated in 34 patients by Wilensky *et al.*[8] Seventy-one percent of patients remained in stable sinus rhythm (SSR) until the time of death (the other 29% developed permanent atrial tachyarrhythmia). In SSR patients, the mean PR interval was nearly normal (180 ± 30 ms) at inclusion in the study but prolonged (210 ± 30 ms; $p < 0.001$) after a mean follow-up of 2.9 years.

In seven studies[1,4,5,9–12] which involved 94 patients considered for pacemaker implantation to treat end-stage CHF, the prevalence of PR intervals >200 ms varied from 30% in Linde *et al.*'s study[4] to 53% in Nishimura *et al.*'s series.[11] Individual values ranged from 100 to 400 ms with an average of 209 ± 40 ms. However, ultra-long PR-interval values are only exceptionally observed in this population.

It has been established that the haemodynamic disorders induced by ultra-long PR intervals may occur in patients without structural heart disease.[13] The early occur-rence of LA contraction during the rapid or the intermediate phase of LV filling results in a complete or partial loss of LA contribution to LV filling. The fusion of the E and A waves on the transmitral flow is a typical Doppler–echocardiographic marker of this phenomenon (Figure 1.2). Simultaneous LV filling time is shortened by the premature atriogenic closure of the mitral valve. Finally, this usually incomplete atriogenic closure and the frequent late reopening of the mitral valve may result in various degrees of end-diastolic mitral regurgitation.[14–16] When these haemodynamic dis-orders are associated with severe symptoms, they may require the implantation of a permanent DDD pacemaker that will correct all these abnormalities provided a properly timed AV delay is programmed.[13]

In DCM patients, several studies – Nishimura *et al.*'s[11] and Scanu *et al.*'s[12] in particular – have clearly shown that moderately prolonged PR intervals (or even nearly normal PR intervals) could have exactly the same haemodynamic conse-quences (Figure 1.3) and hence the same degree of AV dysynchrony in the left heart as ultra-long PR intervals in patients with an apparently normal heart. This apparent paradox can probably be explained by the high prevalence of severe intraventricular conduction block which induces delayed and heterogeneous LV contraction and relaxation in DCM patients.

Intraventricular conduction block

In Wilensky *et al.*'s study,[8] 82% of the patients had significant intraventricular conduction disturbances on the last ECG recorded within 60 days of their death. Among the patients with conduction abnormalities at the first examination, 68% had progressive disturbances in the time period studied. The mean QRS duration increased from 100 ± 20 ms at the first examination to 130 ± 30 ms ($p < 0.0001$) at

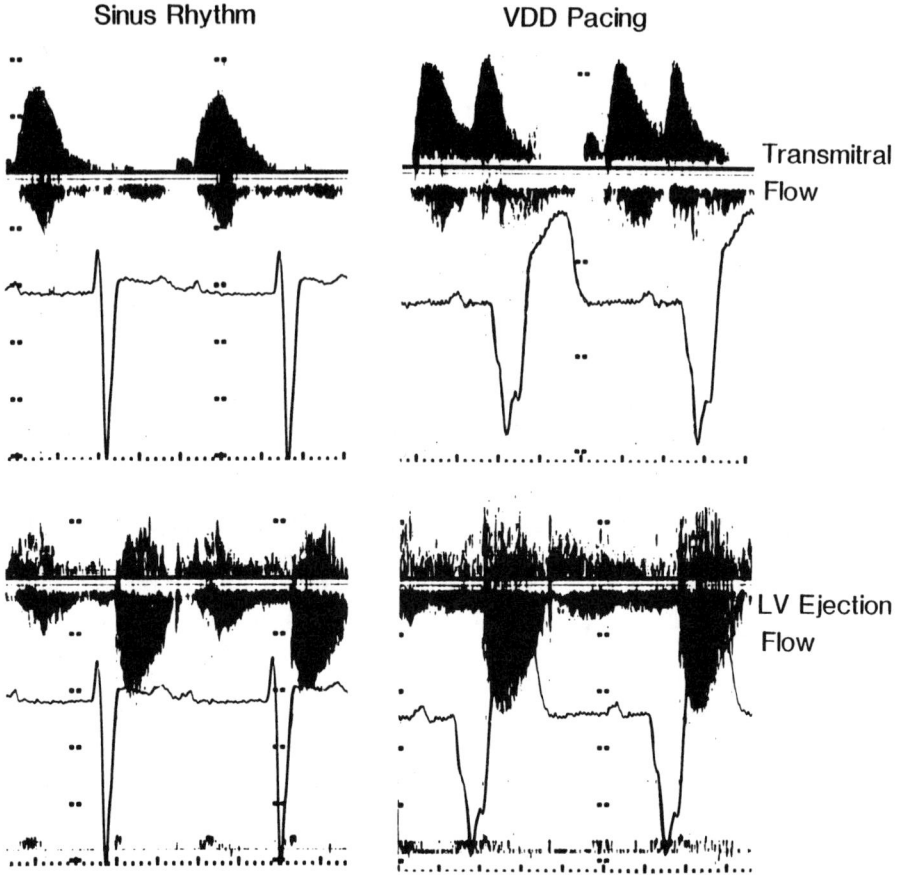

Sinus Rhythm   **VDD Pacing**

Transmitral Flow

LV Ejection Flow

Figure 1.2 Deleterious haemodynamic consequences of ultralong PR interval alone in a patient without structural heart disease. During spontaneous sinus rhythm, the E and A waves of the transmitral Doppler flow are superimposed, resulting in a single summation pulse. Temporary DDD pacing with a 150 ms AV interval normalizes the transmitral flow pattern and produces a significant increase in V_{max} and TVI of the ejection flow.

the end of the follow-up period. Complete bundle branch block was observed in 38% of patients, principally LBBB (29%). RBBB was rare (9%) but in two-thirds of cases it was associated with a left axis deviation, indicative of a probable association to left anterior fascicular block. In the whole group, a left QRS-axis deviation superior to 30 was observed in 65% of the patients.

The haemodynamic consequences of abnormal ventricular activation in DCM patients were extensively studied by Xiao et al.[17–19] who analysed by continuous wave Doppler the characteristics of the LV pressure pulse derived from the time course of functional mitral regurgitation. In 50 DCM patients with QRS duration ranging from normal (70 ms) to extremely long (190 ms), with an average of 110 ms, a positive correlation was found with the overall duration of mitral regurgitation ($r = 0.65$), with the LV contraction time ($r = 0.51$) and with the LV relaxation time

SSR 92 bpm PR = 220 ms   **VDD-P (LV) AVD = 50 ms**

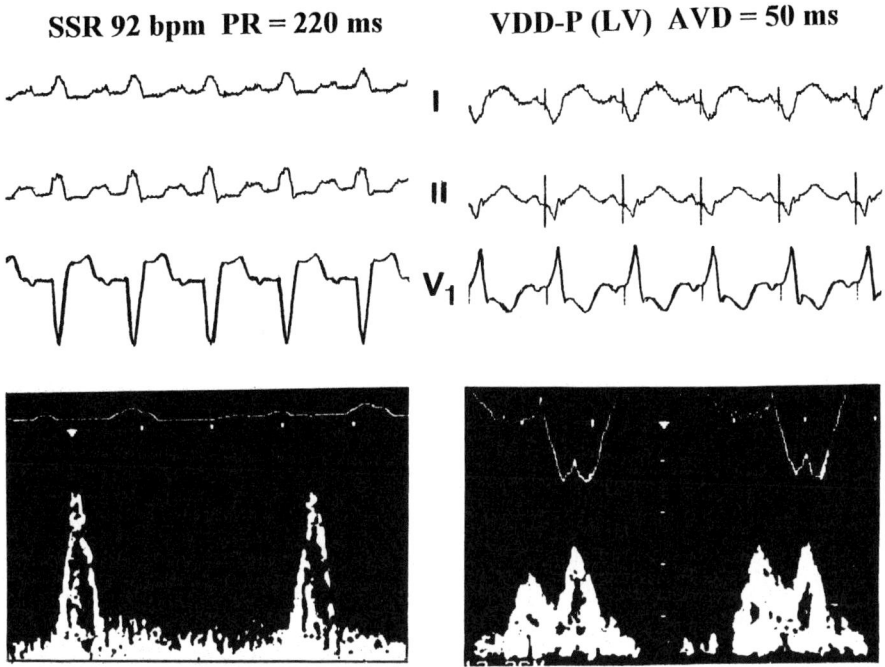

Figure 1.3 Example of 'concealed long PR-interval syndrome' in a NYHA class IV patient with dilated cardiomyopathy. Despite a nearly normal PR interval (220 ms), transmitral Doppler flow analysis shows a single summation pulse with a very shortened diastolic filling time (200 ms). Temporary VDD pacing at a short (50 ms) AV delay makes a large and well-synchronized A wave reappear and increases the diastolic filling time to 400 ms.

($r = 0.52$). The duration of QRS was negatively correlated with the peak rate of LV pressure increase ($+ dP/dt$) ($r = 0.48$) and was positively correlated with the time intervals from Q to peak pressure ($r = 0.49$) and with peak $+ dP/dt$ ($r = 0.72$). The duration of QRS, however, did not directly affect the peak rate of LV pressure decrease ($- dP/dt$), or the isovolumic relaxation time. These data show that the LV contraction and relaxation times will be all the longer, and the LV systolic performance all the poorer, as the QRS complex is wider. Furthermore, extended isovolumic contraction and relaxation times result in a proportional reduction of LV filling time to a critically short threshold of 200 ms or less, in patients with the longest QRS duration.

The morphology (right or left bundle branch block, or undefined intraventricular block) and axis of the QRS complex appear to have no direct influence on the magnitude of the abnormalities observed. However, Xiao et al.[17] noted that left axis deviation was associated with the longest QRS duration values and thus with more severe electromechanical alterations.

The same group also showed[19] that in DCM patients with an electrocardiographic pattern of left bundle branch block or of intraventricular block (QRS duration >120 ms with persistent septal Q wave), the ventricle remained activated through the upper septum, but the onset of mechanical systole was strikingly and symmetrically delayed in both RV and LV free walls. The time intervals from Q wave to septal thickening, from septum to LV posterior wall thickening, from septum to LV free wall thickening and from septum to RV free wall thickening were measured as 43 ± 13 ms, 91 ± 28 ms, 97 ± 30 ms and 65 ± 25 ms, respectively.

All these observations account for the presence of major delay and nonuniformity in contraction and relaxation in patients with poor LV function and high-degree conduction block within the ventricle. Such electromechanical correlations can be explained largely by the fractionate contraction theory.

Individual behaviours

P-wave abnormalities, modifications of the PR interval and intraventricular conduction block may be associated in different ways and to variable degrees in each individual patient. A particular behaviour is that of patients with normal or slightly prolonged P waves, normal (<200 ms) PR interval, but a very wide QRS complex, usually associated with left bundle branch block morphology and left superior axis deviation. Those patients can present with the same haemodynamic disorders as those with a long PR interval, because of a greatly delayed LV activation and contraction that creates severe AV dysynchrony in the left heart. This particular behaviour corresponds to a 'concealed long PR-interval syndrome' and is very specific of DCM patients; it is illustrated in Figures 1.4 and 1.5.

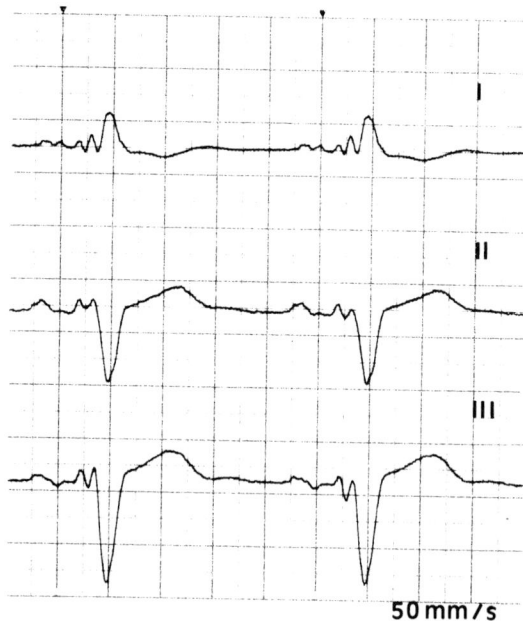

Figure 1.4 Typical ECG example of major intraventricular conduction block in a patient with end-stage dilated cardiomyopathy. The PR interval remains normal (180 ms) but P-wave duration is prolonged (130 ms). There is a major increase in QRS duration (200 ms) with a left bundle branch block and a left axis deviation.

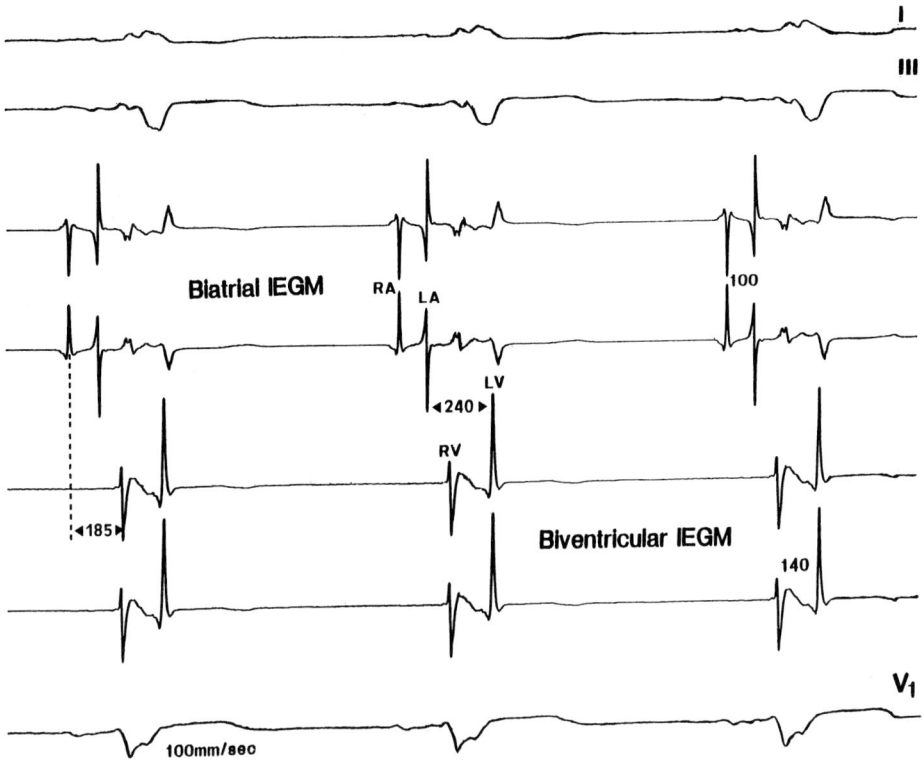

Figure 1.5   Same patient as Figure 1.4. Endocardial mapping using the implanted leads of a 'four-chamber pacemaker'. The interatrial conduction time is 100 ms in spontaneous sinus rhythm. The interventricular conduction time is measured at 140 ms. This discrepancy results in a significant prolongation of the AV conduction time in the left heart (240 ms) while the PR interval is normal (180 ms) on surface ECG. RA = right atrium; LA = left atrium (midpart of the coronary sinus); RV = right ventricle (RVOT); LV = left ventricle (posterolateral vein of the LV free wall).

Optimization of LV Filling by Correcting Mechanical AV Dysynchrony in the Left Heart

Two recent studies have emphasized the critical importance of optimizing AV synchrony, especially in patients with long PR intervals. Nishimura *et al.*[11] acutely investigated 15 patients with severe LV dysfunction (mean LV ejection fraction: 19%) during AV sequential pacing with a ventricular lead classically placed at the RV apex, with variable AV intervals ranging from 60 to 240 ms. Combined Doppler velocity curves and pressures, as obtained by high-fidelity manometer-tipped catheters, and thermodilution cardiac output were used to evaluate the effects of altering AV synchrony. Considering the group of patients as a whole, neither cardiac output nor mean left atrial pressure were significantly different when the baseline haemodynamic variables were compared with those during AV sequential pacing with the various AV intervals. The patients were retrospectively classified into two groups according to the baseline PR interval measured during spontaneous sinus rhythm. In group I (8 patients with PR intervals >200 ms; mean value = 283 ms; range: 230–400 ms) the cardiac output measured at the optimal AV interval in each patient increased by 38% on average, relative to baseline (3.9 ± 0.43 *vs* 3.0 ± 1.0 L/min; *p* = 0.005). The optimal AV interval varied greatly from one patient to another, ranging from 60 to 180 ms. This important observation, albeit evident, highlights the major methodological limitations of the original study published by Hochleitner *et al.*[1] Pacing with optimal AV interval in group I produced a significant increase in LV end-diastolic pressure (from 27.8 ± 6.0 at baseline to 36.9 ± 10.7 mmHg; *p* = 0.03) and in LV diastolic filling time (from 215 ± 58 to 314 ± 102 ms; *p* = 0.03). Meanwhile, the time relation between mechanical left atrial and left ventricular contraction was optimized, as reflected by the frequent normalization of the transmitral flow pattern with the recovery of a well-defined and correctly synchronized A wave (Figure 1.6). Finally, the diastolic mitral regurgitation observed at baseline in 5 out of 8 patients was abolished during AV sequential pacing.

In group II (7 patients with PR intervals <200 ms; mean value = 157 ms; range: 100–200 ms) cardiac output conversely decreased from 4.2 ± 1.8 to 3.4 ± 1.3 L/min on average (*p* < 0.01) and there was no significant change in the diastolic filling period. No patient in this group had diastolic mitral regurgitation.

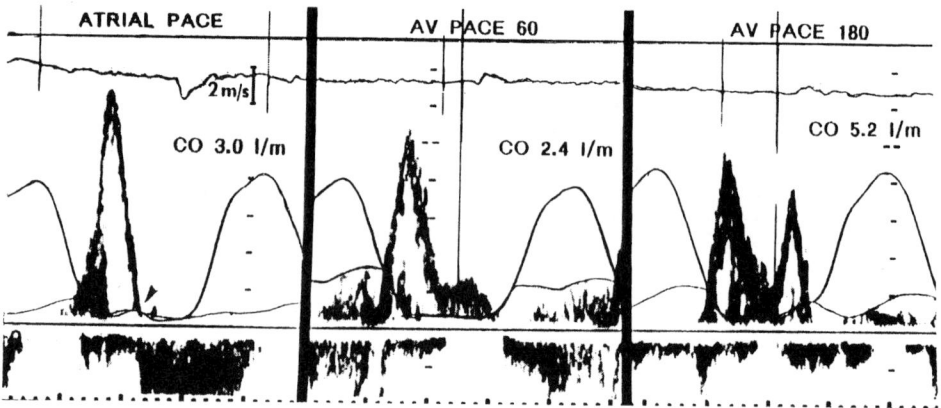

Figure 1.6 Mitral flow velocity curve and simultaneous left atrial (LA) and left ventricular (LV) pressure curves in a patient with severe ischaemic cardiomyopathy. The effects of three different pacing modes at an identical pacing rate are compared. *Left panel:* Atrial pacing with a very long spike–R interval and native conduction. There is an increase in LV pressure above the LA pressure, culminating in a shortening of the diastolic filling time and at the onset of diastolic mitral regurgitation (MR). The E and A waves of the transmitral Doppler flow are superimposed in a single summation pulse. The baseline cardiac output (CO) is 3.0 L/min. *Centre panel:* Sequential AV pacing with a short AV interval (60 ms). Diastolic filling occurs throughout the diastole but there is no evidence of LA contribution due to the simultaneous occurrence of LA contraction and LV contraction, resulting in a significant decrease in CO to 2.4 L/min. At the same time the mean LA pressure increased from 31 to 42 mmHg. *Right panel:* Sequential AV pacing at the optimal AV delay of 180 ms. The relation of LA contraction to LV contraction is now optimal and is illustrated by the normalized pattern of the transmitral Doppler flow. Diastolic filling occurs throughout the entire diastolic filling period. The mean LA pressure is maintained at a relatively low level (34 mmHg) while end-diastolic LV pressure increases to 43 mmHg. Simultaneously, CO is measured at 5.2 L/min, corresponding to a 73% increase on baseline. (Reproduced from reference 11 with the authors' permission)

Nearly identical data have been reported by Scanu *et al.*[12] in a group of 18 DCM patients. The predictors of a significant increase in cardiac output with temporary VDD pacing at the optimal AV interval in each patient were also a short LV filling time (29 ± 8% of the RR interval in 'responder' patients, relative to 44 ± 9% in 'non-responder' patients; $p < 0.01$) and a long PR interval during spontaneous sinus rhythm at baseline.

But, as mentioned above, the occurrence of mechanical AV dysynchrony in the left heart does not imperatively require a long PR interval. Such a behaviour can also be observed in DCM patients with an apparently normal AV conduction time on surface ECG, but with a very wide QRS complex. The so-called 'concealed long PR-interval syndrome' can only be corrected by conventional DDD pacing (ventricular lead at the right ventricular apex) by programming ultrashort AV intervals (Figure 1.3). Optimization of the ventricular activation sequence by using alternative pacing site(s) in the ventricle is of particular importance in this situation and contributes greatly to improving LV filling.

Optimization of the Ventricular Sequence of Activation, Contraction and Relaxation

Electromechanical asynchrony within the ventricle can be either corrected (partially), or unmodified, or even aggravated by ventricular pacing, depending on the selected pacing site. Tradition and facility explain why the RV apex was used in all the studies published so far. However, modern lead technology offers the possibility of permanent ventricular pacing at alternative sites, either in the right ventricle (His-septal pacing, RV outflow tract) or in the left ventricle. Finally, multisite pacing, and especially biventricular pacing, has recently been proposed to achieve the objective of optimal ventricular resynchronization.

Effects of right ventricular apical pacing

The RV apex is unquestionably the worst ventricular pacing site in terms of cardiac performance. By delaying left ventricular activation and inverting the ventricular activation sequence, pacing the right ventricle in the apical region induces asynchronous ventricular contraction and relaxation. The result in a normal heart is a significant modification of both LV systolic function, as demonstrated by Wiggers as early as 1925 on experimental models[20] and by others later,[21–23] and end-systole relaxation and ventricular filling.[24–26] Likewise, myocardial oxygen consumption is reduced by 18% on average and cardiac efficiency (the external-cardiac-work/myocardial-oxygen-consumption ratio) is improved by 41% in AAI compared with rate-equivalent DDD pacing.[27] Finally, histopathology studies conducted in mature or immature dogs have shown that chronic ventricular pacing of the right ventricle apex can lead to cellular lesions of the myocardium.[28,29] These histological lesions might influence LV performance or perhaps lead to long-term impairment of LV function in the so-called 'pacing-induced cardiomyopathies'.

LV asynchrony during right ventricular pacing is greatly aggravated in patients with structural heart disease and especially in ischaemic patients with myocardial infarction scars.[30,31] Vassallo *et al.*,[30] using endocardial mapping studies during apical right ventricular pacing, showed that patients with anterior infarction scars exhibited significantly prolonged earliest LV local activation time (60 ± 15 ms *vs* 40 ± 11 ms; $p < 0.01$), total endocardial activation time (118 ± 30 ms *vs* 76 ± 14 ms; $p < 0.001$) and total duration of LV electrical activity (191 ± 29 ms *vs* 145 ± 17 ms; $p < 0.001$) relatively to patients without infarction. Interestingly, the latest site of activation was the posteroinferior base in the vast majority of patients without infarction or with inferior myocardial scar. In patients with anterior infarction the latest LV activation site varied and was localized in the posteroinferior base in only 20% of cases.

The deleterious electromechanical effects of right ventricular apical pacing may partly explain the failure of DDD pacing to improve haemodynamics in DCM patients, even when AV synchrony is individually optimized.

Alternative pacing sites in the right ventricle

Permanent pacing in the outflow tract. This may be easily and reliably achieved with screw-in leads.[32] Compared with RV apical pacing, RVOT pacing restores a more physiological activation sequence but does not correct interventricular asynchrony, especially the delay in LV activation. Acute studies with temporary pacing[33,34] have shown that RVOT pacing increased cardiac output from 20% to 27% on average in patients without structural heart disease, relative to RV apical pacing. But are these acute results predictive of a long-term haemodynamic benefit? That question remains to be answered.

Likewise, there is currently no evidence that RVOT pacing produces a better haemodynamic performance than RV apical pacing in patients with poor LV function and intraventricular conduction block. Our own experience, however, allows us to assume the superiority for RVOT pacing in the subgroup of patients with complete bundle branch block and left axis deviation.

Septal His–Purkinje pacing. This was investigated in animal models by Karpawich *et al.*[35] in 1991. By capturing the specialized conduction system, this pacing technique has the theoretical advantage of providing near-simultaneous biventricular activation and normal contraction sequences, resulting in a potential improvement of cardiac function. Experimental data reported by Mabo *et al.*[36] are consistent with this hypothesis. By randomly comparing three different pacing modes, atrial pacing preserving normal intrinsic conduction, sequential AV pacing from the His bundle (A–H pacing) and sequential AV pacing from the RV apex (A–RV pacing) at identical pacing rates, these authors showed that the mean aortic pressure was not significantly influenced by the pacing mode in the normal dog heart. But in a dog heart with depressed LV systolic function, the mean aortic pressure was dramatically reduced during A–RV pacing (51 ± 21 mmHg) in comparison with atrial pacing (101 ± 18 mmHg; $p < 0.01$). A–H pacing produced the same haemodynamic performance as atrial pacing (98 ± 20 mmHg; $p = $ NS). These experimental data can be correlated with the results of a clinical study published by Cowell *et al.*[9] in 1994. A comparison was made between the haemodynamic effects of VDD pacing at the optimal AV delay at two different ventricular pacing sites, the RV apex and the septum close to the His bundle region, in 15 patients with poor LV function (LVEF = 33 ± 12%) and chronic CHF. Compared with the baseline state in spontaneous sinus rhythm, RV apical VDD pacing did not significantly increase the cardiac output (4.4 ± 0.7 *vs* 4.1 ± 0.7 L/min; p = NS) whereas septal VDD pacing increased the cardiac output to 4.9 ± 0.8 L/min (p = 0.04).

However, the practical interest of septal His–Purkinje pacing is limited by the widespread diffusion of intraventricular conduction abnormalities in DCM patients with the equivalent of a bilateral bundle branch block in many cases[23] and by the technical feasibility of the method. Karpawich *et al.*[37] in 1992 reported a new endocardial electrode approach using a screw-in lead inserted in the anterior atrial septum just above the tricuspid annulus, but we do not have any information on the long-term performance of this device.

Biventricular pacing

Bakker *et al.*[38] were the first to evaluate the potential role of permanent biventricular pacing in patients with poor LV function and intraventricular conduction block (complete LBBB). In 5 NYHA class III or IV patients, a DDD pacemaker was implanted and connected to two ventricular leads at the ventricular port, one transvenous lead in the right ventricle and one left ventricular epicardial lead. After the implantation the AV delay was optimized in each patient. After 3 months of permanent pacing, 4 patients were improved by at least one NYHA class. The only failure was related to a loss of LV capture from the third postoperative month. In the 4 responder patients, LVEF increased by 8 ± 2% on average. The mean increase in stroke volume was 12 ± 3 mL and the mean increase in diastolic filling time was 90 ± 56 ms. The grade of mitral regurgitation was significantly reduced in two cases. These preliminary results are interesting but questionable because no comparison was made with the effects of single right (or left) ventricular DDD pacing, and we cannot rule out that the haemodynamic benefit observed may have just been the result of AV dysynchrony correction in the left heart, insofar as all patients had a long PR interval in spontaneous sinus rhythm before implantation.

More impressive are the acute observations (temporary pacing) reported by Cazeau *et al.*[39] In 8 NYHA class IV patients with a mean LVEF of 22 ± 8%, four different configurations of ventricular pacing were randomly tested and compared with baseline values in spontaneous rhythm: single RV apical pacing, single RVOT pacing, simultaneous biventricular pacing combining LV and RV apex, and simultaneous biventricular pacing combining LV and RVOT. Patients with spontaneous sinus P waves were paced in the VDD mode (n = 5) at the individually optimized AV delay. Patients with permanent atrial fibrillation (n = 3) were paced in VVI mode. RV apical pacing and RVOT pacing did not induce any significant variation in cardiac output and pulmonary capillary wedge pressure (PCWP). But both configurations of biventricular pacing resulted in a significant haemodynamic improvement. The cardiac output increased by an average of 20% with the LV + RV apex configuration (p = 0.04) and of 25% with the LV + RVOT configuration (p = 0.02). The mean decrease in PCWP peak was 19% (p=NS) with the LV+RV apex combination and 23% (p=0.02) with the LV+RVOT combination. In the optimal biventricular pacing configuration in each patient, the cardiac index increased from 1.8 $\pm$ 0.3 L/min/m^2 to 2.3 $\pm$ 0.3 L/min/m^2 ($p < 0.006$) and the mean PCWP decreased from 31 $\pm$ 10 mmHg to 26 $\pm$ 9 mmHg ($p < 0.01$) (Figure 1.7).

These haemodynamic effects were correlated with modifications of the ventricular activation sequences, as assessed by radionuclide angiography with phase-analysis.[40] Compared with single RV and single LV VDD pacing, biventricular VDD pacing (in the optimal configuration in each patient) reduced LV contraction time by 75 $\pm$ 67 ms, RV contraction time by 65 $\pm$ 62 ms and the overall ventricular contraction time by

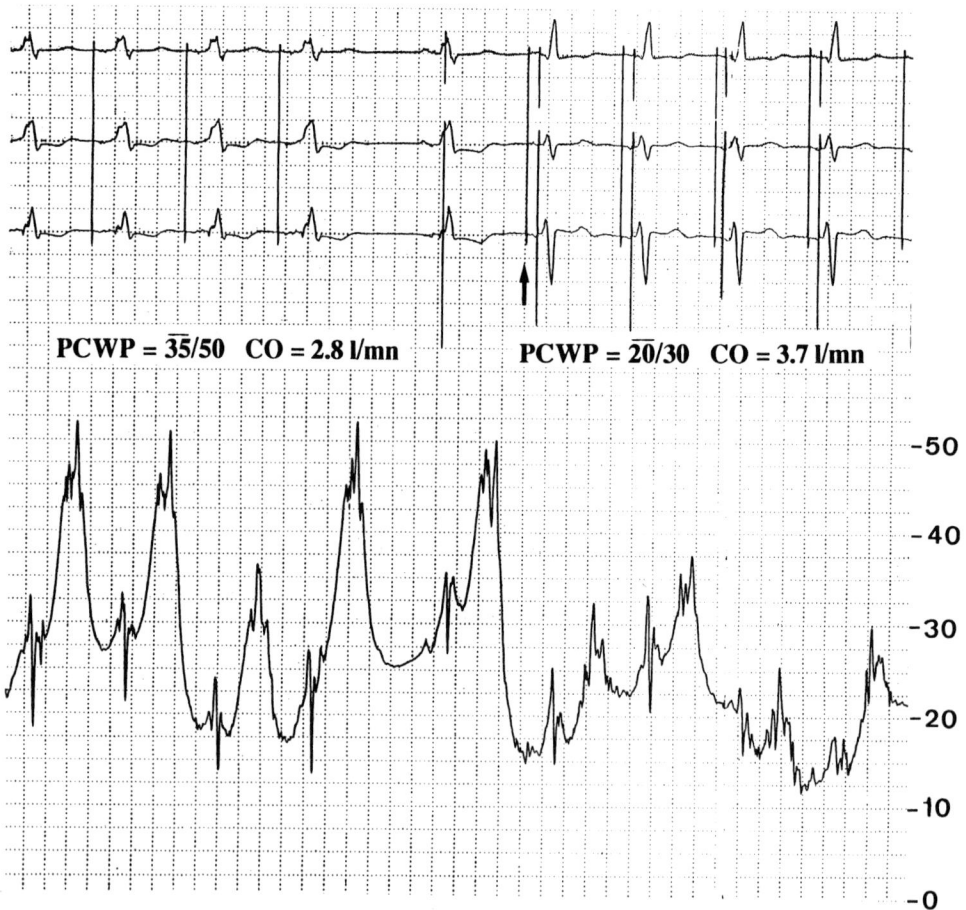

Figure 1.7 Acute haemodynamic effects of biventricular VDD pacing in a NYHA class III patient with idiopathic dilated cardiomyopathy. Switching the device from atrial pacing to VDD instantaneously produces a dramatic decrease in mean (−15 mmHg) and peak (−20 mmHg) pulmonary capillary wedge pressure (PCWP). The cardiac output simultaneously increases by 32%.

99 ± 55 ms. At the same time, LV diastolic filling time was increased by $13 \pm 9\%$. Finally, the LV activation sequence was inverted in all cases.

These data indicate a clear superiority of biventricular pacing over the different configurations of single-site pacing, either in the right or left ventricle, and highlight the key importance of optimally resynchronizing the electromechanical activity within the left ventricle in patients with very poor LV function and major intra-ventricular conduction block.

The same group[41] have recently reported their preliminary experience with chronic pacing. Of the 8 patients who were acutely tested, 7 were implanted with a permanent device corresponding to the optimal configuration defined during the acute study. One patient died during the operation. During a follow-up time ranging from 3 to 17 months, 2 other patients died, 1 from terminal CHF and the other from a noncardiac cause. One patient was transplanted after a long period (17 months) of stabilization in NYHA class II. The other 3 patients were improved by two NYHA classes and were stable in class II. Interestingly, the pacemaker was transiently switched off after 3 months of pacing and that resulted in a significant decrease in the mean cardiac index from 2.4 L/min/m^2 to 2.0 L/min/m^2 ($p < 0.001$).

Selection of Responder Patients

At this time, the selection criteria for pacing therapy in highly symptomatic and drug-refractory DCM patients are still difficult to define. However, we can assume that they should be principally based on indicators of both AV dysynchrony in the left heart and major asynchrony in left ventricular electromechanical activity.

Preselection could probably be achieved on the basis of noninvasive criteria,[42] in particular:

(a) the presence of summation gallup at physical examination;
(b) on 12-lead surface ECG, long PR interval (patients in spontaneous sinus rhythm) and prolonged QRS duration (more than 140 ms?), especially with a pattern of complete left bundle branch block and left axis deviation;
(c) at Doppler–echocardiography examination, functional mitral regurgitation (prolonged to more than 450 ms?) and abnormalities of the diastolic phase with principally a very short LV filling time (less than 200 ms) and secondly the presence of end-diastolic mitral regurgitation.[11]

Another criterion could be the superimposition of the E and A waves of the transmitral Doppler flow in a single summation pulse, although this particular phenomenon may be difficult to differentiate from a simple restrictive filling pattern. Temporary DDD pacing at the optimal AV delay in each patient may be helpful by normalizing transmitral Doppler flow morphology in case of superimposition of the E and A waves (Figures 1.4–1.7).

However, noninvasive markers probably do not suffice to reach the decision of permanent pacemaker implantation. We strongly believe that the final decision has to be conditioned by the individual response (assessed by haemodynamic and/or Doppler–echo measurements) to temporary pacing in the optimal mode for each patient. Different pacing sites in the two ventricles have to be acutely tested separately and in two by two combination. Whenever possible, AV synchrony must also be optimized by pacing in VDD mode at the optimal AV delay for each patient (Figure 1.7). The practical interest of such acute studies was clearly shown by Cazeau *et al.*[39–41] Of the 7 patients who were implanted with a permanent pacemaker, the 4 long-term survivors with stable functional improvement had a mean 48% increase in cardiac output during the acute study before implantation, while the 3 nonresponder patients (early death) had only an average increase of 9% ($p < 0.002$).

Technical Prerequisites to Achieve Optimal Benefit

The optimal pacing configuration is that which best corrects electromechanical asynchrony within the left ventricle and, whenever possible (patients in stable sinus rhythm with a functional left atrium), AV dysynchrony in the left heart. To achieve this objective, the technical requirements vary greatly from one patient to another, but can be predicted from the results of the acute study with temporary pacing.

Biventricular pacing is undoubtedly required in a majority of patients and can be achieved by connecting the two ventricular leads (RV and LV) to the ventricular port of the pacemaker through a double-unipolar Y bifurcated adapter, or better an 'on-line' adapter.

On that basis, three different pacing systems can be considered:

(1) Biventricular pacing alone with a SSIR unit can be proposed for patients with permanent atrial fibrillation. In such cases, radiofrequency catheter ablation may be necessary before the implantation to ensure permanent ventricular pacing and hence permanent capture of the two ventricles.
(2) In patients with stable sinus rhythm and normal interatrial conduction time, a 'triple-chamber' pacemaker is required to provide both optimized AV synchrony (DDD mode) and permanent biventricular pacing. The atrial lead can be classically placed in the upper right atrium or unconventionally in the coronary sinus to sense and to pace the left atrium selectively[43] (Figure 1.8).
(3) The 'four-chamber' pacemaker[44] providing biatrial synchronous pacing plus DDD pacing plus simultaneous biventricular pacing can be indicated in patients with long interatrial conduction time (100 ms), especially in cases of recurrent and drug-refractory atrial tachyarrhythmias. Biatrial synchronous pacing has been shown to prevent arrhythmia recurrences in that particular situation.[45] To achieve this objective, two atrial leads (RA and coronary sinus lead) have to be implanted and a special algorithm of 'atrial resynchronization' has to be loaded into the RAM memory of the DDD or DDD(R) pacemaker (ELA Recherche, le Plessis-Robinson, France).

But the key problem is 'How to permanently pace the left ventricle'. The first implantations for permanent biventricular pacing used LV epicardial leads placed by thoracotomy[38] or thoracoscopy.[46] Unfortunately, this method was associated with a high risk of perioperative and postoperative complications, including death,[46] owing to the extreme weakness of patients. Furthermore, acute pacing thresholds were

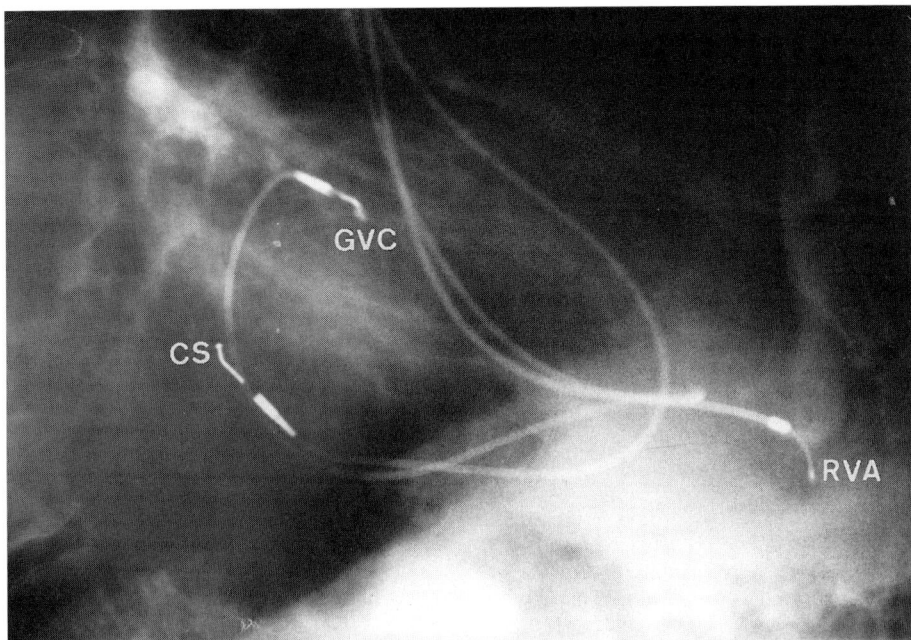

Figure 1.8 Chest X-ray, sagittal view. DDD pacemaker connected to a coronary sinus (CS) lead for left atrial pacing and sensing, and to two ventricular leads placed in the right ventricular apex (RVA) and in the great cardiac vein (GCV) for left ventricular pacing and sensing.

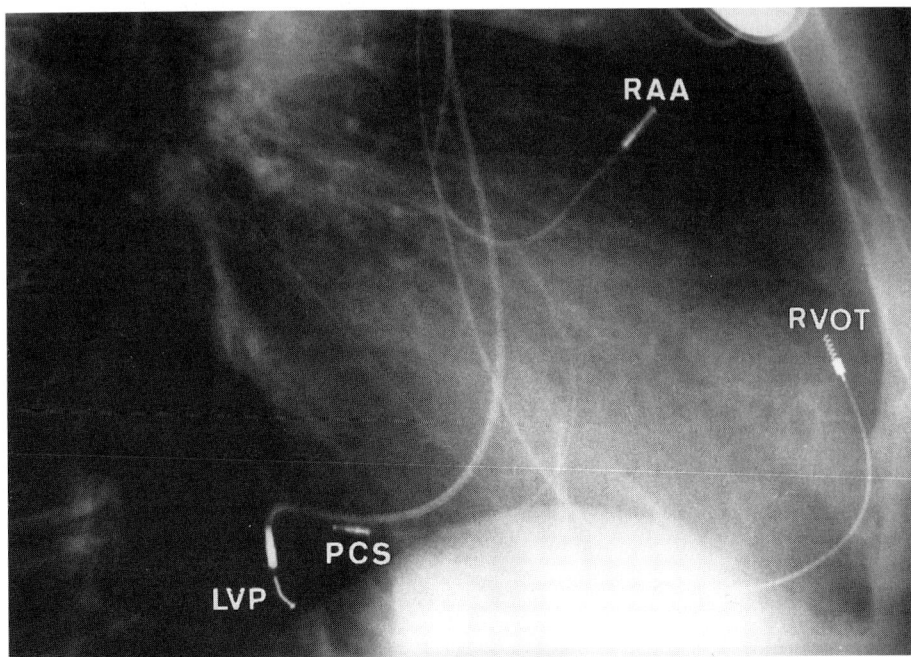

Figure 1.9 Chest X-ray, sagittal view. 'Four-chamber' pacemaker connected to two atrial leads placed in the right atrial appendage (RAA) and in the proximal coronary sinus (PCS), and to two ventricular leads positioned in the right ventricular outflow tract (RVOT) (screw-in lead) and into a posterior vein of the LV free wall (LVP).

usually high, resulting in the risk of secondary loss of LV capture. These major limitations led to moves for a transvenous method. Our group[47] have recently reported their preliminary experience of permanent LV pacing with transvenous leads introduced into the veins of LV free wall through the coronary sinus. By using the same leads as those specifically designed for left atrial pacing,[43] 65% of the attempted procedures were successful. The tip electrode was positioned in a postero-lateral vein (Figure 1.9) or lateral vein (Figure 1.10) in most cases, and occasionally in the great cardiac vein (Figure 1.8) or at the LV apex through the mid-cardiac vein (Figure 1.11). Figure 1.12 summarizes the different pacing sites and corresponding

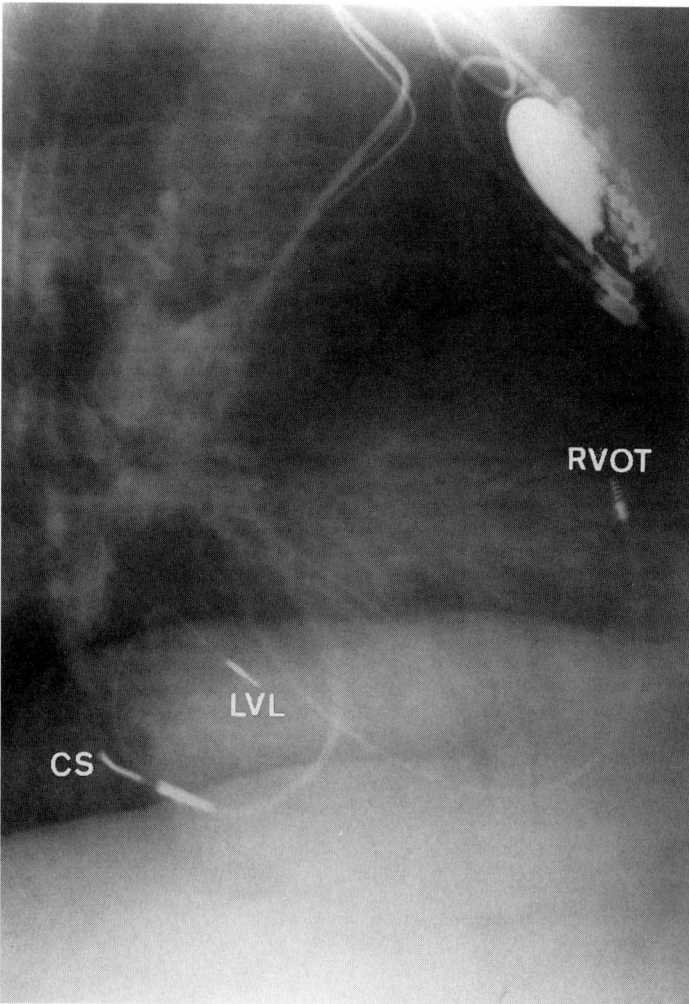

Figure 1.10 Chest X-ray, sagittal view. 'Triple-chamber' pacemaker connected to a coronary sinus (CS) lead for pacing and sensing the left atrium, and to two ventricular leads placed in the right ventricular outflow tract (RVOT) (screw-in lead) and into a lateral vein of the LV free wall (LVL). The tip electrode is anteriorly oriented.

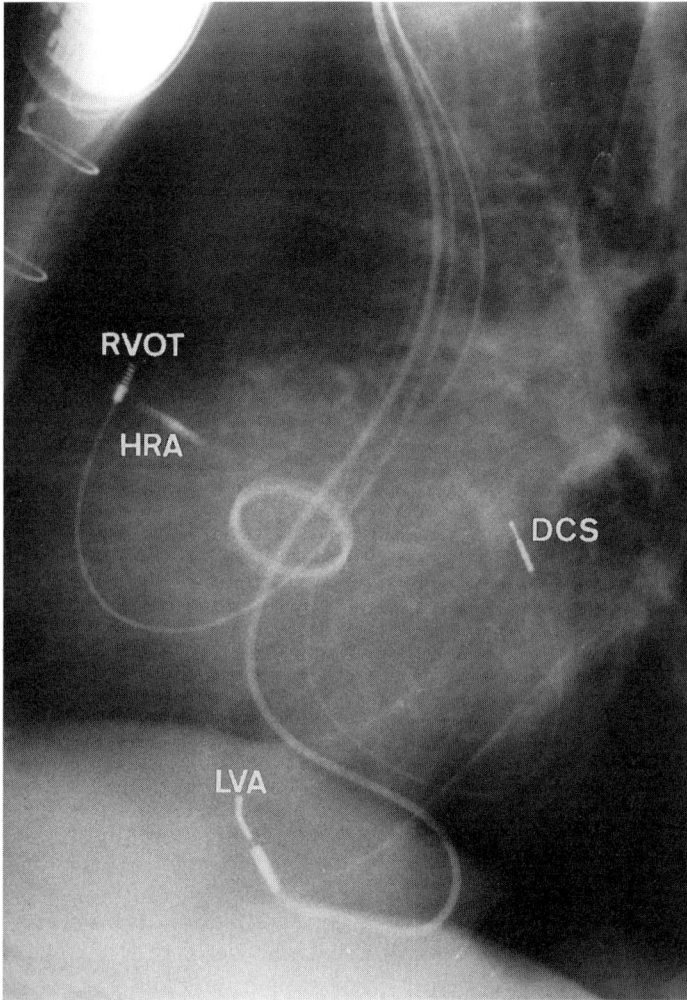

Figure 1.11 Chest X-ray, sagittal view. 'Four-chamber' pacemaker connected to two atrial leads placed in the high right atrium (HRA) and in the distal coronary sinus (DCS), and to two ventricular leads positioned in the right ventricular outflow tract (RVOT) (screw-in lead) and at the LV apex (LVA) through the mid-cardiac vein.

pacing and sensing thresholds. The mean acute pacing threshold was 1.3 ± 1 V and the mean R wave amplitude was 11 ± 6.2 mV. During an average follow-up time of 7 months, only one case of LV capture loss was observed. At the end of follow-up, the mean pacing threshold had increased only slightly (2 ± 1 V) while the mean R-wave amplitude was paradoxically greater (17 ± 5 mV). The success rate of the transvenous method should increase rapidly with new lead designs, best adapted to this particular use.

One question remains: 'Where is the optimal pacing site within the left ventricle?' We can reasonably assume that it is the site of the latest LV activation in the individual

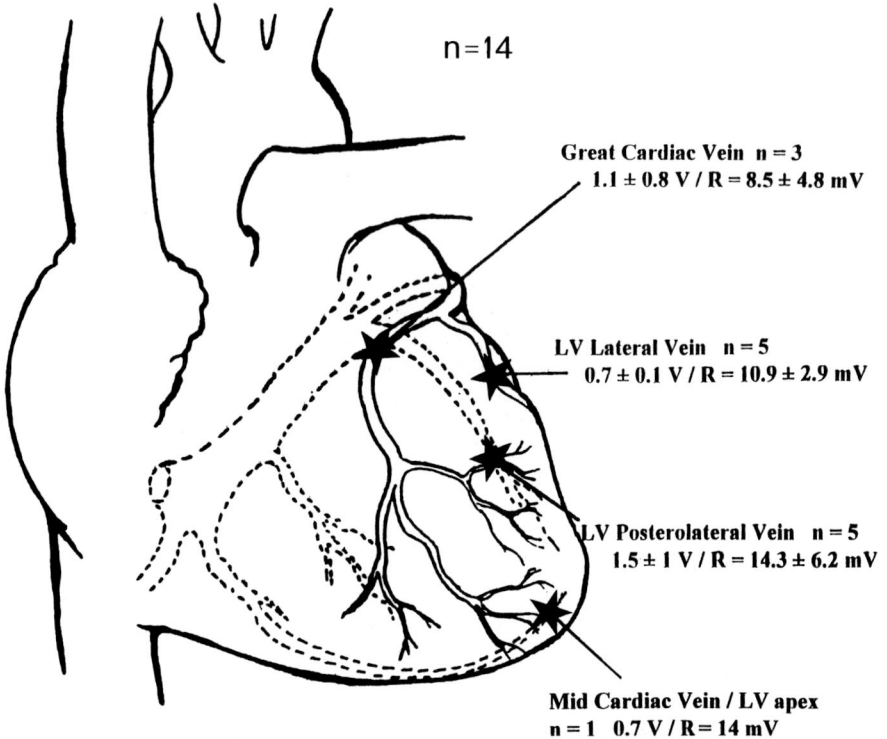

Figure 1.12 Left ventricular pacing sites and the corresponding pacing and sensing thresholds in 14 patients in whom transvenous leads were implanted into the veins of the LV free wall through the coronary sinus.

patient. On the basis of endocardial mapping studies in normal and diseased hearts,[34,35] we know that this site is the LV posteroinferior or posterolateral base in a majority of nonischaemic but also of ischaemic patients. The only exception is represented by patients with anterior myocardial infarction scar, where the site of the latest LV activation is very variable and needs individual evaluation. In practice, we can propose to do an intraoperative mapping of the coronary sinus to locate the area where the latest ventricular electrogram is sensed, then to try to selectively catheterize the adjacent LV vein.

To conclude, the role of pacing therapy for congestive heart failure remains controversial. Conventional DDD pacing, even at the optimal AV delay for each patient, is probably of low interest because of the deleterious effects of apical right ventricular pacing on the sequence of LV activation, contraction and relaxation. By correcting the electromechanical asynchrony within the left ventricle and AV dysynchrony in the left heart whenever possible, multisite pacing in a dual- (ventricular), triple- or four-chamber configuration appears to be capable of providing major and sustained haemodynamic improvement in selected patients. Controlled studies are needed to evaluate the exact value of this new pacing technique and to define more precisely the patient selection criteria as well as the optimal pacing configuration.

Finally, new developments in lead (transvenous LV leads) and adapter technology and in pacemaker algorithms are necessary to extend these new frontiers for cardiac pacing.

References

1. Hochleitner M, Hörtnagl H, Ng C-K, *et al*. Usefulness of physiologic dual-chamber pacing in drug-resistant idiopathic dilated cardiomyopathy. *Am J Cardiol* 1990; **66**: 198–202.
2. Hochleitner M, Hörtnagl H, Hörtnagl H, *et al*. Long-term efficacy of physiologic dual-chamber pacing in the treatment of end-stage idiopathic dilated cardiomyopathy. *Am J Cardiol* 1992; **70**: 1320–5.
3. Brecker SJ, Xiao HB, Sparrow J, Gibson DG. Effects of dual-chamber pacing with short atrioventricular delay in dilated cardiomyopathy. *Lancet* 1992; **340**: 1308–11.
4. Linde C, Gadler F, Edner M, Nordlander R, Rosenqvist M, Ryden L. Results of atrioventricular synchronous pacing with optimized delay in patients with severe congestive heart failure. *Am J Cardiol* 1995; **75**: 919–23.
5. Gold MR, Feliciano Z, Gottlieb SS, Fisher ML. Dual-chamber pacing with a short atrioventricular delay in congestive heart failure: a randomized study. *J Am Coll Cardiol* 1995; **26**: 967–73.
6. Wish M, Fletcher RD, Gottdiener MD, Cohen AI. Importance of left atrial timing in the programming of dual-chamber pacemakers. *Am J Cardiol* 1987; **60**: 566–71.
7. Ramsaran EK, Spodick DH. Electromechanical delay in the left atrium as a consequence of interatrial block. *Am J Cardiol* 1996; **77**: 1132–4.
8. Wilensky RL, Yudelman P, Cohen AI, *et al*. Serial electrocardiographic changes in idiopathic dilated cardiomyopathy confirmed at necropsy. *Am J Cardiol* 1988; **62**: 276–83.
9. Cowell R, Morris-Thurgood J, Isley C, Paul V. Septal short atrioventricular delay pacing: additional hemodynamic improvements in heart failure. *PACE* 1994; **17**: 1980–3.
10. Innes D, Leitch J, Fletcher P. VDD pacing at short atrioventricular intervals does not improve cardiac output in patients with dilated heart failure. *PACE* 1994; **17**: 959–65.
11. Nishimura RA, Hayes DL, Holmes DR, Tajik AJ. Mechanism of hemodynamic improvement by dual-chamber pacing for severe left ventricular dysfunction: an acute Doppler and catheterization study. *J Am Coll Cardiol* 1995; **25**: 281–8.
12. Scanu P, Lécluse E, Michel L, *et al*. Dual-chamber pacing with optimal atrioventricular delay in drug refractory congestive heart failure: predictive factors of acute pacing efficacy (abstract). *Eur Heart J* 1995; **16**: 103.
13. Mabo P, Cazeau S, Forrer A, *et al*. Isolated long PR interval as only indication of permanent DDD pacing (abstract). *J Am Coll Cardiol* 1992; **19**: 66A.
14. Panidis IP, Ross J, Munley B, *et al*. Diastolic mitral regurgitation in patients with atrioventricular conduction abnormalities: a common finding by Doppler echocardiography. *J Am Coll Cardiol* 1986; **7**: 768–74.
15. Appleton CP, Basnight MA, Gonzalez MS, *et al*. Diastolic mitral regurgitation with atrioventricular conduction abnormalities: relation of mitral flow velocity to transmitral pressure gradients in conscious dogs. *J Am Coll Cardiol* 1991; **18**: 843–9.
16. Ishikawa T, Kimura K, Miyazaki N, *et al*. Diastolic mitral regurgitation in patients with first-degree atrioventricular block. *PACE* 1992; **15**: 1927–31.
17. Xiao HB, Brecker SJD, Gibson DG. Effect of abnormal activation on the time course of the left ventricular pressure pulse in dilated cardiomyopathy. *Br Heart J* 1992; **68**: 403–7.
18. Xiao HB, Brecker SJD, Gibson DG. Differing effects of right ventricular pacing and left bundle branch block on left ventricular function. *Br Heart J* 1993; **69**: 166–73.
19. Xiao HB, Roy C, Gibson DG. Nature of ventricular activation in patients with dilated cardiomyopathy: evidence for bilateral bundle branch block. *Br Heart J* 1994; **72**: 167–74.

20. Wiggers C. The muscular reactions of the mammalian ventricles to artificial surface stimuli. *Am J Physiol* 1925; **73C**: 346–78.
21. Finney J. Hemodynamic alterations in left ventricular function consequent to ventricular pacing. *Am J Physiol* 1965; **208H**: 275–82.
22. Badke F, Boinay P, Covell J. Effects of ventricular pacing on regional left ventricular performance in the dog. *Am J Physiol* 1980; **238H**: 858–67.
23. Waltson A, Starr J, Greenfield J. Effects of different epicardial ventricular pacing sites on left ventricular function in awake dogs. *Am J Cardiol* 1973; **32**: 291–4.
24. Grover M, Glantz SA. Endocardial pacing sites affects left ventricular end-diastolic volume and performance in the intact anesthetized dog. *Cir Res* 1983; **53**: 72–85.
25. Park RC, Little LC, O'Rourke RA. Effect of alteration of left ventricular activation sequence on the left ventricular end-systolic pressure–volume relation in closed-chest dogs. *Cir Res* 1985; **57**: 706–17.
26. Litwin W, Gorman G, Huang S. Effects of different pacing modes on left ventricular relaxation in closed-chest dogs. *PACE* 1989; **12**: 1070–6.
27. Baller D, Wolpers HG, Zipfel J, Bretscheider HJ, Hellige G. Comparison of the effects of right atrial, right ventricular apex and atrioventricular sequential pacing on myocardial oxygen consumption and cardiac efficiency: a laboratory investigation. *PACE* 1988; **11**: 394–403.
28. Adomian GE, Beazell J. Myofibrillar disarray produced in normal hearts by electrical cardiac pacing. *Am Heart J* 1986; **112**: 79–84.
29. Karpawich P, Justice C, Cavitt D, Chang C. Developmental sequelae of fixed-rate ventricular pacing in the immature canine heart: an electrophysiologic hemodynamic and histopathologic evaluation. *Am Heart J* 1990; **119**: 1077–82.
30. Vassallo J, Cassidy D, Miller J, *et al*. Left ventricular endocardial activation during right ventricular pacing: effect of underlying heart disease. *J Am Coll Cardiol* 1986; **7**: 1228–33.
31. Hatala R, Savard P, Tremblay G, *et al*. Three different patterns of ventricular activation in infarcted human hearts. *Circulation* 1995; **1**: 1480–94.
32. Barin ES, Jones SM, Ward DE, Camm AJ, Nathan AW. The right ventricular outflow tract as an alternative permanent pacing site: long-term follow-up. *PACE* 1991; **14**: 3–6.
33. Giudici M, Thornburg GA, Buck DL, *et al*. Right ventricular outflow tract permanent pacing provides long-term improvement in cardiac output: evaluation of chronic implants (abstract). *PACE* 1994; **17**: 819.
34. de Cock C, Meyer A, Kamp O, Visser CA. Hemodynamic benefit of right ventricular outflow tract pacing in patients with atrial fibrillation and slow ventricular response selected for VVIR pacing (abstract). *PACE* 1995; **18**: 847.
35. Karpawich PP, Justice CD, Chang CH, *et al*. Septal ventricular pacing in the immature canine heart: a new perspective. *Am Heart J* 1991; **121**: 827–33.
36. Mabo P, Scherlag BJ, Munsif A, *et al*. A technique for stable His-bundle recording and pacing: electrophysiological and hemodynamic correlates. *PACE* 1995; **18**: 1894–901.
37. Karpawich PP, Gates J, Stokes KB. Septal His–Purkinje ventricular pacing in canines: a new endocardial electrode approach. *PACE* 1992; **15**: 2011–15.
38. Bakker PF, Meijburg H, De Jonge N, *et al*. Beneficial effects of biventricular pacing in congestive heart failure (abstract). *PACE* 1994; **17**: 820.
39. Cazeau S, Ritter P, Lazzarus A, Gras D, Mugica J. Hemodynamic improvement provided by biventricular pacing in congestive heart failure: an acute study (abstract). *PACE* 1996; **19**: 568.
40. Ritter P, Cazeau S, Mundler O, *et al*. Modifications of ventricular activation sequences during biventricular pacing in end-stage congestive heart failure (abstract). *Eur J CPE* 1996; **6**: 139.
41. Cazeau S, Ritter P, Lazzarus A, Gras D, Mugica J. Multisite pacing for congestive heart failure (abstract). *PACE* 1996; **19**: 568.
42. Brecker SJD, Gibson DG. What is the role of pacing in dilated cardiomyopathy? *Eur Heart J* 1996; **17**: 819–24.

43. Daubert C, Leclercq C, Gras D, *et al*. Permanent left atrial pacing with a specifically designed coronary sinus lead. *PACE* (in press).
44. Cazeau S, Ritter P, Bakdach S, *et al*. Four chamber pacing in dilated cardiomyopathy. *PACE* 1994; **17**: 1974–9.
45. Daubert C, Gras D, Berder V, *et al*. Resynchronisation atriale permanente par la stimulation biatriale synchrone pour le traitement préventif du flutter auriculaire associé à un bloc interauriculaire de haut degré. *Arch Mal Coeur* 1994; **87**: 1535–46.
46. Ritter P, Bakdach M, Bourgeois Y, *et al*. Implanting techniques for definitive left ventricular pacing (abstract). *PACE* 1996; **19**: 698.
47. Daubert C, Ritter P, Cazeau S, *et al*. Permanent biventricular pacing in dilated cardiomyopathy: is a totally transvenous approach technically feasible? (abstract). *PACE* 1996; **19**: 699.

2

Pacing in Hypertrophic Cardiomyopathy

C. Linde, F. Gadler and L. Rydén

Introduction

Although mentioned by French pathologists in the middle of the nineteenth century, hypertrophic obstructive cardiomyopathy (HOCM) remained incompletely characterized until the descriptions by Tere[1] and Brock[2] in the late 1950s. Using autopsy findings in a group of relatively young males who died suddenly, they described in detail the picture of a concentric left ventricular hypertrophy (LVH) including subaortic obstruction. The condition was usually combined with an anomaly of the mitral valve, and myocardial microscopy revealed a chaotic structure of the myofibrils.

The haemodynamic effect of HOCM was explored during the 1960s in catheterization studies by Braunwald and Ebert,[3] and during the 1970s the use of Doppler echocardiography permitted a more careful exploration of the pathophysiology.[4,5] More recent contributions have focused mainly on the genetic background of hypertrophic cardiomyopathy in the broad sense. In patients with this disease, approximately 30 mutations have been described regarding betamyosine-troponin and tropomyosin in chromosomes 11 and 15.[6–8] It is known that these genetic disturbances are heterogeneous and of variable penetrance, including the clinical manifestation and the risk of sudden death. Within one family the same genotype may create various clinical pictures of the disease. The common denominator is, however, LVH. The localization of this has a definite influence on the symptomatic pattern and partly also on the prognosis. The main type of hypertrophic cardiomyopathy is characterized by a thickening of the interventricular septal wall, affecting the outflow tract of the left ventricle (LV) in particular, although an apical hypertrophy may be present to some extent.

Clinical Manifestations and Diagnostics

The dominating subjective symptoms among patients with HOCM are breathlessness and/or chest pain, which in serious cases may already exist at rest. These symptoms are, however, most typically increased by different amounts of effort. Exercise may also induce various degrees of disturbances in consciousness in the form of dizzy spells and/or fainting attacks. Sudden death may occur. The intensity of the symptoms may vary, reflecting the highly variable LV outflow tract obstruction. The clinical course is somewhat unpredictable. Symptomatic onset at a young age usually reflects a more advanced disease and is considered to carry a higher risk for sudden death. A case history including syncopal attacks is prognostically negative. The disease is usually progressive, although the deterioration of symptoms may be slow, lasting over decades.

Physical examination usually discloses an unspecific systolic murmur, most apparent to the left of the sternal border with a distribution towards the apical region of the heart. A vigorous apical bump dislodged to the left indicates the presence of LVH. In advanced cases, the arterial pulse may appear biphasic as a sign of a mid-systolic outflow tract of obstruction from the LV. It may be difficult to establish a correct diagnosis only by the use of physical findings. The combination of the symptoms described and an unspecific systolic murmur should raise suspicion of HOCM, but further examinations should confirm the diagnosis and the severity of disease.

A resting ECG with signs of LVH increases the suspicion of HOCM, particularly in the presence of marked septal Q waves. Exercise testing may be indicated, although it usually only discloses unspecific information such as a decreased exercise tolerance and possible ECG changes, indicating coronary insufficiency often in combination with a decreasing blood pressure in response to increasing work load.

The technique that firmly establishes the diagnosis is echo–Doppler. Besides disclosing myocardial hypertrophy, this form of investigation provides a dynamic picture of the LV outflow conditions and also reveals the characteristic systolic anterior movement of the anterior mitral leaflet towards the ventricular septum. Patients who have hypertrophy, but only minor or no obstruction of the left ventricle at rest, should be investigated in combination with some type of provocation. This may, for example, be in the form of exercise or isoprenalin infusion. A pronounced outflow tract obstruction may be disclosed during such provocative manoeuvres, illustrating the dynamic character of the disease and explaining effort-induced symptoms.

Drug Therapy and Surgery

Patients with symptomatic HOCM are usually offered pharmacological therapy. Drugs with a negative inotropic effect, such as beta-receptor blockers, calcium channel blockers, and disopyramide are utilized.[9] They may diminish the outflow tract obstruction, and in parallel cause symptomatic relief. Calcium channel blockers have also been considered to at least partly improve the diastolic dysfunction that follows the LVH. It has, however, been recognized that this class of drugs also induces peripheral vasodilatation, which may increase the obstruction and induce signs of heart failure. Side-effects that are fairly common, particularly with the use of high dosages of beta-receptor blockers, are chronotrophic incompetence and leg fatigue.

Treatment with disopyramide is compromised by the frequent, rather unpleasant anticholinergic effect, the understandable reason why this particular type of drug has gained relatively little acceptance. The most commonly used pharmacological treatment seems to be beta-receptor blockers.

Patients who (despite pharmacological therapy) remain symptomatic may be admitted to open heart surgery with myectomy. This procedure has also been combined with mitral valve replacement. A successful myectomy may cause a substantial and long-lasting symptomatic improvement, but it has not been documented to prolong survival. The procedure imposes a relatively small, but nevertheless existing preoperative mortality in the range of 1–2%. Another not unusual complication is high-degree atrioventricular block and an occasional ventricular septal defect.[10–11]

Clinical Experiences of Cardiac Pacing

It has been known that pacing the right ventricle may decrease the outflow tract obstruction on the left side since Hassenstein *et al.*[12] described their initial observations on VVI paced subjects. It was, however, also noted that atrioventricular desynchronization neutralized the beneficial effects on the outflow tract obstruction. This reasonably related to the elimination of the atrial contribution to ventricular filling and to the induction of a pacemaker syndrome, conditions that by physiological reasons should be particularly deleterious for patients with HOCM.[12,13] Technical problems in establishing an appropriate mode of cardiac pacing is the reasonable explanation for the fact that this type of treatment was not further explored until the publications of Jeanrenaud *et al.*[14] and Fananapazir *et al.*[15] during 1992. Since then, cardiac pacing of HOCM has attracted great interest.

Jeanrenaud *et al.* described a series of eight drug-refractory patients with a follow-up of 3–62 months. DDD pacing with programmed sensed AV delays of 50–90 ms improved symptomatology in all patients by at least one functional class. A 50% reduction of LVOT gradients was seen at the long-term follow-up as well as a lower LVOT gradient in SR when pacing was momentarily discontinued. Fananapazir *et al.* reported 44 drug-refractory patients with follow-up of 1–3 months. In this series, LVOT gradients decreased to the same extent as in the previously mentioned study and symptomatology improved, especially regarding angina and impaired consciousness. An improved exercise capacity could also be seen in most patients. The most striking difference between these two studies was Fananapazir's quoted AV delays of 125 ms and longer. In contrast, consequent studies have showed AV delays of ≤100 ms to be necessary to accomplish the desired haemodynamic effects.

Our own experience of cardiac pacing in HOCM originates from 55 patients (69 ± 15 years; 23 males) during the period September 1992 to December 1995. Two of these patients had a previous myectomy and two developed their symptoms of left ventricular obstruction following aortic valvular surgery. Eleven of the patients were in NYHA class IV, 29 in class III and 12 in class II. Thus, all patients were symptomatic and most of them had severe symptoms mainly in the form of dyspnoea and angina pectoris during effort. Syncopal attacks or dizzy spells related to physical exercise were reported by seven of the patients. All of them had been treated with one or several pharmacological agents without clear-cut symptomatic improvement and in some cases with side-effects necessitating the discontinuation of drug treatment. These patients represent a consecutive series of subjects who were referred to our department initially for consideration of myectomy and during the last year also for cardiac pacing. During this period further patients were evaluated without receiving a pacemaker. One of them was referred directly to myectomy and the others were considered suitable for treatment with drugs.

Preoperative Investigations

All our patients underwent preoperative echo–Doppler. The 19 subjects, who in the resting condition had a pressure fall from the left ventricle to aorta below 40 mmHg, were provoked with isoprenalin infusion.[16] During this provocative manoeuvre all of them had a substantial increase in their LV outflow obstruction.

Following the exploration of outflow tract obstruction, pacing was temporarily applied by introducing an electrode into the right ventricular apical portion and in the right atrium. The effect on the outflow tract obstruction of AV synchronous pacing at various AV intervals was evaluated by echo–Doppler. Isoprenalin provocation was repeated in the subjects who disclosed a major obstruction only after this procedure. A reduction of the maximum LV outflow gradient of at least 40 mmHg was needed for permanent pacemaker implantation.

In one study, the importance of the RV lead position was evaluated.[17] A distal apical lead position was compared with a septal position inside the right ventricle in 14 patients. The apical lead position was by far the most superior. In fact, pacing on the septal side in some cases even increased the outflow tract gradient (Figure 2.1). Another factor of paramount importance for a successful decrease of the LV obstruction by pacing is the AV conduction time (Figure 2.2). The programmed AV delay must be shorter than the native PQ interval in order to fully control the RV electrical activation both at rest and during exercise. This means that the AV conduction time must be kept short, and furthermore it must be individually optimized. Too short a conduction time decreases the possibility for ventricular filling and therefore must be avoided. Radiofrequency ablation of the AV node or modification has been attempted among patients in whom it has been difficult to achieve full control over the ventricular activation owing to a spontaneous, fairly short atrial ventricular conduction time, usually below 140 ms.[18] An example of such a procedure is given in Figure 2.3.

Clinical Results

The main results in our series of patients corresponds fairly well with those reported by others. The original resting LV outflow tract gradient of close to 100 mmHg was decreased to a little under 50 mmHg in optimal pacing conditions (Figure 2.4). With regard to long-term results, 41 of the 55 patients were followed for at least 3 months,

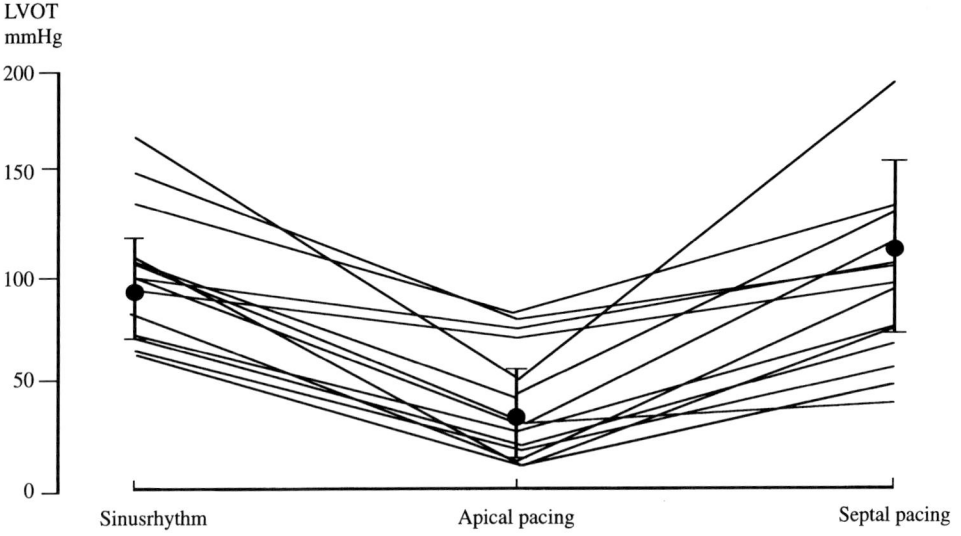

Figure 2.1 Left ventricular outflow tract (LVOT) gradient during sinus rhythm and pacing with optimal AV delay in apical and septal position. Individual patients and mean ± SD.

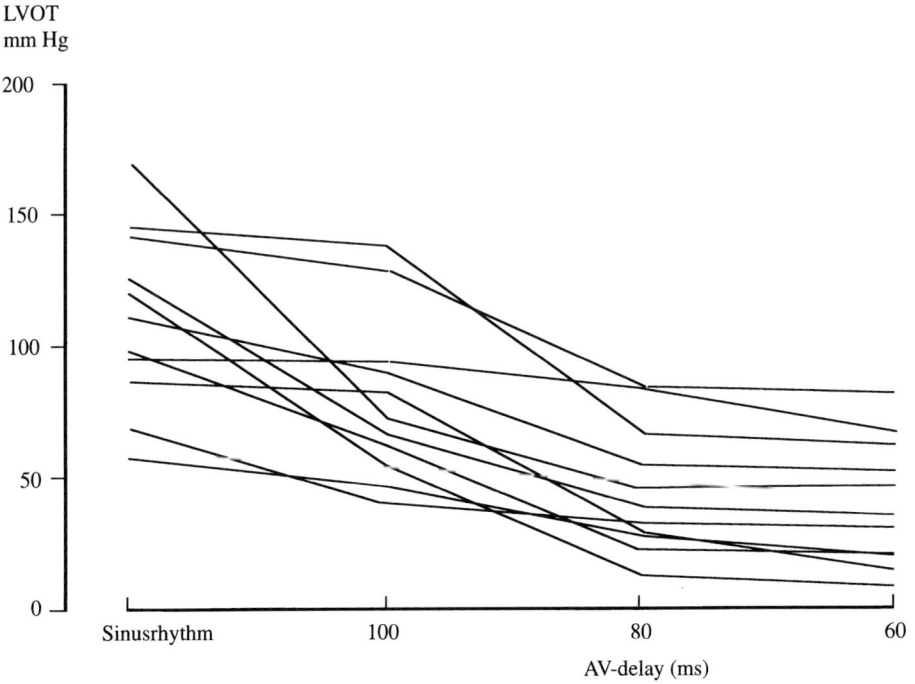

Figure 2.2 Left ventricular outflow tract (LVOT) gradient during sinus rhythm and pacing with different AV delays (sensed), in an individual typical patient.

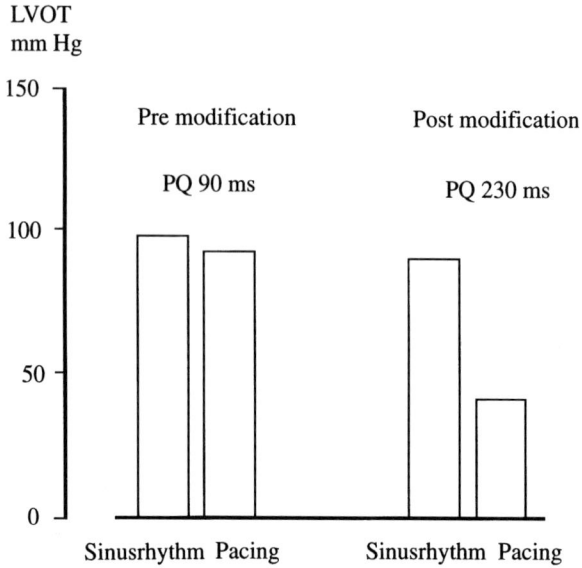

Figure 2.3 Left ventricular outflow tract (LVOT) gradient in one patient during sinus rhythm and pacing before and after AV nodal modification.

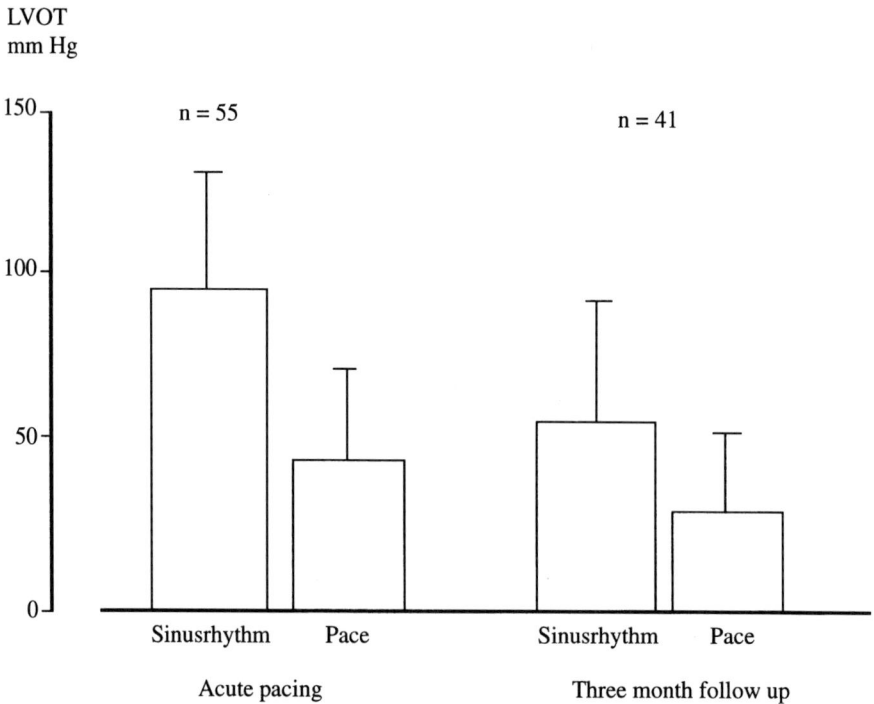

Figure 2.4 Left ventricular outflow tract (LVOT) gradient during sinus rhythm and pacing, acute study and 3-month follow-up.

and the results were long-lasting. An interesting observation was that temporary investigations with a pacemaker made inactive revealed a lower gradient in sinus rhythm, about 50 mmHg, than that observed before pacing was initiated. A similar spontaneous decrease in the LV outflow tract obstruction has been noted also by other investigators.[15,16] In a recent double-blind prospective study of long-term effects of cardiac pacing in 10 subjects who had been paced for at least 3 months, however, we could not document a lasting improvement in the LVOT gradient.[19] Symptoms and the LVOT gradient reappeared 1–13 days after discontinuation of pacing. After reinitialization of pacing, LVOT gradients and symptomatology returned to the same levels as before discontinuation. The pacing-induced effects thus seemed to be dependent on continuous pre-excitation of the apex and no permanent altered activation of the septum took place.

Symptomatic improvement in NYHA class is illustrated in Figure 2.5.[16] Borg ratings during exercise testing revealed that the ratings for chest pain in particular were reduced. This can be noted already at submaximal exercise levels and the results were the same both for patients with spontaneous LV outflow obstruction and for those who revealed a significant gradient only during provocation with isoprenalin. Dyspnoea, frequently the most dominating symptom, was also improved by pacing. In fact, following the initiation of pacemaker treatment more patients were limited by

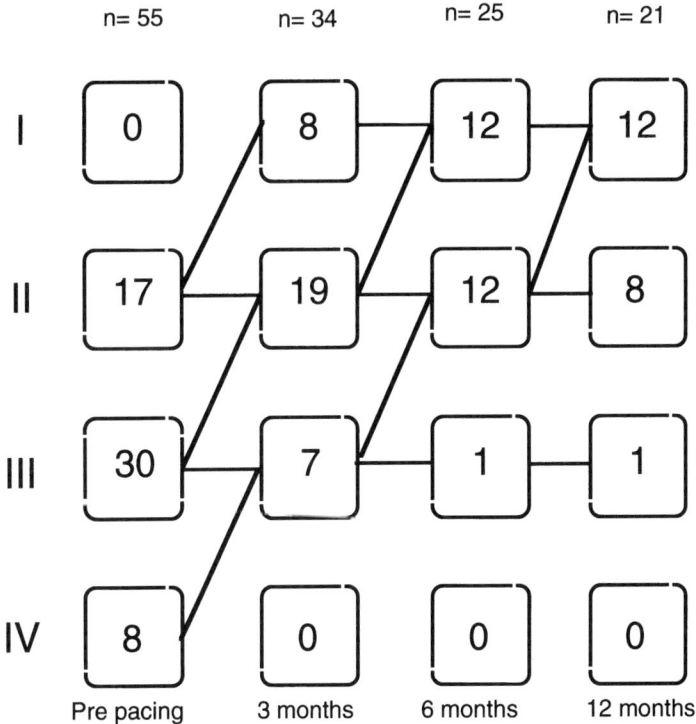

	n= 55	n= 34	n= 25	n= 21
I	0	8	12	12
II	17	19	12	8
III	30	7	1	1
IV	8	0	0	0
	Pre pacing	3 months	6 months	12 months

Figure 2.5 NYHA functional class in patients before pacemaker treatment and after 3, 6 and 12 months of pacing.

general fatigue rather than by chest pain or dyspnoea. One may speculate whether fatigue could be influenced by improved physical training following the institution of cardiac pacing (Figure 2.6).

In our series, seven patients reported loss of consciousness or dizzy spells before pacing, and all were improved in this respect. This observation is in agreement with previous reports.

Of our 55 pacemaker-treated patients, only 3 were subsequently offered myectomy, while the other 52 maintained their improvement with cardiac pacing. In patients with drug-induced side-effects, the pharmacological treatment was either decreased in dosage or sometimes stopped. Presently there is no systematic evaluation of the possibility of eliminating pharmacological therapy for paced HOCM patients. Pacing is therefore at present an additional treatment for patients with drug-refractory symptoms.

Two of the patients who subsequently underwent a surgical procedure had deterioration of angina pectoris which related to progressive coronary artery disease. Thus, myectomy was in those two cases performed at the same time as bypass surgery. The third patient was not improved at all by cardiac pacing. With present knowledge this subject would not have been accepted for permanent pacing: she was the second patient in our series and temporary pacing produced a reduction of her LV outflow tract gradient of only 15 mmHg. Following this experience our criterion for permanent pacemaker implantation was changed to the previously mentioned gradient reduction of 30 mmHg.

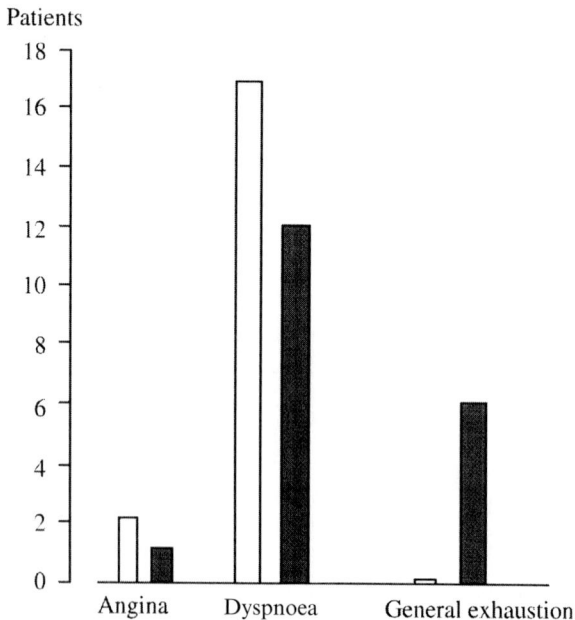

Figure 2.6 Subjective reason for terminating exercise testing in 19 patients before (empty bars) and after (filled bars) 3 months of pacing.

Experiences from Prospective Randomized Studies

The studies reported here represent prospective but uncontrolled investigations. Although promising, these data need confirmation in prospective randomized studies.

Such a study has recently been reported, the PIC multicentre study (unpublished data). In that study, 83 patients with drug-refractory HOCM referred for myectomy and with resting gradients $\geqslant 30$ mmHg were given permanent pacemakers after a temporary test. Patients were randomly assigned to either 3 months of inactive (AAI 30) or active pacing (DDD) after examination with echo–Doppler, Holter, treadmill and Quality-of-Life questionnaire. After 3 months, patients were reprogrammed to the opposite pacing mode and re-evaluated. Seventeen patients required early reprogramming from the inactive to the active pacing mode owing to severe symptoms. The LVOT gradient decreased from 59 ± 35 mmHg (AAI 30) to 31 ± 25 mmHg (DDD, $p < 0.0001$). The mean NYHA class improved from 2.4 ± 0.7 (AAI 30) to 1.6 ± 0.6 (DDD, $p < 0.0001$). Exercise tolerance increased significantly, however, only in the subset of patients with severely limited exercise tolerance at baseline (8.0 ± 1.7 min, AAI 30; 9.8 ± 3.0, DDD: $p = 0.008$). The quality-of-life evaluation revealed significant improvements in alertness, autonomy and tolerance of strenuous physical activity, as well as with regard to self-perceived health and cardiovascular symptoms. Interestingly, pacemaker implantation had a placebo effect, especially regarding chest pain and dyspnoea, observed in those assigned to a first study period of inactive pacing. In these patients, however, symptomatology further and significantly improved when they were reprogrammed to the active mode.

Another randomized blinded study of the effect of cardiac pacing was mentioned earlier in this chapter, in which the effects of a sudden cessation of cardiac pacing in patients who were successfully paced for at least 3 months was evaluated.[19]

Clinical Utility and Future Aspects

It may seem easy to initiate cardiac pacing in patients with HOCM. It should, however, be kept in mind that the results presented have been achieved in very carefully controlled trials. All patients have been assessed preoperatively with Doppler cardiography and temporary pacing. Very careful location of the right ventricular electrode is mandatory. The AV interval must be individually optimized with repeated echo Doppler evaluation. From the present data, supported by controlled trials, cardiac pacing appears to be an important therapeutic possibility for HOCM patients. To avoid negative effects, however, patients must be carefully selected and pacing very meticulously monitored when instituted.

There is scope to simplify the preoperative evaluation. Patients with pronounced LV obstruction at rest could possibly be paced directly with individualization of the pacemaker programming following implantation. Patients without LV obstruction at rest seem to need some form of provocative manoeuvre and temporary pacing before permanent implantation. Centres in which HOCM patients are paced should also be able to perform AV node modification in those individuals in which the pacemaker treatment may be optimized by such a procedure.

There are interesting questions still to be answered. For example, is it possible to stop drug therapy without affecting the cardiac pacing? Does pacing introduced at an earlier stage of the disease diminish the need for subsequent drug therapy? Are the long-term effects of cardiac pacing similar to or better than those of myectomy? A prospective randomized study in which symptomatic, drug-refractory patients are offered either myectomy or cardiac pacing would be of great value. In such a study the question of longevity would be an important parameter. So far, none of the therapeutic models offered to patients with HOCM have been fully evaluated to answer the question whether the treatment influences the vital prognosis of the patient.

References

1. Tere RD. Asymmetrical hypertrophy of the heart in young adults. *Br Heart J* 1958; **20**: 1–8.
2. Brock RC. Functional obstruction of the left ventricle. *Guys Hosp Rep* 1957; **106**: 221–8.
3. Braunwald E, Ebert P. Hemodynamic alterations in idiopathic hypertrophic subaortic stenosis induced by sympathomimetic drugs. *Am J Cardiol* 1962; **10**: 489–95.
4. Maron BJ, Gottdiener JS, Epstein SE. Patterns and significance of left ventricular hypertrophy in hypertrophic cardiomyopathy: a wide angle, two dimensional echocardiographic study of 125 patients. *Am J Cardiol* 1981; **48**: 418–28.
5. Sasson Z, Yock P, Hatle L, *et al.* Doppler echocardiographic determination of the pressure gradient in hypertrophic cardiomyopathy. *JACC* 1988; **1**: 752–6.
6. Watkins H, MacRae C, Thierfelder L, *et al.* A disease locus for familial hypertrophic cardiomyopathy maps to chromosome Iq3. *Nat Gen* 1993; **3**: 333–7.
7. Fananapazir L, Epstein ND. Genotype–phenotype correlations in hypertrophic cardiomyopathy: insights provided by comparisons of kindreds with distinct and identical beta-myosin heavy chain gene mutations. *Circulation* 1994; **89**: 22–32.
8. Watkins H, McKenna WJ, Thierfelder L, *et al.* Mutations in the gene for cardiac troponin-T and alfa-tropomyosin in hypertrophic cardiomyopathy. *N Engl J Med* 1995; **332**: 1058–64.
9. Vigle ED, Rakowski H, Kimball BP, *et al.* Hypertrophic cardiomyopathy: clinical spectrum and treatment. *Circulation* 1995; **92**: 1680–92.
10. Seiler C, Hess OM, Schoenbeck M, *et al.* Long-term follow up of medical versus surgical therapy for hypertrophic cardiomyopathy: a retrospective study. *JACC* 1991; **17**: 634–42.
11. Blanchard DG, Ross J. Hypertrophic cardiomyopathy: prognosis with medical or surgical therapy. *Clin Cardiol* 1991; **14**: 11–19.
12. Hassenstein P, Storch HH, Schmitz W. Erfahrungen mit der Shrittmacherdauerbehandlung bei Patienten mit obstruktiver Kardiomyopathie. *Thoraxkirurgie* 1975; **23**: 496–8.
13. Duck HJ, Hutschenreiter W, Paneau H, *et al.* Vorhofsynchrone Ventrikelstimulation Init Verkürzter AV Verzögerungszeit als Therapieprincip der hypertrophischen obstruktiven Kardiomyopathie. *Z Gesamte Inn Med* 1984; **39**: 437–47.
14. Jeanrenaud X, Goy JJ, Kappenberger L. Effects of dual-chamber pacing in hypertrophic obstructive cardiomyopathy. *Lancet* 1992; **339**: 1318–23.
15. Fananapazir L, Cannon R, Tripodi D, *et al.* Impact of dual-chamber pacing in patients with obstructive hypertrophic cardiomyopathy with symptoms refractory to verapamil and beta-adrenergic-blocker therapy. *Circulation* 1992; **85**: 2149–461.
16. Gadler F, Linde C, Juhlin-Dannfelt A, Ribeiro A, Rydén L. Long-term effects of dual chamber pacing in patients with hypertrophic obstructive cardiomyopathy without outflow obstruction at rest. *Eur Heart J* 1997 (in press).

17. Gadler F, Linde C, Juhlin-Dannfelt A, Ribeiro A, Rydén L. Influence of right ventricular pacing site on left ventricular obstruction in patients with hypertrophic obstructive cardiomyopathy. *JACC* 1996; **27**: 1219–24.
18. Gadler F, Linde C, Darpö B. Radio frequency modification of the atrioventricular conduction as adjunct therapy for patients with hypertrophic obstructive cardiomyopathy treated with pacemakers. Unpublished manuscript.
19. Gadler F, Linde C, Juhlin-Dannfelt A, Ribeiro A, Rydén L. Rapid return of obstruction and symptoms after discontinuation of pacing in patients with hypertrophic obstructive cardiomyopathy: a controlled double-blind study. *Eur Heart J* 1996; **17**: 169.

3

Pacing in Atrial Fibrillation

S. Saksena, I. Giorgberidze, P. Delfaut, A. Prakash, A. N. Munsif and R. B. Krol

Atrial fibrillation (AF) has been recognized, with increasing concern, to be a potentially disabling illness, occurring either as a symptom of many cardiac diseases or as an isolated disorder.[1] It can independently contribute to mortality and morbidity and may have serious prognostic import in acute or chronic cardiac disease.[2] The application of pacing techniques in management of AF has been an important advance in the treatment of these patients. Hitherto, the role of pacing has been dominated by its rate support contribution in the treatment of patients with tachycardia–bradycardia syndrome. More recently, there has been a resurgence of interest in prevention and termination of AF or atrial flutter with atrial pacing methods. Antitachycardia pacing has been employed for reversal of drug-refractory type-1 atrial flutter, but its utility in type-2 atrial flutter and AF is now being explored. This chapter will focus largely on the recent advances in the applications of atrial pacing for prevention and termination of atrial tachyarrhythmias but will initially review the common clinical situations requiring pacing for rate support in AF.

Rate Support in Atrial Fibrillation

There are two potential goals of therapy in AF, control of ventricular rate during tachycardia episodes and restoration of sinus rhythm. The relative effort expended in each goal varies with a number of clinical and arrhythmia characteristics.[3] Selection of a particular goal is confounded by an uncertain state of knowledge which does not conclusively establish the relative benefits of rate control versus rhythm control in the long-term management of these patients.[4] Traditionally, efforts at rate control dominate AF management in two clinical scenarios:

(a) acutely, during an episode of AF with symptomatic rapid ventricular rates;
(b) chronically, in AF patients with either advanced cardiac disease or having failed prior efforts at drug and electrical therapy to restore sinus rhythm.

Both situations may be complicated by intercurrent bradycardia due to the therapy used to reduce ventricular rate (drugs and catheter ablation of the atrioventricular junction). While acute management of such bradycardia requires drug withdrawal with or without the institution of temporary pacing, permanent dual-chamber or ventricular pacemaker insertion is performed in the chronic situation. Similarly, drug-induced bradycardia may complicate efforts at rhythm control, and permanent pacing may be needed for long-term rate support. It is estimated that 133 000 pacemakers were inserted in 1993 in the United States and approximately 50% of these were implanted for sick sinus syndrome. A significant proportion of these implants can be attributed to the bradycardia–tachycardia syndrome.[5] Catheter ablation in the atrioventricular junctional region is an increasing contributor to the need for permanent cardiac pacing for rate support. It has been estimated that approximately 1500 such procedures were performed in the United States in 1991.[6] Atrioventricular nodal modification procedures which attempt rate control without complete transection of atrioventricular conduction can contribute to this number as well since an estimated one-third progress to complete atrioventricular block.[7]

While demand ventricular pacing alone can suffice in some patients after catheter ablation, recent clinical trials have focused on the need for single-chamber rate-responsive pacing versus dual-chamber pacing modes to achieve optimal exercise performance and quality-of-life in these patients.[8] These will be discussed in some detail in a later section of this chapter.

Prevention of Atrial Fibrillation by Pacing

Restoration of atrial rhythm control using atrial-based pacing in patients with AF is now again under active study.[9–11] Initially, the use of permanent pacemakers as adjunctive therapy in patients with bradycardia–tachycardia syndrome produced, as a by-product, observations on the behaviour of AF recurrences. Reduced recurrence rates were reported in paced patients with vagally-mediated bradycardia dependent AF and sick sinus syndrome patients implanted with atrial or dual-chamber pacemakers.[12,13] A variety of potential mechanisms subserving this observation were postulated. It is necessary to review briefly the major electrophysiological changes in AF and consider the potential mechanisms for pacing methods to modify atrial electrophysiology. Clinical trials with atrial fibrillation recurrence end-points using a variety of designs have been reported or are in progress. These will also be reviewed in a later section.

Clinical Electrophysiology of Atrial Fibrillation

Intra-atrial conduction delay and short atrial refractory periods are two of the primary electrophysiological abnormalities reported by many authors in patients with atrial flutter and fibrillation.[14–20] These properties can support the multiple wavelets of electrical excitation hypothesized in AF[21] and recently recorded in animal and human studies.[22,23] In this milieu, multiple local re-entry circuits may be inscribed if a critical wavelength for re-entry is met. Increasing atrial conduction delay may also be mediated by nonuniform anisotropic conduction in a diseased area of atrium, as suggested by Spach *et al.*,[24] or around anatomic obstacles.[25] Cellular uncoupling (nonuniform anisotropy) may result in a conduction block in the propagation parallel to the long axis of the atrial cells, whereas slow conduction may exist in the transverse axis. Thus, re-entry may occur in a very small area of tissue (2–4 mm^2). Recently Papageriou *et al.* noted nonuniform anisotropic properties of atrial conduction in the posterior Triangle of Koch.[26] Atrial conduction delay is often observed in patients with AF and is revealed on surface electrocardiogram by a broad P wave[14–16] and prolonged intra-atrial conduction time.[27] Conduction delays are accentuated by atrial premature beats coupled 10–20 ms beyond the refractory period. Indeed, we have noted such delays exist in the vicinity of the coronary sinus ostium, low-to-mid interatrial septum and crista terminalis when atrial extrastimuli are used to induce AF.[28]

Atrial premature beats can trigger AF[29,30] with critical coupling intervals which typically range from 300 to 500 ms.[31] Propagation of this ectopic wavefront in an abnormal substrate with heterogeneous refractoriness causes conduction block and may induce re-entry.[20] Autonomic nervous system influences can aid in the initiation of AF. Vagal stimulation shortens atrial refractory periods and increases dispersion of atrial refractoriness.[32,33] Sinus bradycardia and atrial cycle length variability are characteristic of vagal influences and have been reported before the onset of AF by several investigators.[31,34–36]

Another important element in AF initiation or maintenance may be a haemodynamic factor. A variety of left and right heart diseases can impede atrial emptying and lead to chamber distension. Mitral or tricuspid valvular dysfunction induced by desynchronization of atrioventricular contraction during AF can result in increased atrial myocardial stretch due to chamber distension. This distension can lead to alterations in conduction and an increase in automaticity.[37] These conditions, as stated before, provide the milieu for AF onset and persistence.

Mechanisms of Atrial Fibrillation Prevention by Pacing

Two major mechanisms by which atrial pacing can prevent atrial arrhythmias are (1) reduction or even elimination of atrial premature beats that initiate intra-atrial re-entry, and (2) alteration of the propagation of premature atrial beats, avoiding intra atrial re-entry.

Suppression of atrial premature beats

Atrial premature beats can emerge during sinus bradycardia. In some patients, occurrence of these atrial premature beats is invariably associated with sinus rates below a critical level.[12] Thus, prevention of slow rates by atrial pacing may reduce atrial premature beats capable of triggering AF and mediate a preventive role for demand atrial pacing. In contrast, the role of overdrive atrial pacing in suppression of atrial premature beats unrelated to sinus bradycardia and, hence, in prevention of AF is not quite as clear. Murgatroyd *et al.* noted that overdrive atrial pacing prevented AF episodes in some patients with atrial premature beats and AF unrelated to brady-cardia, but increased the AF recurrence rate in others.[36] Furthermore, the correlation between heart rates and the frequency of atrial premature beats in the unselected AF patient population has not been well established.

Several mechanisms of spontaneous AF initiation have been proposed and pacing may modify each one. Based on available clinical and experimental data, three potential cellular mechanisms are discussed below:

(1) Atrial premature beats originating from partially depolarized cells with abnormal automaticity may initiate AF.[37] Pacing at faster rates can suppress this type of automaticity by overdrive mechanisms.

(2) Significant variability in atrial cycle length may also predispose to AF initiation. Long–short PP sequences may precede AF initiation. In such cases, rate adaptive pacing may regularize atrial cycle length and eliminate significant cycle length fluctuations.

(3) Initiation of AF and atrial flutter in some clinical settings has been associated with dispersion of refractoriness (and inhomogeneous recovery of excitability) in atria and creation of zones of functional block of conduction as a prerequisite for initiation of re-entry.[15] It has been suggested that the overdrive pacing could reduce the probability of such conduction block by alleviating dispersion of refractoriness. However, dispersion of refractoriness is not significantly altered by overdrive pacing with the rates within the clinically applicable range.[18]

Conversely, overdrive and rate-adaptive pacing has the potential to be proarrhyth-mic. In human atrial fibres, increased pacing rates can produce delayed after-depolarizations which can trigger spontaneous action potentials.[38] Thus, an increased heart rate due to pacing (similar to the sinus tachycardia as seen in Holter data) may favour the initiation of increased spontaneous atrial ectopic activity. El-Sherif and others have shown that re-entrant premature beats can also be facilitated by an increased baseline heart rate.[39]

Alteration of the atrial activation pattern

Atrial premature beat(s) with short coupling interval(s) often encounter local delay and/or conduction block at the site(s) with delayed recovery of excitability (pro-longed refractoriness) or owing to atrial anisotropy. This promotes re-entrant conduction patterns. Altered and earlier excitation of these sites could improve recovery of excitability, reducing conduction delay at this area, and prevent re-entrant excitation from being achieved. By knowing the location of the critical zone of 'slow' conduction or block and the site of origin of premature atrial beats, it could be theoretically possible to optimize the site of preventive pacing.[31,40] A single stimula-tion pattern could suffice. Prevention of AF by single-site pacing is aimed at modification of atrial premature beat propagation at the initial site(s) of re-entrant activation during AF. It requires detailed atrial mapping studies. Reproducibility of re-entrant activation at this site at initiation of AF has to be documented. This may also be studied during AF initiation from different right and left atrial sites. However, the problem is a difficult one since the location of the abnormal atrial substrate and the site of origin of atrial premature beats are usually unknown on routine clinical evaluation. Theoretically, in this case, pre-excitation of many potential abnormal sites can be achieved by pacing both atria simultaneously. This is generally achieved by dual-site pacing methods.

Simultaneous pacing from two sites is performed with transvenous electrodes. The electrophysiological effects of this pacing mode have been extensively studied in our laboratory.[41–43] Acute prevention of AF induction in patients with reproducibly inducible AF with dual-site atrial pacing has been studied.[41] Dual-site atrial pacing has been performed by simultaneous stimulation of the high right atrium and either coronary sinus ostium (dual-site right atrial pacing: DAP) or distal coronary sinus (biatrial pacing: BAP) sites. Pacing and recording sites during computerized endo-cardial catheter mapping are shown schematically in Figure 3.1. Using computerized endocardial or epicardial mapping, we studied atrial activation patterns during single-site pacing from different atrial sites, as well as during dual-site and biatrial pacing.

During single-site pacing, global atrial activation time as reflected in P-wave duration shows minimal differences in single-site pacing compared with sinus rhythm. However, regional atrial activation can differ significantly. A comparison of sinus rhythm and right atrial appendage pacing shows earlier excitation of the atrioventricular nodal–His and adjoining septal regions with the latter mode. The

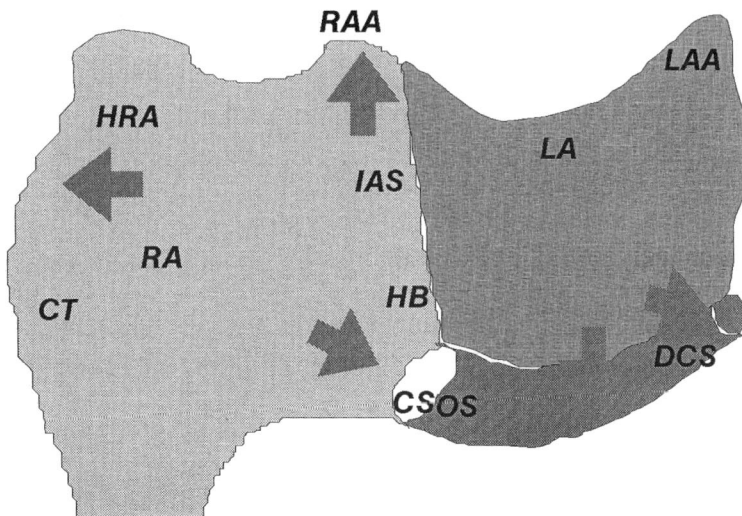

Figure 3.1 Schematic illustrating the sites used for pacing and catheter mapping of atrial activation. Standard 6-Fr decapolar catheters were used for mapping at the crista terminalis and the interatrial septum. Left atrial activation was recorded either by crossing a patent foramen ovale or by positioning a catheter in the lower left pulmonary artery. CSOS = coronary sinus ostium; CT = crista terminalis; DCS = distal coronary sinus; HRA = high right atrium; IAS = interatrial septum; LA = left atrium; LAA = left atrial appendage; RAA = right atrial appendage.

coronary sinus ostial region is, however, rapidly activated during sinus rhythm, perhaps owing to proximity to posterior atrial inputs into the atrioventricular nodal region. Coronary ostial pacing activates the low septal right atrium and the inferior right atrium more rapidly than the inferior left atrium. Distal coronary sinus pacing results in similar conduction delay in the reverse direction, though activation of the atrioventricular nodal–His region often precedes the proximal coronary sinus activation. These pacing data suggest an important role of preferential atrial propagation based either on anatomic obstacles or anisotropic conduction resulting in important regional differences in atrial activation. Consequently, recovery of excitability is altered in similar fashion. This change in atrial activation and recovery of excitability may result potentially in elimination of sites of conduction delay that may be involved in arrhythmogenesis.

Recent studies using catheter mapping during dual-site right atrial and biatrial pacing have raised interesting issues on the feasibility of multisite atrial pacing in prevention of this arrhythmia. Prakash et al. showed that dual-site right atrial pacing in patients with atrial flutter and fibrillation significantly shortens intra-atrial, interatrial and global atrial activation times compared with sinus rhythm, single-site high right atrial and coronary sinus ostial pacing.[42] Both dual-site right atrial and biatrial pacing significantly shorten P-wave duration owing to two simultaneously originating wavefronts and achieve left atrial activation within approximately 40 ms (Figure 3.2). Early activation of the left atrium was also persistently observed during coronary sinus ostial pacing. Munsif et al. showed that in patients with atrial flutter during dual-site right atrial pacing, fusion of two wavefronts occurs in high-to-mid interatrial septum with pre-excitation of mid-to-distal coronary sinus by the wavefront from the coronary sinus ostial pacing electrode.[43] In the region of crista terminalis, fusion occurs predominantly in the mid-cristal area with low crista being pre-excited by the wavefront from the coronary sinus ostial pacing electrode. During biatrial pacing, fusion constantly occurs in the coronary sinus ostial and low crista area with the consistent pre-excitation of the posteroinferior left atrium and the floor of the right atrium. Thus, dual-site atrial pacing, biatrial pacing and coronary sinus ostial pacing achieve the pre-excitation of right and left atrial regions, including low-to-mid intra-atrial septum, posteroinferior left atrium and low crista terminalis. While the role of some of these regions in initiation and maintenance of particular atrial re-entrant rhythms has become well known,[44,45] the importance of others still has to be defined in different clinical settings of this arrhythmia. Furthermore, Prakash et al. found that the propagation of late atrial extrastimuli with coupling intervals of 300–400 ms is not altered by dual-site right atrial or biatrial pacing.[46] However, these two pacing modes significantly reduce the conduction delay that is encountered by closely coupled right atrial extrastimuli in the coronary sinus ostial and low posterior part of the left atrium when compared with single-site high right atrial pacing.[47] These data suggest that the mechanism of AF prevention for the closely coupled atrial premature beat can be the improvement of regional conduction. No definite conclusion about the role of dual-site pacing in the prevention of AF induced by late atrial premature beats can be made. There are currently insufficient data on the efficacy of acute or chronic dual-site pacing for AF prevention in this particular subset of patients.

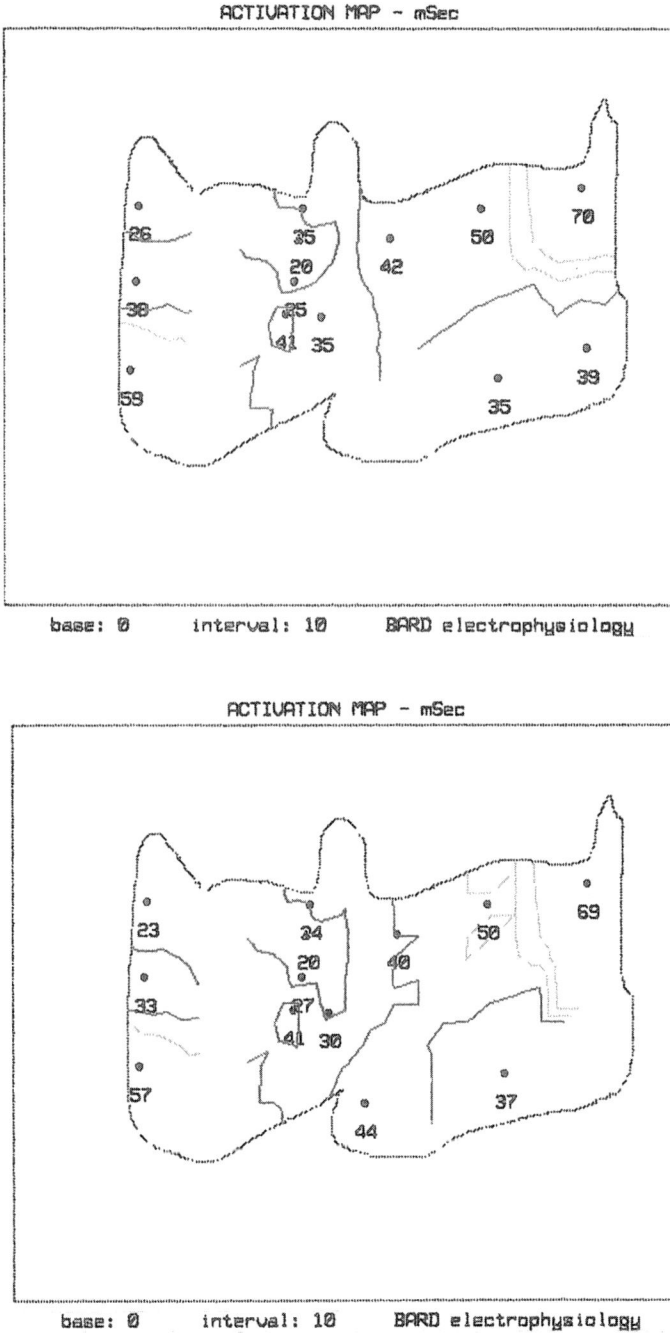

Figure 3.2 Isochronal maps of right and left atrium, depicting regional atrial activation with (*top panel*) dual-site (HRA + CSos) and (*bottom panel*) biatrial (HRA + CS distal) pacing modes. Activation of the inferior and lateral left atrium, His bundle region, crista terminalis and interatrial septum is earlier with both modes of pacing compared with sinus rhythm and high right atrial pacing. This results in an abbreviation of the P-wave duration with both pacing modes compared with sinus rhythm.

Acute studies on prevention of inducible AF with dual-site atrial pacing have shown evidence of benefit. Reproducibly induced atrial flutter or fibrillation, elicited using single to triple extrastimuli during high right atrial pacing drive, can be suppressed in 56% of patients using a dual-site right atrial pacing drive train.[42] This suppression was seen in patients with greater dispersion of refractoriness between the high right atrial and coronary sinus ostial regions, suggesting that a potential mechanism may be related to elimination of this dispersion by altering recovery of excitability. However, a correlation between acute success and results of long-term pacing has yet to be established.

Thus, in the current perspective of permanent preventive atrial pacing, there are two clinical directions to be pursued:

(a) single-site atrial pacing with the implantation of the pacing electrode precisely in the area of AF initiation;
(b) multisite atrial pacing.

The former requires considerable information on intracardiac patterns of AF induction and their reproducibility. Possible involvement of multiple sites in both atria makes this approach currently less feasible. The latter approach requires optimization of the number of pacing sites and long-term pacing modes but is technically relatively easier and has already yielded encouraging results.[44] Electrophysiological remodelling induced by multisite atrial pacing may be of greatest value in the re-establishment of sinus rhythm in the early stages of arrhythmia recurrences. However, the extent of remodelling in a diseased human atrium may be considerably different from that in human or animal atria without organic disease. Short- and long-term results of pacing modalities already implemented in clinical practice for prevention of AF are discussed in the next section.

Clinical Experience with Cardiac Pacing in Prevention of AF

Atrial-Based Versus Ventricular-Based Pacing (Figure 3.3)

A large number of studies, mostly retrospective in nature, have evaluated the benefit of cardiac pacing in prevention of AF recurrences. Most of these reports have compared ventricular pacing and atrial pacing in patients with sick sinus syndrome. In these studies, ventricular pacing was associated with two to four times increased incidence of AF recurrence compared with atrial pacing during a follow-up period of 3–5 years. Rosenqvist noted 9% AF recurrence rates with AAI pacing compared with 69% with VVI pacing in long-term follow-up.[48] Hesselson noted an AF incidence of 7% with DDD pacing and 43% with VVI pacing.[49] Sgarbossa et al.[50] reported a 16% AF recurrence rate at 5 years with DDD pacing compared with a 32% incidence with VVI pacing. What is not clear is whether ventricular pacing is proarrhythmic, whether atrial pacing is antiarrhythmic or both are operative. This is largely due to a lack of a comparison control group of unpaced patients and a prospective randomized study design. Because of the

% PTS IN AF

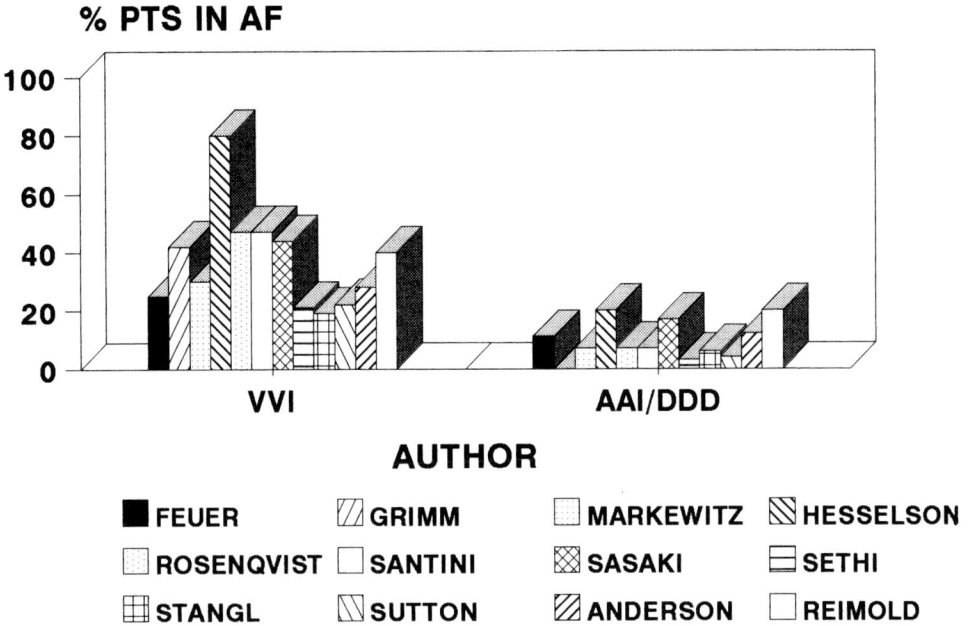

Figure 3.3 A comparison of AF recurrence with VVI and atrial-based pacing in patients with sick sinus syndrome in various series. In all series there is a significant reduction of AF recurrence with atrial-based pacing compared with VVI pacing. The follow-up duration in these series ranged from 2 to 5 years. Note that there is only one prospective study in this analysis. (Based on data in reference 52)

deleterious atrial haemodynamic effects of retrograde ventriculoatrial conduction and atrioventricular asynchrony, ventricular pacing alone may not be an appropriate pacing mode for such patients. A few studies have tried to answer questions unresolved by retrospective observational data. Reimold *et al.* noted that 40% of ventricular-paced patients were in sinus rhythm at 6 months, compared with 55% of unpaced patients and 80% of DDD-paced patients.[51] However, in this study the unpaced control group did not have coexisting bradycardia. In a prospective study using a parallel comparison group, Anderson *et al.* noted 12% incidence of AF recurrence with AAI pacing, compared with 28% with VVI pacing.[52] A prospective randomized trial (the Pacemaker Selection in the Elderly (PASE) trial) reported a reduction in the incidence of AF events with AAI/DDD pacing compared with VVI pacing.[53] While the incidence of AF recurrence seems to be lower when the atrium is paced, the site of atrial pacing may also be important. Based on a retrospective analysis, Seidl suggested that the right appendage may be preferable to pacing at the lateral high right atrium for purposes of AF suppression.[54] Benditt *et al.*[55] noted a lower incidence of recurrent atrial arrhythmias with rate-adaptive atrial pacing than with a nonadaptive mode. Comparable results were reported by Adornato *et al.*[56]

Dual-Site Pacing

Biatrial resynchronization

Correction of advanced interatrial conduction block could potentially eliminate a risk factor for recurrent atrial arrhythmias. Daubert *et al.*[57] utilized a biatrial, rate-adaptive, triggered pacing mode in patients with paroxysmal or chronic atrial flutter or AF. The right and left atrium were simultaneously sensed and paced via high right atrial and coronary sinus electrodes. A screw-in fixation lead was used in the right atrium and a passive fixation lead in the coronary sinus. This pacing system shortened P-wave duration and, after atrioventricular delay optimization, cardiac haemo-dynamics improved particularly in patients with hypertrophic cardiomyopathy. A triggered mode was used to attempt resynchronization of both atria even during early premature beats. Atrial and ventricular rhythms were monitored by a DDDR pacemaker equipped with event storage capability. In a series of 30 patients with drug-refractory atrial arrhythmias and after a mean follow-up of 18 months, significant decrease in tachyarrhythmia episodes were obtained in 15 patients (50%). Coronary sinus lead dislodgement seen in 20% of patients was the major technical problem. A new coronary sinus lead has been under trial to improve fixation.[57] The main limitation of this analysis was the absence of a prospective study design and a randomized or crossover comparison with single-site pacing.

Right atrial dual-site pacing

In a prospectively designed crossover study, Saksena *et al.*[44,59,60] have compared single-site pacing with dual-site right atrial pacing in 30 unselected patients with paroxysmal or chronic drug-refractory AF or atrial flutter. Two screw-in active fixation leads were placed in the high right atrium and at the coronary sinus ostium. The coronary sinus ostium lead was introduced inside the coronary sinus and then withdrawn and fixed to the superior or posterior aspect of the ostium. One cathodal electrode was at the high right atrium in 16 patients and at the coronary sinus ostium in 14 patients. Measurements of thresholds were obtained in bipolar single-site pacing for both sites compared with bipolar dual-site pacing via a Y-connector. The distal pacing electrodes for the two leads were connected via the Y-connector to the atrial output of a bipolar dual-chamber rate-adaptive pulse generator. A ventricular pacing lead was inserted in all patients. Continuous atrial overdrive pacing was established by a high lower rate limit and aggressive rate-response with concomitant but previously ineffective drug therapy. This drug regimen was directed at sinus rate control and modifying incessant or chronic AF. Patients were assigned to dual-site right atrial pacing for the first assigned (phase 1) for 90 days. In consenting patients, pacing was switched to single-site mode for 90 days (phase 2). A second sequence of switching back to dual-site (phase 3) and later again to single-site pacing (phase 4) for 180-day periods in consenting patients has been planned.

All atrial pacing modes showed a significant benefit in arrhythmia-free intervals over a control period of 3 months preceding pacemaker implant. However, the dual-site mode had incremental benefit over the high right atrial and coronary sinus ostial single-site atrial pacing modes. In the first 15 patients, there were no AF recurrences during dual site pacing. Previously ineffective drug therapy was continued. During the single-site pacing (in high right atrium) phase, five AF recurrences occurred in 12 patients. The arrhythmia-free interval before pacing (14 ± 14 days) was significantly prolonged with dual-site pacing (89 ± 7 days) and single-site pacing (76 ± 27 days). Approximately 80% of patients were free from frequent recurrent relapsing or chronic atrial arrhythmias at 1 year. This has allowed a significant decline in antiarrhythmic drug use from a mean of 3.5 drugs before implant to 1.4 drugs during pacing.

In an update, the same group reported on 30 patients. Coronary sinus ostial lead dislodgement occurred in only one patient and high right atrial lead dislodgement in another patient.[60] Both leads were repositioned and remained stable. An unrelated infection of the pacemaker pocket required system explant in one patient. The mean arrhythmia-free interval before pacing was 8.8 ± 10 days and increased to 69 ± 32 days with single-site pacing and 85 ± 17 days with dual-site right atrial pacing. Nine patients experienced AF recurrences (range 1–4, mean 2.1) which were usually self-terminating or occasionally required cardioversion. Nine recurrences occurred initially in the single-site high right atrial pacing mode. Three of these patients also had recurrences in the dual-site mode. Twenty-six of 30 patients remain in atrial-based pacing, with total freedom from recurrent AF in 19 patients and a marked reduction in AF frequency in the other 7 patients.

A benefit in AF prevention of both single-site and dual-site atrial pacing modes in combination with drug therapy is suggested by this pilot study over drug therapy alone. Atrial pacing increases arrhythmia-free periods and dual-site pacing seems to provide additional benefit. This increase in arrhythmia-free intervals also translates into decreased need for cardioversion or drug therapy modification.

Termination of Atrial Fibrillation and Flutter by Pacing

Antitachycardia pacing has been used for reversion of atrial flutter for over 15 years. Waldo and colleagues demonstrated that rapid atrial pacing trains at rates slightly higher than the intrinsic rate of tachycardia can entrain the macro re-entrant right atrial circuit in typical type-1 atrial flutter with acceleration of the local atrial electrograms to the pacing rate.[20] This may be followed either by termination of atrial flutter or its disorganization into AF. This observation was a basis for the concept of entrainment and has been described in detail elsewhere.[61,62] According to this concept, during macro re-entrant atrial flutter, every stimulus impulse of the rapid atrial pacing train engages the flutter circuit via its excitable gap. From the point of entry into the tachycardia circuit, the antidromic wavefront of any subsequent pacing impulse of the stimulation train collides with the orthodromic wavefront of the previous pacing impulse. However, it is the orthodromic wavefront of this sub-sequent impulse that resets the tachycardia. Thus, entrainment is a repetitive, beat-to-beat resetting of the atrial flutter circuit by the orthodromic wavefront of each consecutive pacing impulse of the stimulation train. However, block of the ortho-dromic wavefront – and thus the failure to reset tachycardia – will lead to extinction of the re-entrant circuit and termination of atrial flutter.[62] This is the underlying mechanism of the abrupt (i.e. without transitory AF) termination of atrial flutter by rapid atrial pacing. However, rapid atrial pacing often induces transient and unstable AF which subsequently converts to sinus rhythm. In a number of published series, reversion of atrial flutter via the transitory AF has been considered as a successful endpoint, since the transient AF did not last more than a few minutes.[63–65] In patients pretreated with antiarrhythmic drugs, the acute success rate of rapid atrial pacing for the conversion of type-1 atrial flutter varies from 70% to 80% in clinical series.[65–67] In many centres, rapid atrial pacing has been considered as the first-line therapy for the termination of type-1 atrial flutter because of the simplicity, effectiveness and safety of the procedure. In our and others' experience, a longer cycle length of atrial flutter and shorter duration of arrhythmia episode (<1 month) are the major determinants of success.[65] Prolongation of atrial flutter cycle length by pretreatment with antiarrhythmic drugs improves efficacy.[67]

The efficacy of rapid overdrive atrial pacing in patients with type-2 atrial flutter has reportedly been poor, with the average overall success rate of 10%.[19,20,65] The feasibility of other pacing modalities in termination of type-2 (atypical) atrial flutter or AF remains unclear. The situation is further complicated by the lack of clarity in nomenclature and definitions of atypical atrial flutter.[62] The term 'atypical atrial flutter' has been widely used for atrial flutter with positive F waves in the inferior leads,[68] which may occur simply with clockwise reversal of a macro re-entrant type-1 flutter with preservation of excitable gap, or a much more rapid rhythm without entrainable excitable gap. Such atypical flutter morphology describes arrhythmias that may be right or left atrial or septal in origin or may even be a transitional rhythm to AF. The following discussion will be focused on the effects of pacing on AF and the forms of type-2 atrial flutter in which the re-entrant circuit cannot be clearly defined as of macro re-entrant right atrial origin by conventional catheter mapping in the electrophysiology laboratory.

Unlike type-1 atrial flutter, AF and fast forms of atypical (type-2) atrial flutter for a long time have been considered as the only type of re-entrant arrhythmia which cannot be affected by rapid pacing. However, theoretically, if even the smallest portion of the circuit is free of electrical activation (i.e. the presence of the excitable gap), pacing can succeed in affecting the circuit. In their elegant study using high-density computer mapping, Konings et al. showed that, even during the AF episodes of highest complexity, a particular mapped region of the atrium can be free of electrical activation for about 8% of the entire recording period.[23] Thus, even during the most complex cases of AF, there is a small excitable gap which can be entrained by rapid pacing. Recent studies performed on animals and humans have demonstrated that rapid atrial pacing can affect AF locally. The effects of two different pacing modalities have been studied in experimental and clinical AF and atrial flutter:

(1) One of these modalities is rapid atrial pacing (mostly used in atrial flutter with more organized electrical activity throughout the atria) with the pacing cycle lengths being 10–50 ms shorter than the cycle length of local electrical activity during AF or atrial flutter.[69]
(2) Another method is the high-frequency (ultrarapid) pacing which has been previously applied for termination of sustained ventricular tachycardia.[70] In this

pacing mode, the pacing cycle length is significantly shorter than the cycle length of local electrical activity of the tissue, and varies from 80 to 20 ms in various series.

Each of these methods has particular benefits. One major benefit of rapid atrial pacing could be that it can achieve the entrainment of the adjacent re-entrant circuit with the constant 1:1 capture of the tissue between the pacing site and the actual re-entrant circuit. There is rate-adaptive shortening of the effective refractory period of the paced tissue and facilitation of intra-atrial conduction for every subsequent pacing stimulus in the train. On the other hand, a long distance between the pacing site and actual re-entrant circuit, as well as a small excitable gap of the circuit itself, may prevent this mode of pacing from entraining the circuit. This may result in an unchanged electrogram cycle length at sites in the vicinity of the re-entrant circuit, or, alternatively, degeneration of discrete flutter-like electrical activity into a more complex fibrillatory activity at shorter pacing cycle length owing to the inability of interposed tissue to sustain constant 1:1 response to the pacing. An implied benefit of the high-frequency pacing method is the ability to obtain cellular excitation at the earliest point of recovery of excitability, even in the relative refractory period, and, thus, engage the excitable gap and prevent propagation of the spontaneous tachycardia wavefront. This may be particularly important in faster forms of atypical atrial flutter and AF with higher complexity, in which an 'excitable gap' in re-entrant excitation is considered to be small or to barely exist. On a cell automata model, Peterson has demonstrated the potential ability of high-frequency pacing to destabilize atrial electrogram cycle lengths at multiple locations resulting in arrhythmia termination.[71] However, extremely short pacing cycle lengths – and hence the loss of 1:1 capture – may prevent the capture of a significant mass of atrial tissue and the elimination of re-entrant circuits distant from the pacing site.

Electrophysiological Effects of Pacing During AF

Rapid pacing bursts have been applied in AF experimentally by Kirchhoff *et al.* with regional mapping in segments of the right atrium.[72] They have shown that pacing at cycle lengths equal to the median cycle length of a local atrial electrogram (approximately 90–100 ms) could capture atrial tissue around the pacing site with regional atrial entrainment. Pacing directly affected propagating wavefronts in the right atrial area under the mapping electrode. Capture was demonstrated to result in propagation of the electrical wavefront from the pacing site to sites 4 cm distant from the pacing electrode.[72]

In our clinical series of patients with spontaneous and induced AF or atypical atrial flutter, the capture of local and distant atrial sites was reproducibly observed during the high-frequency pacing train delivery in 80% of patients with atypical atrial flutter.[73] This phenomenon was seen as far away from the pacing site as the lower region of crista terminalis, coronary sinus ostium and low posterior left atrium (Figure 3.4). Thus, capture of substantial regions of both atria can be achieved with high-frequency pacing in atypical atrial flutter. Capucci *et al.* noted transient acceleration of

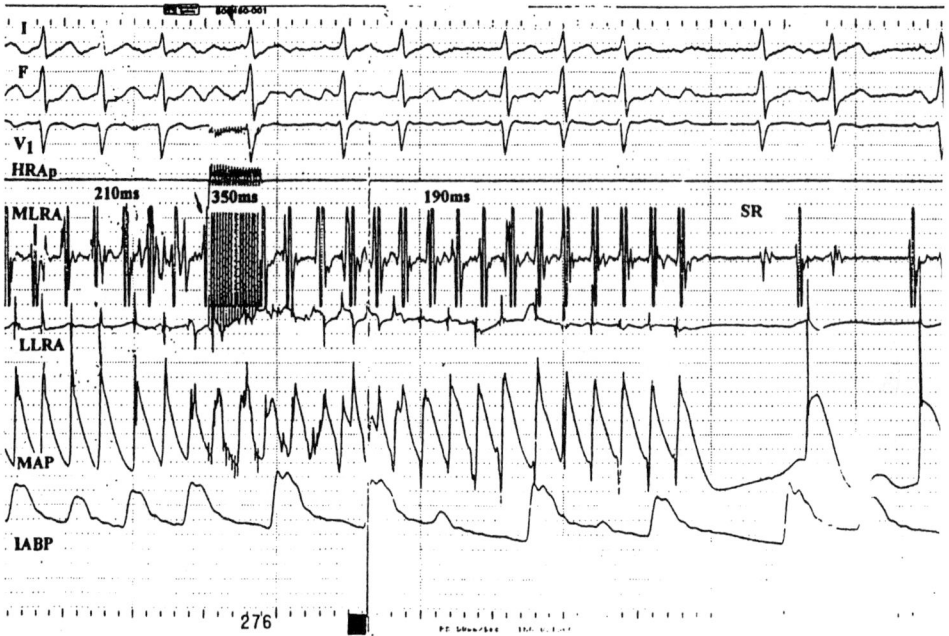

Figure 3.4 Termination of type-2 'atypical' atrial flutter with high-frequency pacing from the high right atrium in a patient with sustained atrial flutter/fibrillation. High-frequency pacing is performed with a cycle length of 20 ms for a duration of 350 ms. Arrhythmia is terminated in 3 seconds after termination of the pacing train. HRAp = high right atrial pacing channel; IABP = intra-atrial blood pressure recording; I, F, V_1 indicate surface ECG leads; LLRA = low lateral right atrial recording site; MAP = monophasic action potential recording from the low right atrial region. Termination of atrial arrhythmia is preceded by acceleration of local electrical activity. Transient disorganization and a marked change in the bipolar electrogram and monophasic action potential morphology can be noted at the distant low atrial recording site after cessation of the pacing train. (Reprinted from reference 75 with permission)

local atrial electrograms by ultrarapid atrial pacing in patients with atrial fibrillation.[69] However, this can only be observed at or near pacing sites with discrete atrial electrograms.[73]

Termination of AF with Atrial Pacing

Initially, this appears less feasible owing to the electrophysiological properties of the atrial fibrillatory milieu, which includes:

(a) a very small or virtually nonexistent excitable gap, impairing penetration of the circuit by pacing;

(b) depressed conduction properties of atrial tissue with great numbers of arcs of conduction block and zones of slow conduction (isochrone clumping) preventing access of the paced wavefront to the circuit;

(c) unpredictable location of the pacing site owing to the inability to precisely localize the circuit with the excitable gap.

Obviously, these difficulties become more prominent with the increase of fibrillatory complexity. In animal mapping studies, AF was not terminated by rapid atrial pacing. This was due to (1) entrainment of only a limited area of atrial mass, insufficient for the termination of fibrillatory activity; and (2) loss of capture due to acceleration of AF during rapid pacing at very short cycle lengths.[72] However, the results of high-frequency atrial pacing in AF with more organized local electrical activity (type-2 atrial flutter and type-1 AF) are more encouraging. In a recent report from our laboratory,[73] high-frequency atrial pacing terminated type-2 atrial flutter in 60% of cases after transient acceleration of local atrial activity (Figure 3.4). The mechanism of termination remains unclear, though one may assume that:

(a) the pacing may eliminate the re-entrant circuit of a single broad wavefront with subsequent self-extinction of daughter wavelets; or
(b) a long-lasting pacing train may capture most or part of the atria at one point, creating multiple 'wandering' leading circuits, which self-terminate shortly upon the cessation of pacing.

Insights from electrogram recordings suggest that capture of distant atrial sites by the pacing train can be a harbinger of successful capture of the circuit and bystander regions with subsequent destabilization and termination of arrhythmia.

Thus, the effects of the single-site ultrarapid pacing modality in AF is limited to alteration of local electrical activity with minimal or no distant atrial effects.[73] This can account for the absence of efficacy in termination of established AF. Termination of AF with high-frequency pacing should be pursued and may become possible by increasing the amount of simultaneous atrial capture. With regard to this, selection of different pacing sites (e.g. the coronary sinus ostium) and modalities (dual-site or multisite atrial pacing) may increase the success of ultrarapid atrial pacing.

Current and Future Clinical Trials of Pacing in AF

Several retrospective studies as previously mentioned have reported the benefit of atrial pacing over ventricular pacing in patients with sick sinus syndrome. The main end-point of these studies has been the development of chronic AF, although other clinical events such as heart failure and death have also been addressed. This benefit has also been observed in a prospective parallel single-centre study from Denmark. This study included 225 consecutive patients with sick sinus syndrome randomized to atrial (110 patients) or ventricular (115 patients) pacing, one of which was exclusively used at two collaborating institutions.[52] At 18 months of follow-up, 23% of patients had developed chronic AF in the ventricular-paced group, compared with 14% in the group with atrial pacing. Thromboembolism occurred in 20 patients in the ventricular-paced group, compared with six patients in the atrial-paced group ($p = 0.008$). There was, however, no significant difference in mortality. These observations, though important, are not randomized and hence may be biased by the selection of the two populations. The first question that arises is whether maintenance of sinus rhythm is desirable. The second is the preferred pacing mode. Several multicentre studies are now under way in Europe and the United States looking at these unresolved issues.

Lamas suggested that to identify the true benefit there was a need for prospective randomized multicentre studies looking at end-points like mortality, thromboembolism and quality-of-life in addition to AF recurrence. Furthermore, an important issue that needs to be resolved is whether maintenance of sinus rhythm is of incremental benefit as compared with AF with a controlled ventricular rate.

The PASE study (PAcemaker Selection in the Elderly)

This was a prospective randomized multicentre study comparing DDDR and VVIR modes of pacing in patients over 65 years of age.[53] The clinical end-points of the study were AF, pacemaker syndrome, all-cause mortality, stroke and heart failure. Preliminary results have been reported and have served as pilot data for the MOST study (see later). Four-hundred and three patients (mean age 76 years, 59% males) from 29 centres were included in the study. Patients had either sinus node dysfunction (36%), atrioventricular nodal disease (49%) or both (8%). At 3 months the overall incidence of pacemaker syndrome was 11%, stroke 1.5%, heart failure 5%, AF 9%, and 11 patients (2.7%) had died. Twenty-eight percent of patients reported an improvement in their specific activity scale (based on a quality-of-life questionnaire) and 32% reported an improvement in their general health. During longer follow-up at the end of 1 year, in patients with sinus node dysfunction the mortality was 12% with VVIR and 6% with DDR pacing. The incidence of stroke was 4% with VVIR and 2% with DDDR pacing. There was a trend towards favourable results with DDDR pacing, though the difference was not statistically significant. At a follow-up of 19 months, the incidence of AF was 14.4% in the DDDR group and 11.9% in the VVIR-paced patients. This difference was statistically significant. Pre-implant AF was the strongest predictor of development of AF.[74]

The AFFIRM study (Atrial Fibrillation/Flutter In Rhythm Management)

The AFFIRM study is sponsored by the National Institutes of Health. It is a multicentre prospective randomized study comparing two treatment strategies, rate control or rhythm control. Sixty-five centres in the United States and Canada are involved in the study with the two major end-points being total mortality and the incidence of stroke. The hypothesis is that rhythm control is superior to rate control. Future multicentre studies comparing pacing modes have similar objectives in comparing atrial-based pacing with ventricular pacing.

The MOST study (Mode Optimization and Survival Trial)

The MOST study is sponsored by the National Institutes of Health to address the second question of optimal pacing mode. This study will probably be the largest study on this issue, aiming to recruit 2000 patients in three years to compare VVIR and DDDR pacing. The study population will include patients over 21 years of age and hence will not have a bias towards the elderly. Total mortality and a composite end-point consisting of the first occurrence of stroke, heart failure, hospitalization or death will constitute important secondary end-points. A very important aspect, cost effectiveness of the pacing mode, is also being addressed in this study.

The CTOPP study (Canadian Trial Of Physiological Pacing)

Another similar study is the CTOPP study. This is a multicentre, prospective, randomized, unblinded study being conducted in Canada. The inclusion criteria are all patients over the age of 18 years with an indication for pacemaker implantation. The study aims at recruiting 2550 patients and intends to have an average follow-up of 3.5 years. The primary end-points are either cardiac mortality or stroke, with secondary end-points being all-cause mortality, AF, admission for congestive heart failure, arterial embolism and changes in pacemaker mode because of pacemaker syndrome. Though this study is similar to the MOST study, there are certain differences. The CTOPP is a generator randomization study as opposed to mode randomization. This would allow patients with pacemaker syndrome to be excluded from the study and thereby limit follow-up. In addition, the MOST study allows modulation of rate response on the assumption that rate response by itself could affect both the primary and secondary outcomes. CTOPP is designed on the assumption that rate response modulation would not affect any of the end-points. This will need to be analysed as an important variable. In summary, CTOPP examines at all pacemaker implants while MOST requires patients to have sinus node dysfunction.

The Stop-AF study

This is a multicentre, prospective, randomized, controlled, sequential study with the primary aim of determining the recurrence of AF in VVI versus DDD-paced patients. The study is being conducted in the United Kingdom. A secondary objective of the study is to determine whether signal-averaging of the P wave can predict the development of AF. The intended recruitment is of 350 patients within 1 year with a 2-year follow-up.

The DAPPAFF study (Dual-site Atrial Pacing in Prevention of Atrial Fibrillation and Flutter)

The study design is shown in Figure 3.5. Our pilot data demonstrate the benefit of atrial pacing modes in AF prevention, quantitate this benefit in terms of arrhythmia-free intervals for patients with paroxysmal AF and bradycardia, and confirm the feasibility of long-term dual-site right atrial pacing. The suitability of the coronary ostial site for long-term pacing is established by our study. The pilot had a prospective sequential study design and was not randomized for mode. A larger prospective multicentre study is now being initiated to compare rate support, single-site and dual-site right atrial rate responsive pacing modes in a prospective crossover trial. This is a prospective, randomized study being sponsored in part by Medtronic Inc. (Minneapolis, MN). Four US and one Canadian centre are initiating the study. These include the Eastern Heart Institute in Passaic, New Jersey, the Mayo Clinic in Rochester, Minnesota, the University of Alabama at Birmingham in Alabama, the Henry Ford

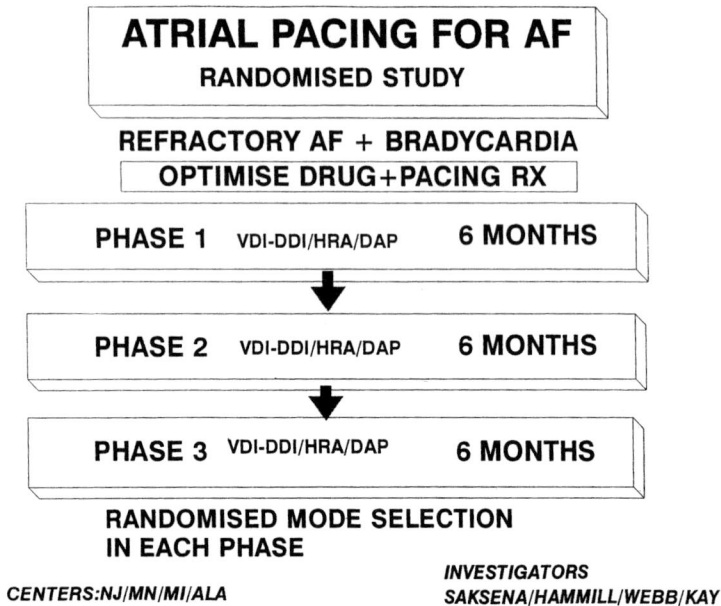

Figure 3.5 Study design of the DAPPAFF study. Illustrated are the phases of the study with duration of each phase of 6 months' duration, randomized pacing modes used in the study, and the participating centres.

Hospital in Detroit, Michigan and the University of Calgary in Alberta. The study will enroll 120 patients, each being randomly assigned to all three pacing modes. Clinical, electrocardiographic and device-based end-points to detect symptomatic, sustained AF recurrences will be employed. All patients will have a minimum follow-up of 18 months. Quality-of-life, cardioversion and other interventions and drug therapy will be monitored. The study is expected to be completed by 1998.

References

1. Lie JT, Falk RH. Pathology of atrial fibrillation: insight from autopsy studies. In: Falk RH, Podrid PJ (eds), *Atrial Fibrillation: Mechanisms and Management*. New York: Raven Press, 1992: 1–14.
2. Kannel WB, Wolf PA. Epidemiology of atrial fibrillation. In: Falk RA, Podrid PJ (eds), *Atrial Fibrillation: Mechanisms and Management*. New York: Raven Press, 1992: 81–92.
3. Horowitz LN. Atrial fibrillation. In: Horowitz LN (ed), *Current Management of Arrhythmias*. Philadelphia: Decker Inc., 1991: 51–7.
4. The NHLBI AFFIRM Investigators. Atrial fibrillation follow-up investigation of rhythm management: the AFFIRM study design. (Submitted for publication 1996).
5. Bernstein AD, Parsonnet V. Survey of cardiac pacing and defibrillation in the United States. *Am J Cardiol* 1996; **78**: 187–96.
6. Scheinman MM. NASPE survey on radiofrequency catheter ablation: implications of clinicians, third party insurance and government regulatory agencies. *PACE* 1992; **15**: 2228–31.

7. Kuck K-H, Kunze K-P, Schluter M, Duckeck W, Engelstein ED, Geiger M. Transcatheter modulation by radiofrequency current of atrioventricular nodal conduction in patients with atrial fibrillation or flutter. In: Saksena S, Luderitz B (eds), *Interventional Electrophysiology*, 2nd edn. Armonk, NY: Futura, 1996: 271.

8. ABLATE and PACE Trials (Canada).

9. Zipes DP, Wallace AG, Sealy WC, Floyd WL. Artificial atrial and ventricular pacing in the treatment of arrhythmias. *Ann Int Med* 1969; **70**: 885.

10. Daubert C, Cazeau S, Limousin M, Remy M, Ritter P, Mabo P. Atrial resynchronization: a new algorithm in DDD pacing. *Eur J CPE* 1994; **4**(172): 41.

11. Prakash A, Saksena S, Berg J, *et al.* Dual site atrial pacing for the acute and chronic prevention of atrial fibrillation/flutter: a prospective study (abstract). *JACC* 1995; **25**: 230A.

12. Coumel P, Friocourt P, Majica J, Attuel P, Leclercq JF. Long-term prevention of vagal atrial arrhythmias by atrial pacing at 90/minute: experience with 6 cases. *PACE* 1983; **6**: 552.

13. Attuel P, Pellerin D, Mugica J, *et al.* DDD pacing: an effective treatment modality for recurrent atrial arrhythmias. *PACE* 1988; **11**: 1647.

14. Simpson RJ, Foster JR, Gettes LS. Atrial excitability and conduction in patients prone to atrial fibrillation (abstract). *Am J Cardiol* 1981; **47**: 496.

15. Cosio FG, Palacios J, Vidal JM, *et al.* Electrophysiologic studies in atrial fibrillation: slow conduction of premature impulses: a possible manifestation of the background for reentry. *Am J Cardiol* 1983; **51**: 122.

16. Buxton AE, Waxman HL, Marchlinski FE, *et al.* Atrial conduction: effects of extrastimuli with and without atrial dysrhythmias. *Am J Cardiol* 1984; **54**: 755.

17. Josephson ME. Atrial flutter and fibrillation. In: *Clinical Cardiac Electrophysiology: Techniques and Interpretations*. Philadelphia: Lea & Febiger, 1993: 275–310.

18. Luck JC, Engel TR. Dispersion of atrial refractoriness in patients with sinus node dysfunction. *Circulation* 1979; **60**: 404–11.

19. Watson RM, Josephson ME. Atrial flutter. I: Electrophysiologic substrates and modes of initiation and termination. *Am J Cardiol* 1980; **45**: 732–41.

20. Waldo AL, Plumb VJ, Henthorn RW. Observations on the mechanism of atrial flutter. In: Surawicz B, Reddy P, Prystowsky EN (eds), *Tachycardias*. The Hague: Martinus Nijhoff, 1984: 213–29.

21. Moe GK. On the multiple wavelet hypothesis of atrial fibrillation. *Arch Int Pharmacodyn Ther* 1962; **140**: 183–8.

22. Allessie MA, Lammers WJEP, Bonke FIM, Hollen J. Experimental evaluation of Moe's multiple wavelet hypothesis of atrial fibrillation. In: Zipes DP, Jalife J (eds), *Cardiac Arrhythmias*. New York: Grune & Stratton, 1985: 265–76.

23. Konings KTS, Kirchhof CJHJ, Smeets JRLM, Wellens HJJ, Penn OC, Allessie MA. High density mapping of electrically induced atrial fibrillation in humans. *Circulation* 1994; **89**: 1665–80.

24. Spach MS, Miller WT, Geselowitz DB, Barr RC, Kootsey JM, Johnson EA. The discontinuous nature of propagation in normal canine cardiac muscle. *Circ Res* 1981; **48**: 39–54.

25. Boineau JP, Schuessler RB, Mooney, *et al.* Natural and evoked atrial flutter due to circus movement in dogs: role of abnormal atrial pathways, slow conduction, nonuniform refractory period distribution and premature beats. *Am J Cardiol* 1980; **45**: 1167.

26. Papageorgiou P, Monahan K, Boyle NG, *et al.* Site-dependent intra-atrial conduction delay: relationship to initiation of atrial fibrillation. *Circulation* 1996; **94**: 384.

27. Josephson ME, Kastor JA, Morganroth J. Electrocardiographic left atrial enlargement. *Am J Cardiol* 1977; **39**: 967.

28. Saksena S, Giorgberidze, Prakash A, *et al.* Endocardial catheter mapping of induced atrial fibrillation (abstract). *Circulation* 1996; **94**: 1–555.

29. Killip T, Gault JH. Mode of onset of atrial fibrillation in man. *Am Heart J* 1965; **70**: 172.

30. Bennett MA, Petecost BL. The pattern of onset and spontaneous cessation of atrial fibrillation in man. *Circulation* 1970; **41**: 981–8.

31. Mehra R, Hill MRS. Prevention of atrial fibrillation/flutter by pacing techniques. In:

Saksena S, Luderitz B (eds), *Interventional Electrophysiology*, 2nd edn. Armonk, NY: Futura, 1996: 521.

32. Tsuji H, Fujhjiki A, Tani M, *et al.* Quantitative relationship between atrial refractoriness and the dispersion of refractoriness in atrial vulnerability. *PACE* 1992; **15**: 403.

33. Ninomyia I. Direct evidence of nonuniform distribution of vagal effects on dog atria. *Circ Res* 1966; **19**: 576.

34. Coumel P. Neural aspects of paroxysmal atrial fibrillation. In: Falk R, Podrid PJ (eds), *Atrial Fibrillation: Mechanisms and Management*. New York: Raven Press, 1992: 109–26.

35. Capucci A, Santarelli A, Boriani G, Magnani B. Atrial premature beats coupling interval determines lone paroxysmal atrial fibrillation onset. *Int J Cardiol* 1992; **36**: 87.

36. Murgatroyd F, Slade A, Nitzsche R, *et al.* A new pacing algorithm for the suppression of atrial fibrillation. *PACE* 1994; **17**: 863.

37. Kimura T, Imanishi S, Arita M, *et al.* Two different mechanisms of automaticity in diseased human atrial fibers. *Jpn J Physiol* 1988; **38**: 851.

38. Mary-Arabine L, Hordof AJ, Danilo P, Malm JR, Rosen MR. Mechanisms for impulse initiation in isolated human atrial fibers. *Circ Res* 1980; **47**: 267.

39. El-Sherif N, Gough WB, Zeiler RH, Hariman R. Reentrant ventricular arrhythmias in the late myocardial infarction period. 12: Spontaneous versus induced reentry and intra-mural versus epicardial circuit. *JACC* 1985; **6**: 124.

40. Mehra R, Santel D. Electrical preexcitation of ischemic tissue for prevention of ventricular tachyarrhythmias. *PACE* 1986; **9**: 282.

41. Prakash A, Saksena S, Krol RB, *et al.* Electrophysiology of acute prevention of atrial fibrillation and flutter with dual site right atrial pacing. *PACE* 1995; **18**(II): 803.

42. Prakash A, Saksena S, Kaushik R, Krol RB, Munsif AN, Mathew P. Right and left atrial activation patterns during dual site atrial pacing in man: comparison with single site pacing. *PACE* 1996; **19**(II): 697.

43. Munsif AN, Prakash A, Krol RB, Mathew P, Lewis C, Saksena S. Crista terminalis, atrial septal and coronary sinus activation during single and dual site atrial pacing. *PACE* 1996; **19**(II): 578.

44. Saksena S, Prakash A, Hill M, *et al.* Prevention of recurrent atrial fibrillation with chronic dual site right atrial pacing. *JACC* 1996; **28**: 687–694.

45. Olgin JE, Kalman JM, Lee RJ, Saxon L, Lesh MD. Induction of human atrial flutter: mechanism of initiating block and direction of rotation (abstract). *PACE* 1996; **19**: 593.

46. Prakash A, Hill M, Giorgberidze I, *et al.* Propagation of atrial premature beats during atrial pacing: insights from regional atrial mapping. *PACE* 1996; **19**(II): 642.

47. Prakash A, Munsif A, Krol R, *et al.* Regional atrial conduction delays vary for short coupled premature beats during single and dual site atrial pacing (abstract). *JACC* 1997; **29**: 253A.

48. Rosenqvist M, Brandt J, Schuller H. Long-term pacing in sinus node disease: effect of stimulation mode on cardiovascular mortality and morbidity. *Am Heart J* 1988; **116**: 16–22.

49. Hesselson AB, Parsonet V, Bernstein AD, Bonavita G. Deleterious effect of long term single chamber ventricular pacing in patients with sick sinus syndrome: the hidden benefits of dual chamber pacing. *JACC* 1992; **19**: 1542–9.

50. Sgarbossa EB, Pinski SL, Maloney JD, *et al.* Chronic atrial fibrillation and stroke in paced patients with sick sinus syndrome: relevance of clinical characteristics and pacing modalities. *Circulation* 1993; **88**: 1045–53.

51. Reimold SC, Lamas GA, Cantillon CO, Antman EM. Risk factors for the development of recurrent atrial fibrillation: role of pacing and clinical variables. *Am Heart J* 1995; **129**: 1127–32.

52. Anderson HR, Thuesen L, Bagger JP, Vesterlund T, Thomsen PEB. Prospective randomized trial of atrial versus ventricular pacing in sick sinus syndrome. *Lancet* 1994; **344**: 1523–8.

53. Estes NAM, Griffin J, Wang PJ, *et al.* Morbidity and mortality of permanent dual chamber pacemaker implantation in the elderly (abstract). *PACE* 1995; **18**: 841.

54. Seidl K, Hauer B, Schwick N, Buchele T, Senges J. Is the site of atrial lead implantation in dual chamber pacing of importance for preventing atrial fibrillation? The hidden benefits of lead implantation in the right atrial appendix (abstract). *PACE* 1995; **18**: 810.
55. Benditt D, Wilbert L, Hansen R, *et al.* Late follow-up of dual-chamber rate-adaptive pacing. *Am J Cardiol* 1993; **71**: 714–19.
56 Adornato E, Monea P, Pangallo A, Adornato EMF, Consolo A. Comparative evaluation of DDD-R and DDD pacing modes in the prevention of atrial fibrillation (abstract). *PACE* 1993; **16**(II): 1145.
57. Daubert C, Mabo P, Berder V. Arrhythmia prevention by permanent atrial resynchronization in advanced interatrial block. *Eur Heart J* 1990; **11**: 237.
58. Daubert C, Gras D, Ritter P, Leclercq C, Baisset M, Mabo P. Experience with a new coronary sinus lead specifically designed for permanent left atrial pacing (abstract). *PACE* 1995; **18**: 825.
59. Saksena S, Prakash A, Madan N, *et al.* Prevention of atrial fibrillation by pacing. In: Barold SS, Mugica J (eds). *Recent Advances in Cardiac Pacing: Goals for the 21st century.* 1997 (in press).
60. Prakash A, Saksena S, Hill M, *et al.* Long-term results with dual and single site atrial pacing for prevention of refractory atrial fibrillation (abstract). *Circulation* 1996; **94**: 1–68.
61. Waldo AL, Plumb VJ, Arciniegas JG, *et al.* Transient entrainment and interruption of the atrioventricular bypass pathway type of paroxysmal atrial tachycardia: a model for understanding and identifying reentrant arrhythmias. *Circulation* 1983; **67**: 73–83.
62. Waldo AL. Some observations concerning atrial flutter in man. *PACE* 1983; **6**: 1181–9.
63. Della Bella P, Tondo C, Marenzi G, *et al.* Facilitating influence of disopyramide on atrial flutter termination by overdrive pacing. *Am J Cardiol* 1988; **61**: 1046–9.
64. Gloor HO, Fromer M, Kappenberger L. Endocardial conversion of atrial flutter: success rate of various stimulation protocols. *Clin Prog Electrophysiol Pacing* 1986; **4**: 67–75.
65. Baeriswyl G, Zimmermann M, Adamec R. Efficacy of rapid atrial pacing for conversion of atrial flutter in medically treated patients. *Clin Cardiol* 1994; **17**: 246–50.
66. Greenberg ML, Kelly TA, Lerman BB, DiMarco JP. Atrial pacing for conversion of atrial flutter. *Am J Cardiol* 1986; **58**: 95–9.
67. Camm J, Ward D, Spurrel R. Response of atrial flutter to overdrive atrial pacing and intravenous disopyramide phosphate, singly and in combination. *Br Heart J* 1980; **44**: 240–7.
68. Lesh MD, Kalman JM. To fumble flutter or tackle 'tach'? Toward updated classifiers for atrial tachyarrhythmias. *J Cardiovasc Electrophysiol* 1996; **7**: 460–6.
69. Capucci A, Biffi M, Boriani G, *et al.* Dynamic electrophysiological behavior of human atria during paroxysmal atrial fibrillation. *Circulation* 1995; **92**: 1193–202.
70. Fisher JD, Ostrow E, Kim SG, Matos JA. Ultrarapid single-capture train stimulation for termination of ventricular tachycardia. *Am J Cardiol* 1983; **51**: 1334–8.
71. Peterson DK. High frequency burst pace termination of atrial flutter and atrial fibrillation in a two dimensional cell automata model (abstract). *PACE* 1996; **19**: 697.
72. Kirchhof CJHJ, Chorro F, Scheffer GJ, *et al.* Regional entrainment of atrial fibrillation studied by high resolution mapping in open-chest dogs. *Circulation* 1993; **88**: 736–49.
73. Giorgberidze I, Krol RB, Mongeon L, Munsif AN, Mathew P, Saksena S. Electrocardio graphic and intracardiac atrial electrogram findings in 'atypical' type 2 atrial flutter. *Eur JCPE* 1996; **6**: 19.
74. Stambler B, Ellenbogen K, Pinsky S, *et al.* Development of post-implant atrial fibrillation (AFIB) during DDDR versus VVIR pacing in the PASE trial (abstract). *PACE* 1996; **19**: 619.
75. Saksena S, Luderitz B (eds). *Interventional Electrophysiology*, 2nd edn. Armonk, NY: Futura, 1996.

4

Algorithms for Management of Atrial Fibrillation in Patients with Dual-Chamber Pacing Systems

G. N. Kay and R. S. Bubien

Patients with bradyarrhythmias who require pacemaker implantation ideally receive a device that provides both rate response and AV synchrony. For patients with intact sinus node function, the VDD and DDD pacing modes provide appropriate rate response as well as AV synchrony. For individuals with impaired sinus node function, these combined goals of pacemaker therapy are typically achieved with AAI(R) pacing (provided that the AV connection system is intact), DDD(R) pacing (in the presence of impaired AV conduction), or VVI(R) pacing (in the presence of chronic atrial fibrillation).

For patients with intermittent supraventricular arrhythmias, the VDD, DDD and DDD(R) pacing modes all are limited by the potential for rapid ventricular pacing as a result of tracking pathological atrial electrograms. Patients with paroxysmal supraventricular arrhythmias may become markedly symptomatic in the presence of rapid ventricular rates owing to inappropriate atrial tracking. In order to provide tracking of the sinus node during the periods of sinus rhythm while avoiding inappropriate tracking of atrial arrhythmias, a wide variety of algorithms have been created. These algorithms range from very simple to very complex. The more recently developed algorithms offer the capability to change the mode of response to sensed atrial events from a tracking to a nontracking mode. Thus, if the atrial rhythm exceeds a programmable detection rate for a sufficient number of intervals, the ventricle will not be paced at an inappropriately rapid rate. In most cases, the ventricles will be paced at a rate determined by a rate-adaptive sensor during the nontracking mode of operation. The purpose of this review is to describe the wide variety of algorithms available in dual-chamber pacemakers that have been designed to recognize and respond to atrial tachyarrhythmias and to compare their relative strengths and weaknesses. This discussion will start with the assumption that, whenever possible, all patients require both AV synchrony and rate response.

In order to understand mode switching, several features of atrial sensing must be appreciated. First, the atrial electrogram must be of sufficient amplitude and slew rate

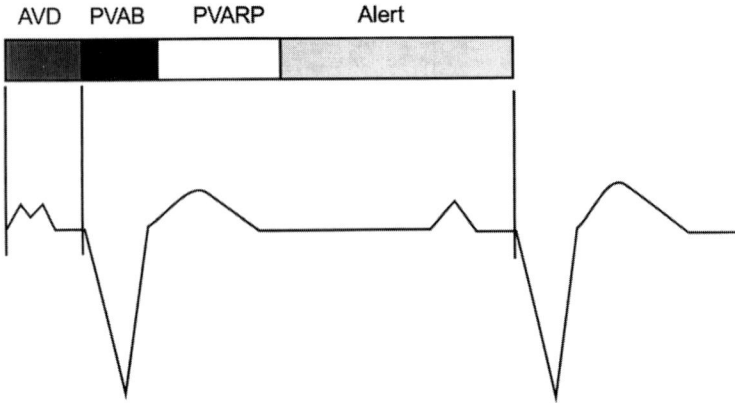

Figure 4.1   Atrial timing cycle of dual-chamber pacing system. During the AV delay (AVD), sensing in the atrium is inactivated. For most pacemakers, atrial sensing is inactivated for the entire AV delay. However, for some newer models of pacing systems, sensing is allowed following the 100 ms of the AV delay. During the PVAB period atrial sensing is not possible. This interval is designed to prevent atrial sensing of far-field R waves. Atrial events that occur within the PVAR period will be sensed if they fall beyond the end of the PVAB period but within the PVAR period. However, these events will not be tracked by the ventricular channel. Atrial events that occur following the end of the PVAR period before the next atrial escape interval (alert period) are tracked and generate an AV delay. In order for sensing of atrial arrhythmias to be optimized, the AV delay should be as short as possible during high atrial rates in order to minimize the total blanking period for atrial sensing (AV delay plus PVAB period).

to be sensed by the sensing amplifier. Although an atrial electrogram may be of excellent quality during sinus rhythm, the amplitude typically decreases during atrial arrhythmias. Therefore, a high level of sensitivity (low sensing threshold) is required. This generally requires the use of a bipolar sensing lead in order to reject myopotentials and other interfering signals and yet detects atrial activity during atrial fibrillation. It must be recognized that sensing is not possible during the post ventricular atrial blanking (PVAB) period which occurs immediately following a paced or sensed ventricular complex and during the initial portion of the AV interval (Figure 4.1). Thus, in order for sensing of atrial tachycardias to occur, the AV interval and PVAB period should be as short as possible and yet long enough to prevent inappropriate far-field sensing. In order for the sensing window to be optimized (opened), the AV interval should also shorten in response to an increasing atrial rate (Figure 4.2). This is particularly challenging for the detection of atrial flutter in which every other cycle may be unrecognized if it falls within the PVAB period and neither be sensed nor cause shortening of the AV interval (Figure 4.3).

VVI(R), AAI(R) and DDI(R) Pacing Modes

In the presence of chronic atrial arrhythmias with impaired AV conduction, the VVI(R) mode provides rate response and is the only feasible pacing mode. In this situation, AV synchrony is not possible and the VVI(R) pacing mode is the standard of

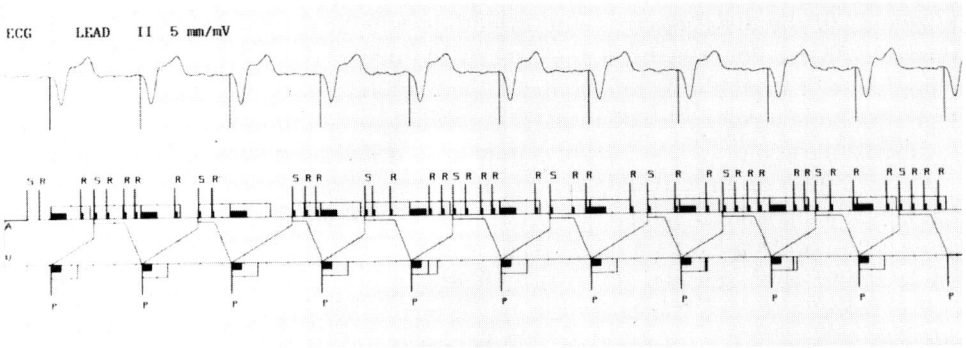

Figure 4.2 This figure demonstrates appropriate mode-switching during an episode of atrial fibrillation. Sensed events falling outside of the PVAR period (S) generate a new atrial blanking period. Events falling within the PVAR period (R) also generate a new atrial blanking period. Note that there is significant dropout of signals during atrial fibrillation owing to loss of atrial sensing. Also note that there is no sensing possible during the PVAB period. This illustrates the importance of minimizing the total duration that the sensing amplifier cannot sense in order to allow appropriate recognition of atrial fibrillation.

care. However, for patients in whom the AV conduction system is intact, the AAI(R) pacing mode is an elegant solution to the problem of inappropriate tracking of paroxysmal atrial arrhythmias. In such patients, AAI(R) pacing provides both rate response and AV synchrony without the risk of tracking pathological atrial arrhythmias. The risk of developing AV block in patients with sinus node dysfunction who have a narrow QRS complex and do not demonstrate AV Wenckebach conduction at pacing rates less than 120 bpm has been shown to be quite low (<4% per year).[1] For such individuals, AAI(R) pacing is the preferred mode. In the presence of atrial fibrillation or atrial flutter, atrial pacing will be inhibited (provided that the atrial electrogram amplitude and slew rate exceed the programmed atrial sensitivity

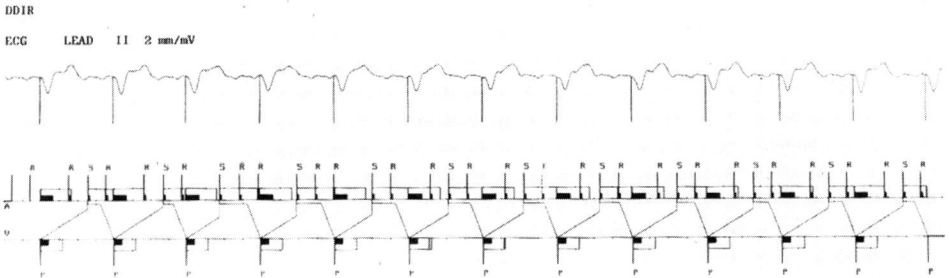

Figure 4.3 Example of atrial flutter as sensed by a Medtronic Thera™ pacemaker with appropriate mode-switching. Note that there is dropout of sensing of the atrial electrogram during the PVAB period denoted by the black rectangle in the atrial marker channel. If every other atrial electrogram falls within the atrial blanking period, atrial flutter may not be appropriately sensed and mode-switching may not occur. However, in this example, mode-switching was appropriate. (Reproduced with permission)

threshold). If the atrial electrogram amplitude falls below the programmed atrial sensitivity threshold, asynchronous atrial pacing may occur. This is of no concern in the presence of atrial fibrillation, though asynchronous pacing may potentially trigger degeneration of atrial flutter or atrial tachycardia to atrial fibrillation. Thus, the atrial sensitivity threshold should be programmed to a low amplitude to ensure appropriate inhibition of atrial pacing during atrial arrhythmias. Generally, this requires that a bipolar atrial lead be used for atrial sensing. A limitation of the AAI(R) pacing mode is the requirement for a relatively long atrial refractory period to avoid far-field R-wave and T-wave sensing. This may limit sensing during pacing near the upper rate limit of the sensor when the atrial cycle length may be less than the programmed atrial refractory period. Thus, at rapid rates it is possible for functional AOOR pacing to occur with the AAI(R) pacing mode.

The DDI(R) pacing mode overcomes one of the limitations of AAI(R) pacing. In the presence of intact AV nodal function, ventricular pacing is largely inhibited in the DDI(R) mode as the device essentially functions as an atrial rate-responsive pacing system with ventricular backup should AV block or conduction delay occur. However, in the presence of impaired AV conduction, if the atrial rate exceeds the sensor-indicated rate, AV synchrony will be lost and the device essentially functions in the VVI(R) mode. Thus, DDI(R) pacing has limited utility in the presence of AV block unless there is such severe dysfunction of the sinus node that intrinsic atrial activity would not be anticipated. This mode may be especially useful for patients in whom AV conduction is normal, but there is a suspicion of disease within the bundle branch system in whom the later development of AV block is possible.[2]

Simple Algorithms for DDD(R) Pacing

Several pacemakers have utilized relatively simple algorithms to respond to the occurrence of intermittent atrial tachyarrhythmias while providing tracking of sinus node function. Perhaps the simplest of these algorithms has been the VDD(R) or DDD(R) pacing mode in which the atrial sensitivity threshold is programmed to a relatively high amplitude (relatively insensitive) so that the atrial electrogram during sinus rhythm is sensed appropriately while a lower-amplitude atrial electrogram during atrial fibrillation or atrial flutter will not be sensed.[3] Wood et al.[4] observed a decrease in the atrial electrogram amplitude during electrophysiological testing, between atrial flutter compared with sinus rhythm and atrial fibrillation compared with sinus rhythm. Ricci et al.[5] reported that the bipolar electrogram amplitude during atrial fibrillation was 65% of the amplitude during sinus rhythm ($R = 0.85$) in patients who had an implanted Thera[TM] DR pacemaker. For example, if the atrial electrogram measures 3 mV during sinus rhythm and only 1 mV during atrial flutter, programming the atrial sensitivity threshold to 2 mV would allow the sinus node to be tracked appropriately while the device would ignore the atrial electrogram during atrial flutter and pace at the programmed lower rate (essentially in the DVI(R) mode). Such a strategy may be very effective for patients with large atrial electrograms during sinus rhythm. However, since many patients with paroxysmal atrial arrhythmias have diffuse atrial disease, the atrial electrogram in sinus rhythm may be of relatively poor quality, requiring that the atrial sensitivity threshold be programmed to a more sensitive value. In these individuals, it may not be possible to find an atrial sensitivity threshold that will discriminate the atrial electrogram in sinus rhythm from the electrogram during atrial tachyarrhythmias.

Separately Programmable Upper Tracking and Upper Sensor Rates

A relatively simple method for managing paroxysmal atrial arrhythmias has been to programme the upper tracking limit of a DDD(R) pacing system to a lower rate than the upper sensor rate.[6-8] Thus, in the presence of sinus rhythm, appropriate tracking of the atrial activity would occur up to the programmed upper tracking limit. Once the upper tracking limit has been exceeded, pacemaker Wenckebach or 2:1 block would occur with the ventricle paced at the sensor-indicated rate. If the sensor-indicated rate is slightly faster than the normal sinus rate since the atrium is paced, AV synchrony will be maintained above the upper tracking limit. Such a method for managing atrial arrhythmias has proven useful and can be applied to most newer DDD(R) pacemakers.

This strategy has the disadvantage of limiting the upper tracking rate. Thus, if the patient has developed sinus tachycardia without an appropriate increase in the sensor-indicated rate, pacemaker Wenckebach block may occur that may be symptomatic. Secondly, when an atrial tachyarrhythmia does occur, the ventricle will be paced at the upper tracking limit which may also be sensed by the patient as inappropriately rapid.

Fallback Algorithms

Several manufacturers (CPI, Vitatron and ELA) offer 'fallback' algorithms to respond to atrial arrhythmias.[9-12] Fallback is designed to desynchronize the ventricles from rapid atrial activity during tachyarrhythmias. The ELA Chorus™ pacemakers provide for fallback to a programmed fallback rate once the atrial electrogram occurs at a rate faster than the upper tracking limit (Figure 4.4). For example, if the atrial pacing rate exceeds the upper tracking limit, pacemaker Wenckebach behaviour will occur for a programmable number of cycles (10, 100, 500, 1000 or 2000). If the atrial rate remains above the programmed upper rate, the pacemaker gradually prolongs the ventricular pacing cycle length by 31 ms every eight cycles until the programmed fallback rate is reached. Once the atrial sensed rate falls below the upper tracking limit, this algorithm shortens the ventricular pacing cycle length by 63 ms for every eight cycles, allowing resynchronization of the atria and ventricles. In the ELA Chorus™ RM rate-responsive pacing system, fallback occurs to the sensor-indicated rate which allows for rate response during the fallback sequence. A limitation of this algorithm has been the lack of sensing during the post ventricular atrial refractory (PVAR) period. Thus, if a very rapid atrial rate occurs such as during atrial flutter (in which every other atrial cycle occurs within the PVAR period), fallback may not

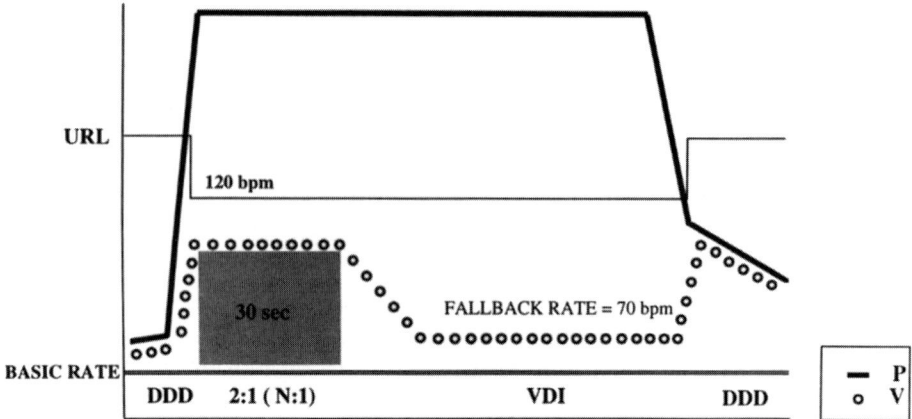

Figure 4.4 Fallback algorithm of the ELA Chorus™ pacemaker. The programmed lower rate (basic rate), upper tracking rate limit (URL) and atrial rate (dark line) are shown. Note that normal DDD function occurs during atrial rates below the upper tracking limit. However, once the upper rate limit has been exceeded the device functions at a fallback rate of 120 bpm with AV Wenckebach function for 30 seconds. The device then gradually prolongs the ventricular pacing cycle length until the fallback rate of 70 bpm is reached and maintained as long as the atrial rate exceeds the upper rate limit. During fallback the device functions in the VDI mode. Once the atrial rate decreases below 120 bpm, the device gradually decreases the ventricular cycle length as it resynchronizes in the DDD pacing mode. (Reproduced with permission)

occur. Thus, this algorithm has a complex relationship between the upper rate limit for tracking and the 2:1 point. In order for this algorithm to function, the PVAR period must be short enough for the 2:1 rate to be significantly faster than the upper tracking limit. The second limitation is that the device requires careful programming of the upper tracking limit so as to avoid inappropriate fallback during sinus tachycardia. This algorithm is characterized by relatively slow onset of fallback pacing following the onset of an atrial tachyarrhythmia with the likelihood for the patient to experience palpitations prior to the onset of fallback pacing. Because of the requirement for a short PVAR period and a 2:1 block rate that is at least 30–50 bpm faster than the upper tracking rate, devices offering this method for managing atrial arrhythmias also require an effective algorithm to limit pacemaker-mediated tachycardia.

Since a short PVAR period is necessary, the ELA Chorus™ II pacemaker offers a more sophisticated algorithm utilizing a 'window of atrial rate acceleration detection' (WARAD). The WARAD is defined as the previous sensed PP interval × 0.75, or the average of the last eight atrial intervals if paced. If an atrial event occurs within WARAD, the AV delay is shortened to 31 ms (Figure 4.5), thereby limiting the change in ventricular pacing rate. If the atrial events continue to occur within WARAD for 30 seconds, the Chorus™ II device switches to fallback with pacing in the VDI mode with the ventricular escape interval lengthened by 31 ms every eight cycles until the fallback rate is reached. In the presence of a gradually increasing atrial rate such as sinus tachycardia, the previously described fallback algorithm occurs if the atrial rate exceeds the upper tracking limit. Thus, the WARAD interval serves to differentiate a sudden change in the atrial rate (typical of atrial tachy-

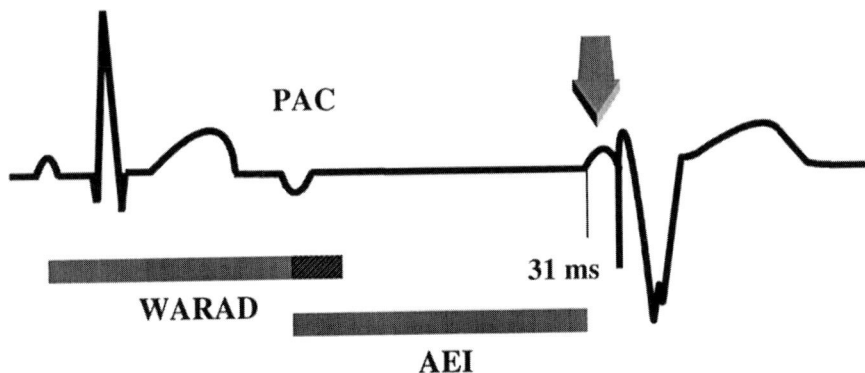

Figure 4.5 Function of the 'window of atrial rate acceleration detection' (WARAD) of the ELA Chorus™ II pacemaker. The WARAD is calculated as the previous PP interval multiplied by 0.75. If an atrial event occurs within the WARAD as shown by the premature atrial contraction (PAC), the premature beat is not tracked. Rather the next AV interval is shortened by 31 ms (large arrow). This feature prevents tracking of a sudden change in atrial rate by continuously comparing the atrial cycle length with the preceding PP interval. (Reproduced with permission)

arrhythmias) from sinus tachycardia (in which a more gradual increase in pacing rate would be expected).

Conditional Ventricular Tracking Limit

Intermedics has introduced a relatively simple method for managing rapid atrial rates that is known as the 'conditional ventricular tracking limit' (CVTL).[2,13–15] This algorithm provides continuous adjustment of the upper tracking limit based on the output of a rate-adaptive sensor. Pacemakers utilizing CVTL limit the upper tracking rate to 35 bpm faster than the sensor-indicated rate. In the presence of sinus tachycardia without an increase in the sensor rate, pacemaker Wenckebach block will occur at relatively low rates. However, if the sensor-indicated rate increases appropriately in response to exercise, the upper tracking limit increases such that pacemaker Wenckebach behaviour occurs only at the programmed tracking limit.

The Intermedics Marathon™ pacemaker incorporates 'SmarTracking' in which the slope of the relationship between the sensor-indicated rate and the upper tracking limit is programmable (Figure 4.6). Thus, if an aggressive curve is chosen, small changes in the sensor-indicated rate allow the upper tracking limit to increase rapidly. In contrast, if a relatively conservative slope is programmed, the upper tracking limit increases only gradually in response to a change in the sensor-indicated rate. The difference between the upper rate limit and the sensor-indicated rate is programmable. This device provides a more sophisticated mode-switching algorithm that can be programmed in addition to SmarTracking, allowing a high degree of refinement in the response to atrial arrhythmias.

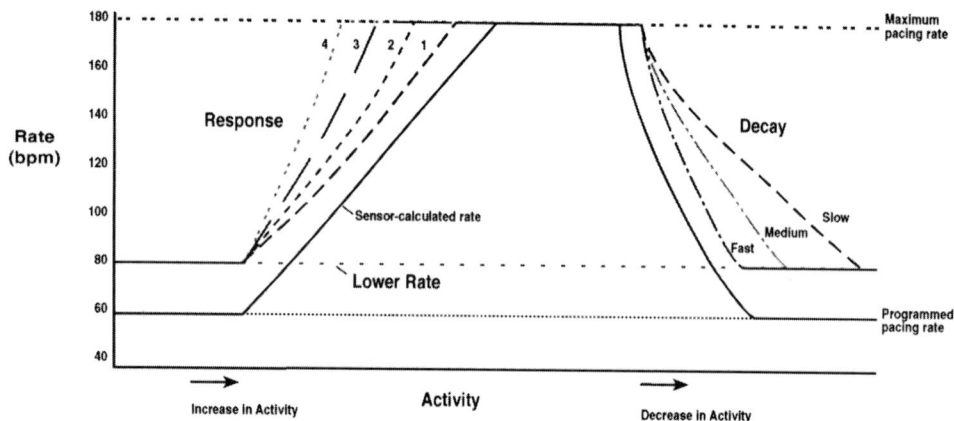

Figure 4.6 SmarTracking of the Intermedics Marathon™ pacemaker. The programmed pacing rate is 50 bpm with an upper tracking limit of 180 bpm. The upper tracking limit is continuously adjusted to the sensor calculated rate. If there is no change in the sensor calculated rate, the AV Wenckebach rate will be limited, in this case to 80 bpm. However, the slope of the curve relating the sensor calculated rate to the upper rate limit is programmable from a value of 1 (the least responsive) to 4 (the most responsive). Similarly, the decay is also programmable to slow, medium or fast. This feature prevents tracking of rapid atrial rates unless the sensor indicates that the patient is active. (Reproduced with permission)

A disadvantage of CVTL and SmarTracking is the requirement that the rate-responsive sensor be accurately programmed to avoid pacemaker Wenckebach at inappropriately low pacing rates.

Mode-Switching Algorithms for Management of Atrial Tachyarrhythmias (Table 4.1)

Telectronics pacemakers

The Telectronics Meta™ DDDR 1250H pacing system introduced the first automatic mode-switching (AMS™) algorithm. In the DDDR mode, the AV interval and the PVAR period decreased in response to a change in the sensor-indicated rate based on an MV (Minute Ventilation™) sensor. The device, which is no longer commercially available, functioned with a very long PVAR period at the lower rate limit (PVAR-period base) and a PVAR period that shortened in response to the MV sensor. Atrial events occurring after the end of the PVAR period but before the sensor indicated VA escape were tracked.[2,16–18] However, atrial events occurring within the PVAR period caused an atrial rate monitor to increment from a value of 0 to a value of 1 (Figure 4.7). Successive atrial events within the PVAR period resulted in further incrementing of the atrial rate monitor until it reached a value of 3 and automatic mode-switching occurred. During mode-switching the device changed from the DDD(R) to the VVI(R) pacing mode. Resynchronization to the DDD(R) mode occurred when the atrial rate monitor had returned to 0 or if no P wave was sensed within 2 seconds. The post ventricular atrial blanking (PVAB) period of this device was a fixed value of 100 ms.

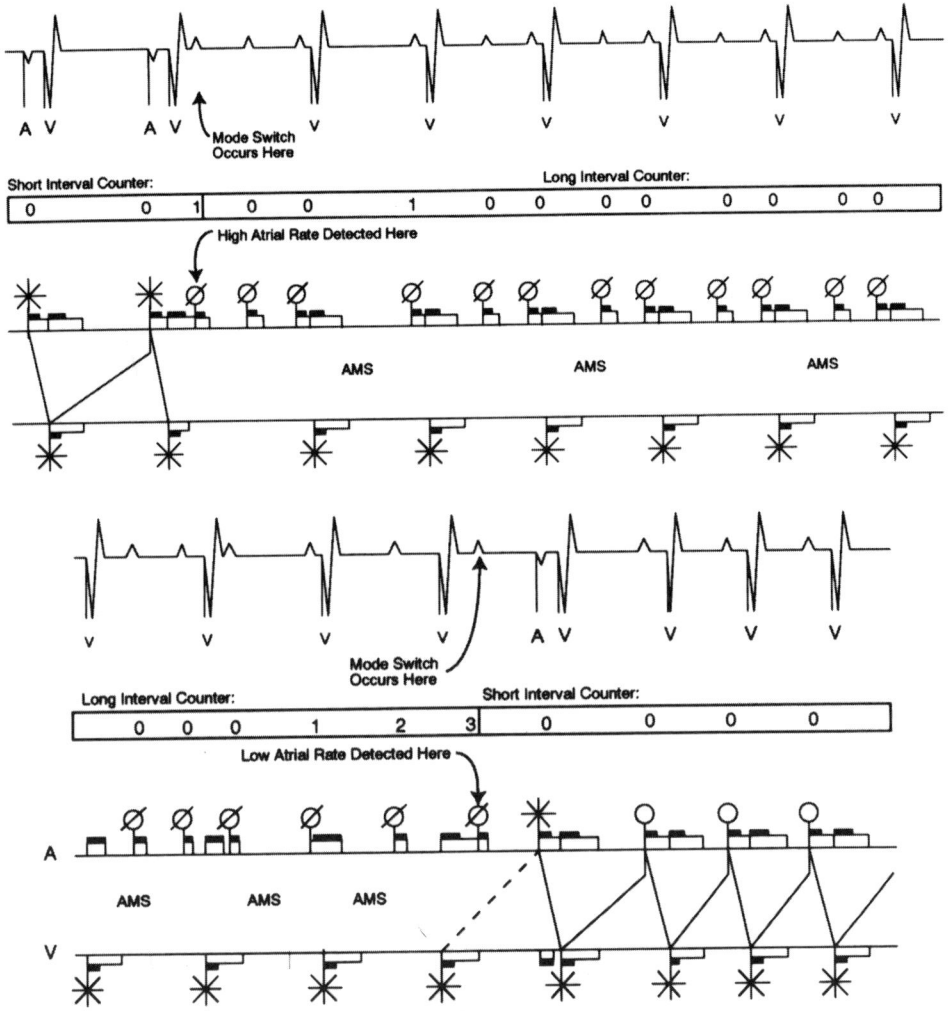

Figure 4.7 The automatic mode-switching algorithm of the Telectronics Meta™ DDDR 1250H pacemaker. This device used a short-interval counter that was initiated when a single atrial event was sensed within the PVAR period (*top panel*). The short-interval counter was incremented by 1 for each atrial event within the PVAR period. The long-interval counter detected sensing following the end of the PVAR period. When the long-interval counter reached 3, mode-switching reverted the device back to the DDDR tracking mode (*bottom panel*). Note that in this example, there is one atrial event that occurred outside the PVAR period denoted by the long-interval counter of 1. The long-interval counter was decreased to 0 by subsequent atrial events occurring within the PVAR period. This device was extremely sensitive to the onset of atrial arrhythmias, but the specificity for pathological arrhythmias was relatively poor, resulting in inappropriate mode-switching in many cases. (Reproduced with permission)

Because of this short PVAB period, far-field R-wave sensing could trigger inappropriate mode-switching ('reverse crosstalk').[19]

The Meta™ DDDR 1250H pacemaker was very sensitive to the onset of atrial arrhythmias with rapid mode-switching. However, the very long PVAR-period base

Table 4.1 Mode-switching algorithms in various pacemakers

Generator	Mode from:	Mode to:	Conversion	Reversion	PVARP blanking	Atrial safety window	Comments
Chorus™ RM	DDD(R) DDD/VVI(R) DDD	VVI(R) VVI(R) VVI	Atrial rate > max rate for 50 to 2000 WB cycles, then fallback begins (+ 31 ms every eighth cycle)	Atrial rate < max rate at which time fallup begins (− 63 ms every eighth cycle) until the sinus rate is met	172 ms (141–359 ms)	No	Slow mode switch and long fallback (1.43 min) and fallup (15 s) times; MTR must be > MSR resulting in high rate tracking prior to mode switch; fixed PVARP can limit upper tracking rates; no competitive atrial pacing protection
Marathon™ DR	DDD(R) VDD(R) DDD VDD	VVI(R)* VVI(R)* VVI* VVI*	'Run' of atrial events (1, 2, 3, 4, 5, 6, or 7) > 'rate' criteria (95–300 bpm) * Mode switches to SmarTracking rate (if ON) vs the sensor or min. rate Mode switch timed to ventricular events	1 atrial event < rate criteria, or an atrial paced event Mode switch timed to ventricular events	? ms	Only if programmed to an aggressive AMS sensitivity of just 1 atrial event	Mode switches to inappropriately high SmarTracking rate if ON; fast mode switch, but nonspecific when run criteria = 1; reversion criteria of only 1 event can cause frequent mode switch; no consistent protection against competitive atrial pacing; nonphysiological sensor rate may result in inappropriate SmarTracking and VVI(R) rates; long PVARPs or AV delays limit upper rates
META™ DDDR 1254	DDD(R) VDD(R) DDD VDD	VVI(R) VVI(R) VVI VVI	5 or 11 atrial events > 150, 175 or 200 bpm AMS timed to ventricular events	3 atrial events < AMS rate, or 1 second atrial asystole AMS timed to ventricular events	150 ms	Yes; atrial protection interval (API) = 30% operating pacing interval	Fast mode switch with specificity and longer PVARP blanking; mode switch timed to ventricular events; API introduced to protect from competitive atrial pacing; long PVARPs allowed owing to adaptive algorithm
META™ DDDR 1256 1256D 1256B	DDD(R) VDD(R) DDD VDD	VVI(R) VVI(R) VVI VVI	3, 4, 5, 6, 7, 8, 9, 10 or 11 events > 130, 140, 150, 160, 170, 180, 190, or 200 bpm AMS timed to atrial events	3 atrial events < AMS rate, or 1 second atrial asystole AMS timed to atrial events	150 ms	Yes; atrial protection interval (API) = 30% operating pacing interval	Fast mode switch with expanded options; lower rates and counts improves sensitivity to slow atrial flutter; mode switch timed to atrial events for faster initial switch and resumption of AV synchrony; API maintained; long PVARPs allowed owing to adaptive algorithm
Thera™ DR and Thera i™ DR	DDD(R) DDD VDD	DDI(R) DDI(R) VVI(R)	Mean atrial rate ('fast' P to P interval = − 24 ms from running average; 'slow' P to P interval = +8 ms) until > 120, 125, 130 to 175, 185, 190 bpm, then fallback begins with +40 ms each cycle until sensor rate met	Mean atrial rate < programmed maximum rate (from 200 ms to 500 ms = 13 seconds in DDIR) at which time fallup begins (− 40 ms each cycle) to the sinus rate; or five consecutive atrial paced events	150 ms with mode switch ON	Yes; non-competitive atrial pacing (NCAP) of 300 ms	Slower time for mode switch to occur to and from DDIR mode; additional fallback time to sensor rate post switch; AV delay must be ≤ 160 ms; aggressive AV delay shortening algorithm; PVARP must be ≤ 310 ms; USR must be = UTR; NCAP creates erratic behaviour and is OFF during mode switch to DDIR; other restrictions apply

Device	Mode	Mode	Detection	Restoration	Value	API	Comments
Trilogy™ DR+	DDD(R) DDD	DDI(R) DDI	If the sensed atrial rate is at or above the programmed ATDR (atrial tachy detect rate) for 5–10 s, mode-switching will occur. ADTR is programmable; 20 beats above the higher or max sensor or max tracking rate to 300 bpm	When the atrial rate drops below the maximum tracking rate, the original mode will be restored	50–200 ms in 25 ms steps	No	Slower time to mode switch and no anti-atrial competition feature (i.e. API); paroxysmal atrial arrhythmias above the 2:1 block rate will not result in a mode switch
Vigor™ DR	DDD(R) VDD(R) DDD VDD	VVI(R) VVI(R) VVI VVI	8 atrial events > max rate starts Wenckebach duration counter of 10, 20, 40, 60, 80, 100, 2000 ventricular cycles and then fallback begins of 1, 2, 3, 4 or 5 min to the sensor rate	Atrial rate < max rate for 8 events (consecutive?), atrial asystole for 8 events, or VVI(R) pacing above the tachycardia rate	80 ms	No	Mode switch rate = max rate; slower mode switch; fallback to sensor rate post mode switch is ≥ 1 min; short fixed PVARP blanking may cause far-field R-wave sensing and mode switch; fixed PVARP can limit upper tracking rates; no competitive atrial pacing protection
META™ DDDR 1250H	DDD(R) DDI(R) VDD(R)	VVI(R) VVI(R) VVI(R)	P-wave in PVARP; or atrial interval < operating TARP; or atrial interval < max rate (TARP equal to max rate at max sensor-driven rates) AMS timed to ventricular events	Based on number of fast atrial events which caused AMS: up to 3 'slow' events (>TARP); 2 s atrial asystole; or 8 consecutive events in PVARP with atrial rate monitor (i.e. short interval counter) = 0	100 ms	Yes; any P-wave in PVARP prevents atrial output (VVI(R))	First ever device with mode switch; fast, nonspecific mode switch; AMS always ON; AMS tied to max rate and operating TARP; short PVARP blanking could result in far-field R-wave sensing and AMS; very early PACs or PVCs with retrograde conduction could initiate AMS; mode switch timed to ventricular events; long PVARP allowed owing to adaptive algorithm; AV delays restricted to 175 ms or less
META™ DDDR 1254	DDD(R) VDD(R) DDD VDD	VVI(R) VVI(R) VVI VVI	5 or 11 atrial events > 150, 175 or 200 bpm AMS timed to ventricular events	3 atrial events < AMS rate or 1 s atrial asystole	150 ms	Yes; atrial protection interval (API) = 30% operating pacing interval	Fast mode switch with specificity and longer PVARP blanking; mode switch timed to ventricular events; API introduced to protect from competitive atrial pacing; long PVARPs allowed owing to adaptive algorithm
META™ DDDR 1256 1256D 1256B	DDD(R) VDD(R) DDD VDD	VVI(R) VVI(R) VVI VVI	3, 4, 5, 6, 7, 8, 9, 10 or 11 events > 130, 140, 150, 160, 170, 180, 190 or 200 bpm AMS timed to atrial events	3 atrial events < AMS rate or 1 s atrial asystole	150 ms	Yes; atrial protection interval (API) = 30% operating pacing interval	Fast mode switch with expanded options; lower rates and counts improves sensitivity to slow atrial flutter; mode switch timed to atrial events for faster initial switch and resumption of AV synchrony; API maintained; long PVARPs allowed owing to adaptive algorithm

values resulted in the potential for mode-switching to VVI(R) pacing to occur in the presence of sinus tachycardia. Initial clinical studies showed a very high occurrence of inappropriate mode-switching. A significant limitation of this device was the inability to programme automatic mode-switching 'off' when the DDD(R) pacing mode was selected. This often resulted in abandonment of DDD(R) pacing to the DDD mode in patients in whom inappropriate loss of AV synchrony produced troublesome symptoms.

The Meta™ DDDR 1254 pacing system (also no longer commercially available) offered significant improvement in the automatic mode-switching algorithm.[2,20] First, the PVAR period could be programmed to shorter values which prevented sinus tachycardia from triggering inappropriate mode-switching in most cases. Second, the automatic mode-switch rate became programmable. Third, the number of intervals required to exceed the mode-switch detection rate was programmable to either five or eleven beats (Figure 4.8). Fourth, the PVAB period was increased to 150 ms, preventing inappropriate mode-switching from far-field R waves. Fifth, mode-switching was from the DDD(R) mode to the DDI(R) mode. Resynchronization from the DDI(R) mode back to DDD(R) occurred after three PP intervals slower than the automatic mode switch detection rate or after 1 second without a detectable P wave within the atrium. The modified Meta™ DDDR algorithm proved to be far better tolerated with a lower occurrence of inappropriate mode-switching. The ability to programme this feature 'off' was also added. Although this device offered far better specificity, there was some decrease in the sensitivity to detection of atrial tachyarrhythmias and a slower response time before the onset of mode-switching.

The current Meta™ DDDR 1256 pacemaker allows the mode-switch detection rate to be programmed from 130 to 200 bpm with 3–11 atrial sensed events. As with the model 1254 pacemaker, the high rate events do not have to be consecutive.

Medtronic pacemakers

The Medtronic Thera™ and Thera-i™ pacemakers provide mode-switching from the DDD(R) to the DDI(R) pacing mode in response to atrial tachyarrhythmias.[5,21] A mean atrial interval (MAI) is continually calculated to track beat-to-beat changes in atrial cycle length (Figures 4.9 and 4.10). If the measured atrial cycle length is less than the mode-switch detection interval, the MAI is reduced by 24 ms. However, if the atrial cycle length is greater than the MAI, the MAI is increased by 8 ms. If the MAI becomes less than the programmable atrial detection interval, mode-switching occurs to the sensor-indicated rate. The mode-switch detection rate is programmable from 120 to 190 bpm in increments of 5 bpm. This detection rate is independent of the programmed upper tracking rate. At the onset of an atrial tachyarrhythmia, the pacemaker exhibits typical Wenckebach or 2:1 block behaviour as the MAI is continually updated. At the termination of an atrial tachyarrhythmia, the MAI is gradually increased until resynchronization occurs when the MAI exceeds the mode-switch detection interval. Since the increment in MAI (8 ms) is less than the decrement in MAI (24 ms), this device tends to remain mode-switched appropriately during atrial fibrillation even when undersensing of the electrogram occurs. However, the

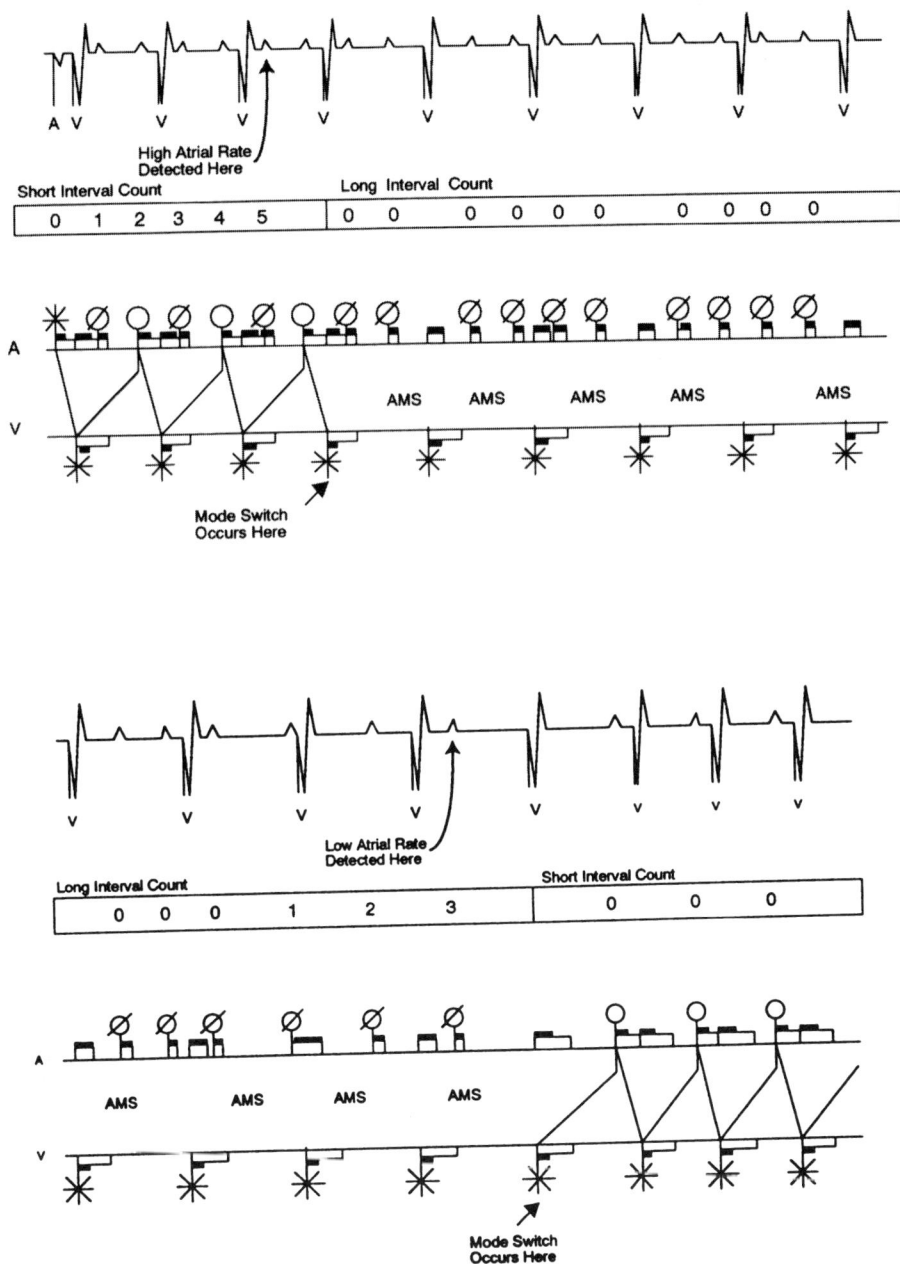

Figure 4.8 The automatic mode-switching algorithm of the Meta™ DDDR 1254 pacemaker. The number of beats required to occur at a rate greater than the programmed detection rate could be set to a value of 5 or 11 (*top panel*). In this case with a programmed detection criterion of five beats, atrial events occurring outside the PVAB period resulted in incrementing of the short-interval counter. After five intervals had been detected at a high rate, automatic mode-switching (AMS™) occurred. Automatic mode-switching was terminated when three long intervals at a cycle length greater than that of the high atrial rate-detection rate interval resulted in incrementing of the long-interval counter. When the long-interval counter had reached 3, the device reverted back to the DDDR tracking mode (*bottom panel*). (Reproduced with permission)

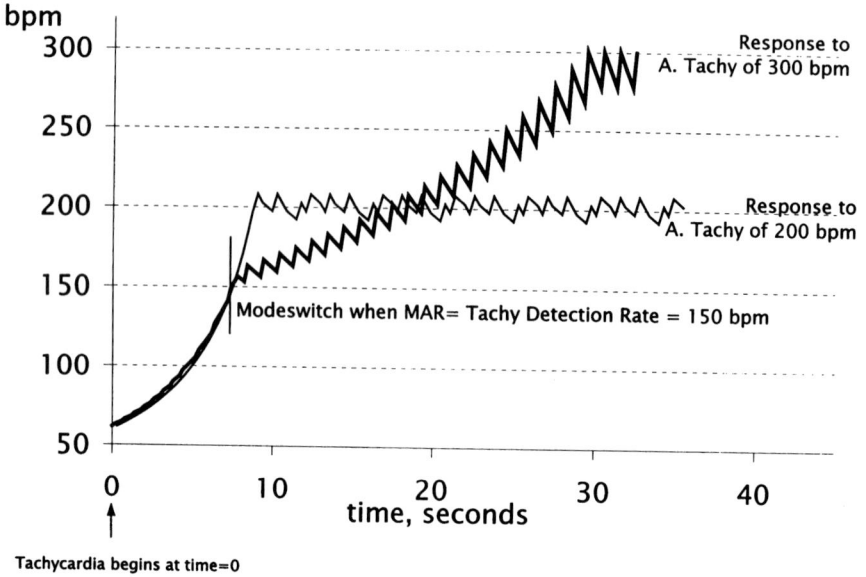

Tachycardia begins at time=0

Figure 4.9 Mode-switching detection feature of the Medtronic Thera-i™ pacemaker. Sensing of the atrium allows calculation of a mean atrial interval. The mean atrial interval is continually updated by the sensed atrial cycle length. If atrial events occur at a rate faster than a programmable tachycardia detection rate (horizontal line), pacing occurs at the upper tracking limit with a standard AV Wenckebach behaviour. When the mean atrial interval becomes less than that calculated for the programmed tachycardia detection rate, the device switches to the DDIR pacing mode. (Reproduced with permission)

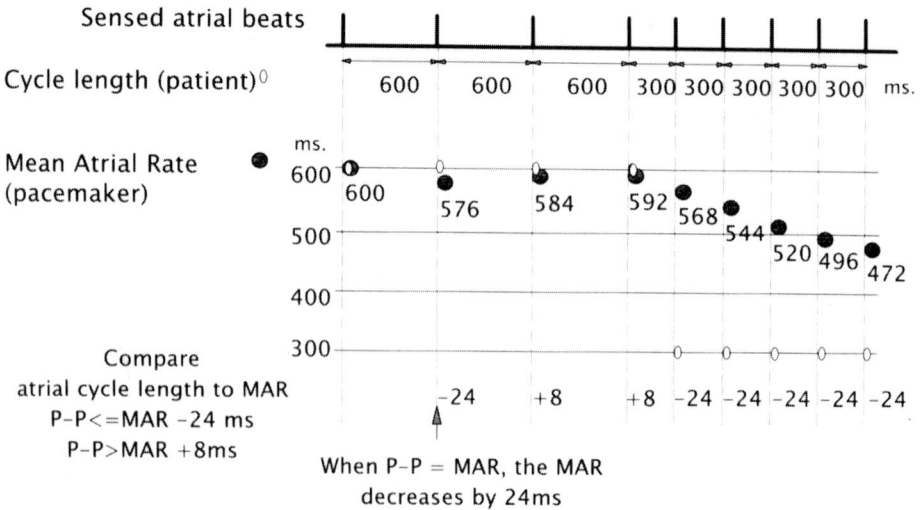

Figure 4.10 Example of the mean atrial interval. Note that at the onset of an atrial tachycardia at a cycle length of 300 ms, the mean atrial interval is decremented by 24 ms if the PP interval is less than the mean atrial interval. Resynchronization occurs when the PP interval is greater than the mean atrial interval with the mean atrial interval incremented by 8 ms for each longer interval. When the mean atrial interval exceeds that calculated for the tachycardia detection rate, resynchronization occurs with normal DDD pacing. (Reproduced with permission)

onset of mode-switching can be prolonged for up to 30 atrial cycles, especially if there is undersensing of the atrial electrogram during atrial fibrillation.

Biotronik pacemakers

The Biotronik Gemnos™ and Dromos™ pacemakers provide for automatic mode-switching through the use of a retriggerable atrial refractory period[11] (Figure 4.11). Atrial events which occur within the programmable total atrial refractory (TAR) period are sensed, but do not initiate an AV delay. Such a sensed event within the atrial refractory period resets the atrial refractory period by an amount equal to the programmed TAR period. If further atrial events are sensed within the new TAR period, the refractory period is further extended until an atrial event occurs outside of refractoriness (in which case it is tracked) or the lower rate limit has been reached and an atrial paced event is initiated. Thus, these devices switch from the DDD(R) pacing mode to the DVI(R) mode in the presence of atrial tachyarrhythmias. This algorithm has the advantages of being quite simple to implement and understand, of allowing sensing within the TAR period, and the potential for underdrive termination of a re-entrant atrial arrhythmia from asynchronous pacing. The Gemnos™ and Dromos™ pacemakers featuring dual-demand automatic mode-switching respond rapidly to

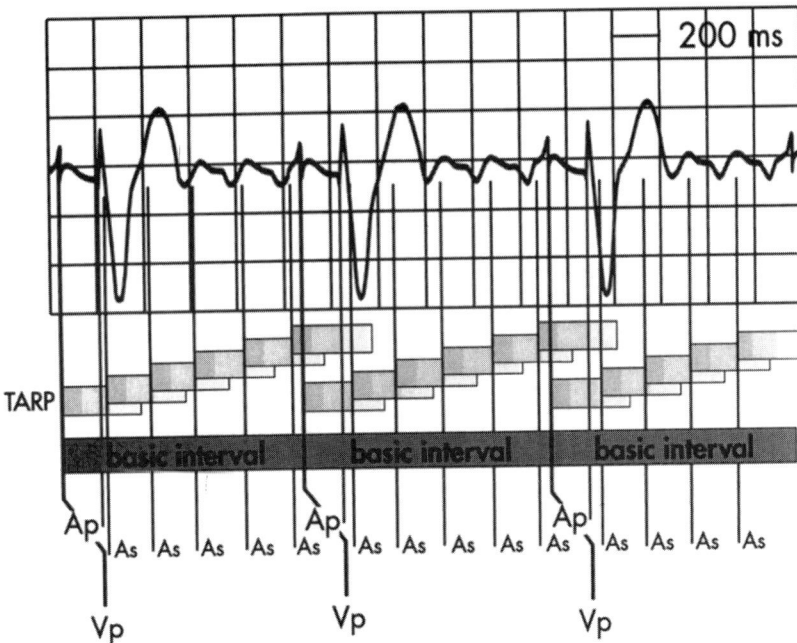

Figure 4.11 Function of the Biotronik Gemnos™ and Dromos™ pacemakers with a retriggerable atrial refractory period ('dual demand pacing'). When an atrial event occurs within the total atrial refractory (TAR) period, a new TAR period is reset. Atrial sensing during the reset TAR period produces a new TAR period until the lower pacing limit is reached. The device then delivers atrial pacing stimuli in the DVIR pacing mode at the lower rate limit (DDD pacing) or the sensor-indicated rate (DDDR pacing). (Reproduced with permission)

the onset and termination of atrial tachyarrhythmias. A disadvantage of this algorithm is the potential to trigger atrial fibrillation by asynchronous pacing in the DVI(R) mode.

CPI pacemaker

The CPI Vigor™ pacemaker offers an 'atrial tachy response' that allows the device to switch from the DDD(R) to the VVI(R) pacing mode in the presence of atrial tachyarrhythmias (Figure 4.12). This device requires sensing of eight cycles at a rate greater than the upper tracking limit to confirm detection of a tachycardia. During this period, tracking of the atrial events results in pacemaker Wenckebach or 2:1 block behaviour. Following detection of the tachyarrhythmia, pacing is allowed at the upper rate limit for a programmable duration of 10 to 2000 ventricular cycles. Following this, fallback occurs over a period of 1–5 minutes from the AV Wenckebach rate to the VVI(R) pacing mode.

Resynchronization occurs once eight atrial cycles have occurred at a rate less than the upper tracking limit. This device allows rate smoothing to be programmed to decrease the beat-to-beat change in pacing rate prior to mode-switching as well when resynchronizing to the dual-chamber tracking mode following cessation of an atrial arrhythmia. Since eight cycles are required for detection as well as a minimum of 10 ventricular cycles prior to onset of the fallback function, this device is relatively slow to mode-switch following the onset of a tachyarrhythmia, but is unlikely to become inappropriately unswitched during a sustained atrial arrhythmia.

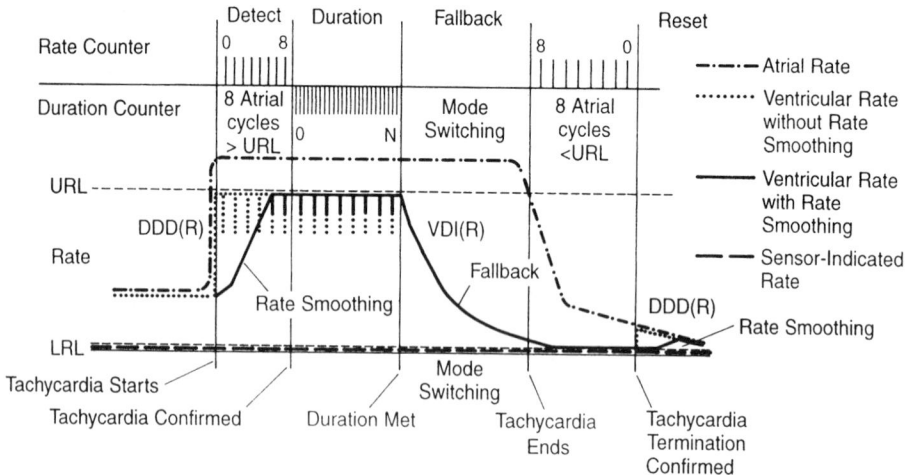

Figure 4.12 Atrial tachy response feature of the CPI Vigor™ pacemaker. During the onset of a tachycardia, if the atrial rate exceeds the upper tracking limit for eight cycles, ventricular pacing occurs at the upper rate limit for a programmable duration from 10 to 2000 cycles. Following this, there is fallback to the VVIR pacing mode at the sensor-indicated rate. When eight cycles occur at a rate less than the upper tracking limit, resynchronization to the DDDR pacing mode occurs. This feature can be used in conjunction with rate-smoothing to smooth transitions prior to mode-switching and when returning to the DDDR pacing mode. (Reproduced with permission)

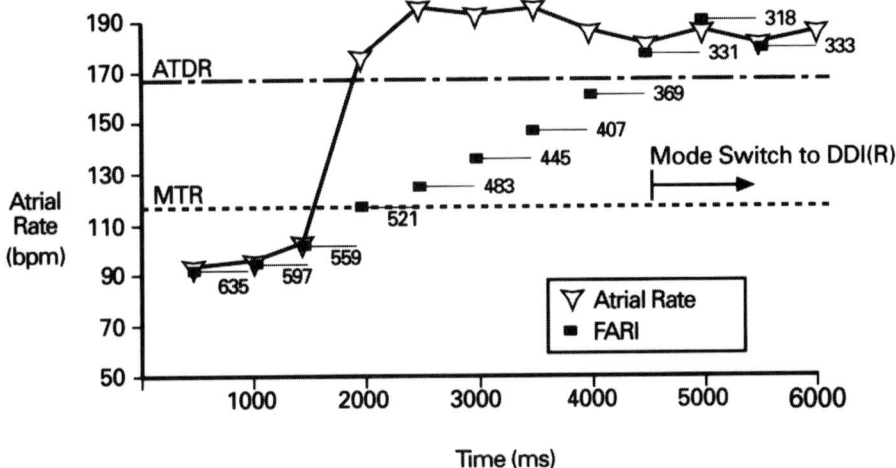

Figure 4.13 Function of the Pacesetter Triology™ DR + auto mode-switch function. This device has a maximum tracking rate as well as an atrial tachycardia detection rate that is programmable. When the atrial rate exceeds the atrial detection rate interval, a filtered atrial rate interval (FARI) is decreased by up to 38 ms per interval. Once the filtered atrial rate interval corresponds to a rate faster than the atrial tachycardia detection rate (ATDR), mode-switching occurs to the DDIR pacing mode. (Reproduced with permission)

Pacesetter pacemaker

The Pacesetter Trilogy™ DR+ allows a programmable atrial tachycardia detection rate (ATDR) and a filtered atrial rate interval (FARI) to determine the onset and termination of mode-switching.[22] If the atrial cycle length is shorter than the FARI, the FARI is automatically decreased by up to 38 ms (Figures 4.13 and 4.14). If the atrial rate remains faster than the ATDR, further shortening of the FARI occurs until mode-switching is activated. Once the atrial cycle length exceeds the FARI, the FARI is increased by up to 25 ms. Mode-switching occurs from the DDD(R) to the DDI(R) mode. Mode-switching is also available in the DDD to DDI sense during atrial arrhythmias. The Triology™ DR+ atrial tachycardia detection rate is programmable from at least 20 bpm faster than the maximum tracking rate up to 300 bpm. Mode-switching occurs rapidly, with the interval for detection dependent on the ATDR. The PVAB period is programmable from 50 to 200 ms. In addition, sensing is allowed after the first 100 ms of the AV delay. The Trilogy™ DR+ allows independently program-mable atrial tachycardia detection rates, maximum tracking rate, and maximum sensor rate.

Intermedics pacemaker

The Intermedics Marathon™ DDD(R) pacemaker provides a 'programmable mode-switching' feature as well as the SmarTracking feature described previously. Mode-switching is based on a programmable rate-detection criterion as well as the number of beats exceeding the rate criterion (Figure 4.15). The mode-switching detection rate can be programmed from 10 bpm above the maximum pacing rate up to 300 bpm in

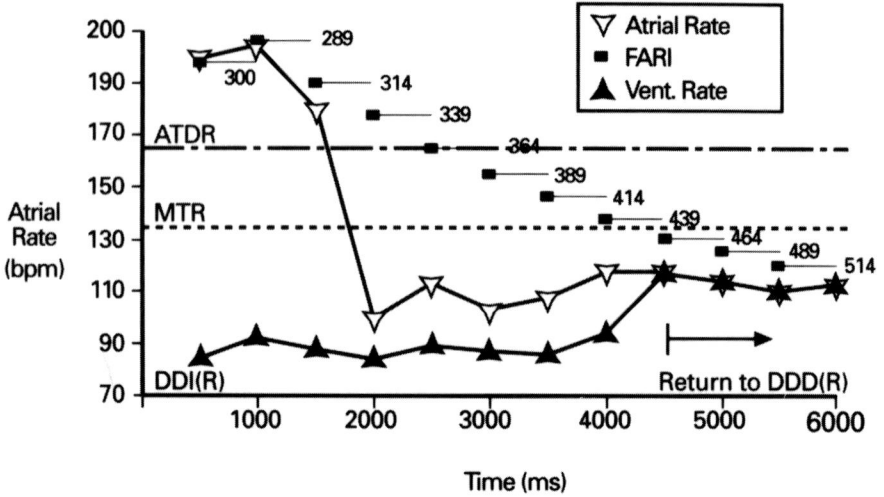

Figure 4.14 Resynchronization using the Pacesetter Triology™ DR + auto mode-switch feature. When the atrial rate is lower than the atrial tachycardia detection rate (ATDR), the filtered atrial rate interval (FARI) is increased by 25 ms per cycle until resynchronization occurs. The PVAB period is programmable from 50 to 200 ms in this device and sensing is allowed after the first 100 ms of the AV interval. (Reproduced with permission)

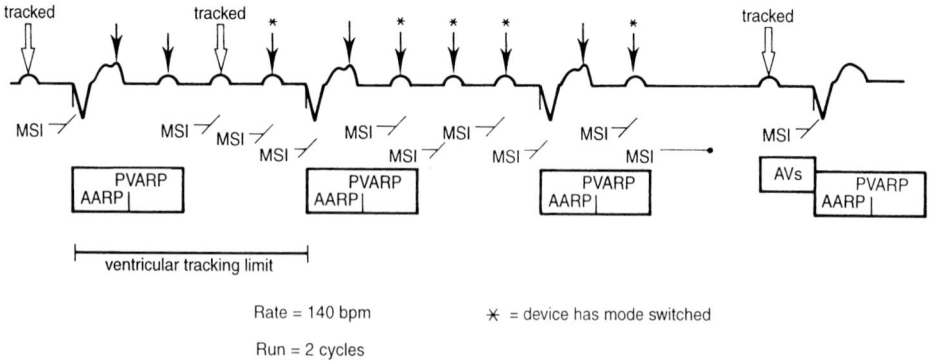

Figure 4.15 Programmable mode-switching feature of the Intermediate Marathon™. Following the first atrial beat sensed within the atrium, shown at the far left, a mode-switching interval (MSI) begins. Following this, there is tracking of the atrium stimulus with the ventricle paced at the ventricular tracking limit. Following each sensed atrial event, a new mode switch interval is initiated. If an atrial event occurs within the mode-switch interval, a new mode-switch interval is started. Once the number of cycles (run) has reached the programmed detection criterion (1–7 cycles) mode-switching occurs (*) and the ventricle is paced at the sensor-indicated rate. Following termination of the tachycardia, if no atrial event occurs within the mode-switch interval, the next atrial event will be tracked in the usual DDD(R) pacing mode (last atrial complex of tracings). (Reproduced with permission)

increments of 5 bpm. The programmable range of beats for detection is from 1 to 7 cycles. A mode switching interval is activated after every sensed atrial event that does not fall within the PVAB period. The PVAB period has a duration of 100 ms. The duration of the mode-switching interval is determined by the mode-switching detection rate. If a sensed atrial event occurs within the mode-switching interval, a new mode-switching interval is triggered and the run counter incremented by 1. If another event occurs within the mode-switching interval, the run counter is incremented by one cycle and a new mode-switching interval is triggered. Mode-switching occurs to the DDI(R) pacing mode. Resynchronization occurs once no atrial event occurs within the mode-switching interval.

This algorithm allows very rapid detection of atrial arrhythmias and prompt mode-switching within as little as one ventricular cycle. However, atrial undersensing during atrial fibrillation may result in the device becoming inappropriately unswitched. Thus, a very sensitive atrial sensitivity threshold should be programmed to prevent undersensing of atrial fibrillation. The combined use of SmarTracking and 'programmable mode-switching' can be used to provide a smooth transition in pacing rates at the onset and end of mode-switching.

Vitatron pacemaker

The Vitatron Diamond™ DDD(R) pacing system utilizes a 'physiological' band of rates to distinguish sinus tachycardia from pathological arrhythmias.[3,23] The physiological band is calculated from the atrial rate whether it is sensed or paced. This feature allows a 'physiological' band to be calculated which is defined as 15 bpm above and below the average atrial rate (Figure 4.16). If an atrial event occurs above the physiological band, the device switches to the DDI(R) pacing mode. A single premature atrial event that occurs above the physiological band is not tracked. The ventricular escape interval is calculated by the sensor rate or lower limit of the physiological band. The pacemaker may also provide an additional atrial pacing stimulus (atrial synchronization pace) following a premature atrial contraction to prevent an irregular ventricular rate. Mode-switching can be programmed to either a fixed mode or an automatic mode. If the automatic mode is programmed, the dynamic upper tracking rate varies with the physiological rate. At rest, the upper tracking rate has a minimum value of 100 bpm and changes as a result of the continually updated physiological rate. When programmed to the fixed mode, the upper limit of the physiological band is equal to the maximum tracking rate and mode-switching occurs when the atrial rate exceeds the maximum tracking rate.

This algorithm provides for very rapid detection of atrial tachyarrhythmias. The Diamond™ pacemaker also offers a fallback mechanism to minimize change in the ventricular pacing cycle length when mode-switching occurs.

Characteristics of Ideal Mode-Switching Algorithms

Although the algorithms described above have markedly improved the response of dual-chamber pacing systems to atrial tachyarrhythmias, none of the algorithms is

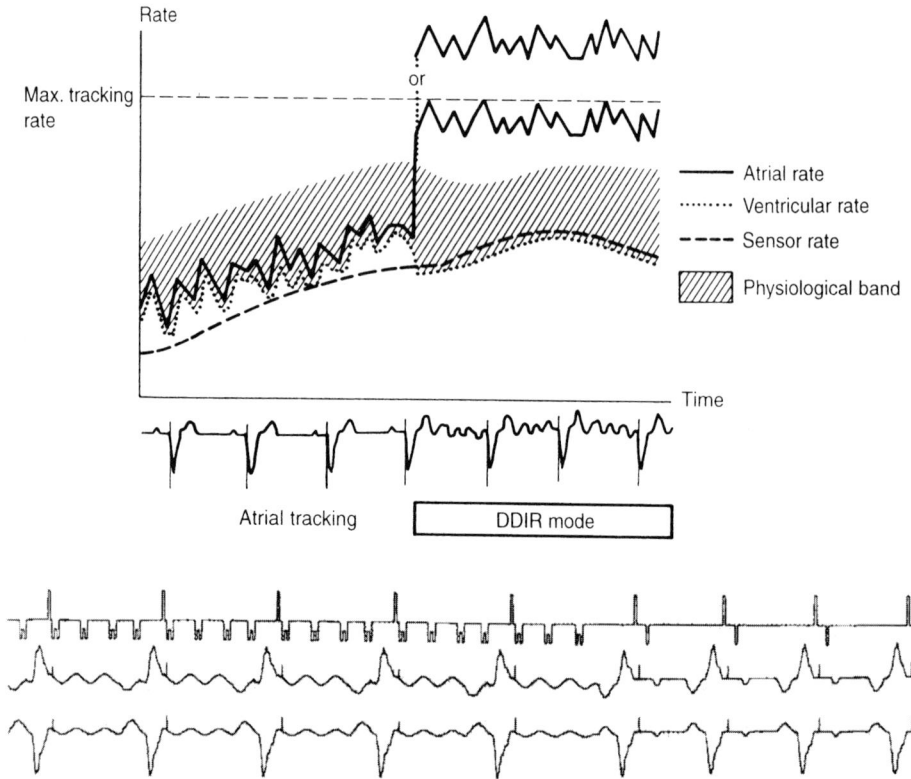

Figure 4.16 Mode-switching with the Vitatron Diamond™ pacemaker. Since atrial tachyarrhythmias are usually characterized by an abrupt increase in atrial rate at the onset, this device calculates a physiological band or heart rate that is defined as 15 bpm greater than and less than the sensed atrial rate. If the atrial rate exceeds the physiological band, switching occurs to the DDI(R) pacing mode. If there is a gradual increase in atrial rate beyond the maximum tracking limit, standard DDD(R) pacing with AV Wenckebach operation occurs. This device allows mode-switching to occur within one atrial cycle if the atrial cycle exceeds the physiological band. Resynchronization occurs when the atrial rate falls within the physiological band as indicated by the sensor. (Reproduced with permission)

perfect. However, the following conclusions can be reached regarding the ideal characteristics of a mode-switching algorithm.

(1) The sensing amplifier should be sufficiently sensitive to prevent dropout of atrial electrograms during atrial fibrillation. This generally requires that bipolar sensing be used in order to reject far-field R waves, myopotentials, and other electrical interference.

(2) The atrial sensitivity threshold should be 0.25 mV or less.

(3) The duration of blanking in the atrial sensing circuit should be minimized to allow the greatest possible chance to sense pathological atrial electrograms. This requires that the sensed AV interval be shortened aggressively in response to an increasing atrial rate, or that sensing be allowed within the terminal portion of the AV interval.

(4) Since atrial undersensing may occur during atrial fibrillation, all of the algorithms may allow inappropriate unswitching to occur. Because of this, the upper tracking limit should be programmed rather conservatively to avoid inappropriate tracking of pathological atrial arrhythmias.

The ideal algorithm should provide a wide range of programmable atrial sensitivity values, flexibility in the rate and number of cycles required for detection of atrial arrhythmias, and separately programmable upper tracking and sensor-indicated rate limits.

Effective detection of and response to atrial arrhythmias offers physicians the option for programming the upper rate of a dual-chamber pacemaker to a more physiological value. Each of the algorithms discussed above offers significant improvement in symptoms related to inappropriate tracking of atrial arrhythmias.

References

1. Sutton R, Kenny RA. The natural history of sick sinus syndrome. *PACE* 1986; **9**: 1110–14.
2. Mond HG, Barold SS. Dual chamber, rate adaptive pacing in patients with paroxysmal supraventricular tachyarrhythmias: protective measures for rate control. *PACE* 1993; **16**: 2168–85.
3. Boute W, Albers BA, Giele V. Avoiding atrial undersensing by assessment of P wave amplitude histogram data. *PACE* 1994; **17**: 1878–82.
4. Wood MA, Moskovljevic P, Stambler BS, *et al.* Comparison of bipolar atrial electrogram amplitude in sinus rhythm, atrial fibrillation, and atrial flutter. *PACE* 1996; **19**: 150–6.
5. Ricci R, Puglisi A, Azzolini P, *et al.* Reliability of a new algorithm for automatic mode switching from DDDR to DDIR pacing mode in sinus node disease patients with chronotropic incompetence and recurrent paroxysmal atrial fibrillation. *PACE* 1996; **19**: 1719–23.
6. Hanich RF, Midel MG, McElroy BP, *et al.* Circumvention of maximum tracking limitations with a rate modulated dual chamber pacemaker. *PACE* 1989; **12**: 392–7.
7. Higano ST, Hayes DL, Eisinger G. Advantage of discrepant upper rate limits in a DDDR pacemaker. *Mayo Clin Proc* 1989; **64**: 932–9.
8. Higano ST, Hayes DL. P wave tracking above the maximum tracking rate in a DDDR pacemaker. *PACE* 1989; **12**: 1044–8.
9. Van Wyhe G, Sra J, Rovang K, *et al.* Maintenance of atrioventricular sequence after His-bundle ablation for paroxysmal supraventricular rhythm disorders: a unique use of the fallback mode in dual chamber pacemakers. *PACE* 1991; **14**: 410–14.
10. Mayumi H, Uchida T, Shinozaki K, *et al.* Use of a dual chamber pacemaker with a novel fallback algorithm as an effective treatment for sick sinus syndrome associated with transient supraventricular tachyarrhythmia. *PACE* 1993; **16**: 992–1000.
11. Barold SS, Mond HG. Fallback responses to dual chamber (DDD and DDDR) pacemakers: a proposed classification. *PACE* 1994; **17**: 1160–5.
12. Johnson NJ. Inconsistent response to rapid atrial rhythms in a DDD pacemaker with the fallback feature. *PACE* 1995; **18**: 1458–62.
13. Lee MT, Adkins A, Woodson D, *et al.* A new feature for control of inappropriate high rate tracking in DDDR pacemakers. *PACE* 1990; **13**: 1852–5.
14. Lau CP, Tai YT, Fong PC, *et al.* Clinical experience with an activity sensing DDDR pacemaker using an accelerometer sensor. *PACE* 1992; **15**: 334–43.
15. Leung SK, Lau CP, Leung WH, *et al.* Apparent extension of the atrioventricular interval due to sensor-based algorithm against supraventricular tachyarrhythmias. *PACE* 1994; **17**: 321–30.

16. Lau CP, Tai YU, Fong PC, *et al*. Atrial arrhythmia management with sensor controlled atrial refractory period and automatic mode switching in patients with minute ventilation sensing dual chamber rate adaptive pacemakers. *PACE* 1992; **15**: 1504–14.
17. Pitney MR, May CD, Davis MJ. Undesirable mode switching with a dual chamber rate responsive pacemaker. *PACE* 1993; **16**: 729–37.
18. Wagshal AB, Dansereau LJ, Mittleman RS, *et al*. Undesirable mode switching with a Telectronics 1250 META DDDR pacemaker (letter, comment). *PACE* 1993; **16**: 2212–13.
19. Sweesy M, Batey R, Forney R, *et al*. Automatic mode change in a DDDR pacemaker for supraventricular tachyarrhythmias (abstract). *PACE* 1991; **14**: 737.
20. Provenier F, Jordaens L, Verstraeten T, *et al*. The 'automatic mode switch' function in successive generations of minute ventilation sensing dual chamber rate responsive pacemakers. *PACE* 1994; **17**(II): 1913–19.
21. Ovsyshcher IE, Katz A, Bondy C. Initial experience with a new algorithm for automatic mode switching from DDDR to DDIR mode. *PACE* 1994; **17**(II): 1908–12.
22. Levine PA, Bornzin GA, Barlow J, *et al*. A new automode switch algorithm for supraventricular tachycardias. *PACE* 1994; **17**(II): 1895–9.
23. den Dulk K, Dijkman B, Pieterse M, *et al*. Initial experience with mode switching in a dual sensor, dual chamber pacemaker in patients with paroxysmal atrial tachyarrhythmias. *PACE* 1994; **17**(II): 1900–7.

5

Optimal Pacing in Sick Sinus Syndrome

H. R. Andersen

The first pacemaker treatment for sinus node disease in man was performed in 1968 by Silverman who paced the right atrium using an epicardial atrial electrode.[1] Subsequently, development of transvenous leads allowed implantation of permanent atrial leads.[2] Following that early period the tremendous development of pacing leads, with both passive and active fixation, allowed physicians to select freely where to insert the leads in the heart. For patients with sick sinus syndrome (SSS) the choice is between single-lead atrial pacing (AAI), single-lead ventricular pacing (VVI), and dual-chamber pacing (DDD). (In this chapter DDD pacing represents all pacemaker modalities with a lead in both the atrium and the ventricle.) The advantages and disadvantages of stimulation in the atrium, in the ventricle or in both chambers, and the various clinical outcomes that can be expected, should always be considered when choosing a specific pacemaker for an individual patient.

AAI and DDD pacing more closely resembles the normal physiology of cardiac activation and haemodynamics than does VVI pacing, because both maintain the synchrony of atrial and ventricular contractions. However, VVI pacing is still used in approximately 50% of patients,[3–6] in spite of analyses documenting that DDD pacing is both clinical and cost-effective compared with VVI pacing.[7] The reluctance to implant more physiological pacemakers may be related to the initial higher device cost and more complex programming and follow-up of DDD pacemakers. Furthermore, the lack of large-scale prospective randomized trials to document which pacing mode is superior may also contribute significantly. Our present knowledge about the long-term clinical outcomes which can be expected with the various pacing modes relies on carefully conducted observational studies and only one minor randomized trial.

Long-Term Effects of VVI and AAI/DDD Pacing

Atrial Fibrillation

Paroxysmal atrial fibrillation, atrial flutter and supraventricular tachycardia are common findings in SSS patients. Shaw et al.[8] observed that in unpaced patients the prevalence of atrial fibrillation rises to 50% if one considers only patients with paroxysmal tachyarrhythmias. Thus, atrial fibrillation is a part of the natural history of SSS. The impact of different pacing modalities on the development of chronic atrial fibrillation has been reported in several studies. Observational data comparing VVI with AAI/DDD pacing reported a significantly higher incidence of atrial fibrillation in the VVI group (Table 5.1).

In a review of the literature up to 1986, Sutton and Kenny[9] estimated that in a $2\frac{1}{2}$-year follow-up period, the incidence of atrial fibrillation during VVI pacing was 22.3% compared with 3.9% in the AAI group ($p < 0.001$). The most carefully conducted observational study performed by Rosenqvist et al.[15] reported similar results: in a 4-year follow-up the incidence of chronic atrial fibrillation was 47% in the VVI group and 6.7% in the AAI group. Sgarbossa et al.,[21] in a large observational study of 507 patients treated with AAI/DDD pacemaker ($n = 395$) or VVI pacemaker ($n = 112$), observed chronic atrial fibrillation in 17% of patients after a mean follow-up of 59 months. Independent predictors of chronic atrial fibrillation were: prior history of paroxysmal atrial fibrillation ($p < 0.001$); use of preimplant antiarrhythmic drug ($p < 0.001$); VVI pacing mode ($p = 0.003$); age ($p = 0.005$); and valvular heart disease ($p < 0.001$). Andersen et al.[22] did a prospective randomized trial of 225 patients and compared AAI with VVI pacing. After a mean follow-up of 40 months, 23% of the VVI-paced patients had atrial fibrillation at one or more ambulatory visits, compared with 14% in the AAI group ($p = 0.12$). Chronic atrial fibrillation developed in 13% of the VVI group, and in 7% of the AAI group ($p = 0.24$).

The presence of paroxysmal supraventricular tachyarrhythmias ('tachy-brady syndrome') prior to pacemaker implantation is an important factor that further influences the likelihood of developing chronic atrial fibrillation. Rosenqvist et al.[15] found atrial fibrillation in 69% of VVI-paced patients with 'tachy-brady syndrome' and in 18% of VVI-paced patients without the syndrome. The modality of pacing also

Table 5.1 Effect of pacing mode on development of atrial fibrillation in nonrandomized trials

	No. of patients		Mean follow-up (months)		Atrial fibrillation (% per year)[a]	
	AAI/DDD	VVI	AAI/DDD	VVI	AAI/DDD	VVI
Sutton and Kenny (1986) (review)[9]	410/0	651	33	39	1.4	6.9
Santini et al. (1990)[10]	135/79	125	60	60	1.9	11.9
Bianconi et al. (1989)[11]	153	150	44	59	4.8	7.9
Markewitz et al. (1986)[12]	67/69	87	32	32	3.1	10.0
Feuer et al. (1989)[13]	0/110	110	40	48	2.4	4.5
Sasaki et al. (1988)[14]	12/12	25	20	35	0	12.3
Rosenqvist et al. (1988)[15]	89/0	79	44	47	1.8	12.1
Zanini et al. (1989)[16]	53/0	57	45	40	1.0	5.3
Stangl et al. (1990)[17]	110/0	112	40	33	1.8	6.9
Grimm et al. (1990)[18]	0/41	203	32	69	4.5	5.6
Sasaki et al. (1991)[19]	17/24	34	62	39	3.3	13.6
Hesselson et al. (1992)[20b]	0/366	193	42	44	1.6	7.1

[a] Mean for AAI/DDD: 2.3%; for VVI: 8.7%.
[b] Follow-up period was reported for a total study population of 950 patients of which 559 patients (59%) has SSS.

influenced the outcome: in AAI-paced patients the incidence fell to 9% in patients with 'tachy-brady syndrome' and to 3% in those without. Sgarbossa *et al.*[21] observed that in patients with a preimplant history of paroxysmal atrial fibrillation, independent predictors of chronic atrial fibrillation were: prolonged episodes (>1 hour) of paroxysmal atrial fibrillation ($p < 0.001$); long history (>5 years) of paroxysmal atrial fibrillation ($p = 0.004$); VVI pacing mode ($p = 0.025$); use of antiarrhythmic drugs before pacemaker implant ($p = 0.024$); and age ($p = 0.04$). In patients without a history of paroxysmal atrial fibrillation the incidence of chronic atrial fibrillation was 0% during the first 5 years of follow-up for both pacing modalities. In the randomized trial, chronic atrial fibrillation developed in 17% of the VVI patients and in 9% of the AAI patients with 'tachy-brady syndrome' prior to implantation.[22] In patients without the syndrome the figures were 6% for VVI pacing and 4% for AAI pacing, respectively. Multivariate analysis identified 'tachy-brady syndrome' at the time of randomization as the only independent factor significantly correlated ($p < 0.02$) with an increased risk of developing chronic atrial fibrillation during follow-up.

Thus, based on these results, it seems evident that VVI pacing is associated with an increased risk of atrial fibrillation in patients with sick sinus syndrome compared with AAI/DDD pacing. The risk is particularly high in patients with 'tachy-brady syndrome'. The exact mechanisms which link VVI pacing with the development of chronic atrial fibrillation is unknown. VVI pacing may predispose or AAI/DDD pacing may prevent or delay the natural evolution of SSS to chronic atrial fibrillation. The explanation might be related to atrial overdrive pacing eliminating sinus bradycardia with concomitant homogenization of atrial refractory periods, or to preserved AV synchrony, or both. However, the observations strongly indicate that the atrium should be sensed and paced in patients with sick sinus syndrome.

Thromboembolism

There is a definite risk of thromboembolism in patients with SSS, both before and after implantation of a pacemaker.[20,21,23,24] In nonrandomized observational studies comparing VVI pacing with AAI/DDD pacing, the incidence of thromboembolic events is higher after implantation of a VVI pacemaker than after implantation of an AAI/DDD pacemaker (Table 5.2).

In their review, Sutton and Kenny[9] found that the incidence of thromboembolism in patients with SSS was 13% in the VVI patients ($n = 532$) but only 1.6% in the AAI patients ($n = 321$) ($p < 0.001$). In the randomized trial[22] by Andersen *et al.*, 17.4% of VVI-paced patients and 5.5% of AAI-paced patients developed arterial thromboembolism after a mean follow-up of 40 months ($p = 0.0083$). In patients without atrial fibrillation before randomization and during follow-up, thromboembolism occurred in 12% of the VVI group, versus 5% of the atrial group ($p = 0.25$). Multivariate analysis identified randomization to VVI pacing as the only variable significantly associated with an increased risk of a thromboembolic event during follow-up ($p = 0.04$). Recently, preliminary data from an ongoing randomized trial comparing VVI(R) with DDD(R) pacing in 163 patients with SSS was reported and showed 4% stroke in the VVI(R) group versus 2% stroke in the DDD(R) group after 1 year follow-up.[29]

Table 5.2 Effect of pacing mode on development of stroke and thromboembolism in nonrandomized trials with more than 50 patients

Author	Number	Follow-up[a] (months)	Stroke/ thromboembolism (%)
Curzi et al. (1985)[25]	n = 164	NR	12
	VVI = 120	NR	17
	AAI = 44	46	0
Sasaki et al. (1983)[26]	n = 78	NR	21.8
	VVI = 42	NR	38.1
	AAI = 36	NR	2.8
Sethi et al. (1990)[27]	n = 87	49	6.9
	VVI = 47		10.6
	DDD = 40		2.5
Nürnberg et al. (1991)[28]	n = 130	41	7.7
	VVI = 93	NR	11
	AAI = 15	NR	0
	DDD = 22	NR	0
Rosenqvist et al. (1988)[15]	n = 168	NR	13.7
	VVI = 79	47	15
	AAI = 89	44	12
Bianconi et al. (1989)[11]	n = 303	NR	8.6
	VVI = 150	59	11
	DDD = 153	44	6
Zanini et al. (1989)[16]	n = 110	NR	—
	VVI = 57	45	7.0
	AAI = 53	40	—
Sasaki et al. (1991)[19b]	n = 75	NR	
	VVI = 34	39	26
	AAI = 17	—	—
	DDD = 24	62	2
Santini et al. (1990)[10]	n = 339	60	5.3
	VVI = 125	NR	10.4
	AAI = 135	NR	2.2
	DDD = 79	NR	2.5

[a] NR = not reported.
[b] Only one cumulative figure for stroke/thromboembolism (2%) and follow-up period (62 months) was reported for the 41 patients with a physiological pacemaker (AAI and DDD).

In the randomized trial by Andersen et al.[22] the 5.5% annual rate of thromboembolism in the VVI group was unusually high, whereas the 1.6% annual rate in the AAI group was similar to that reported in a meta-analysis of the five recent large randomized trials of antithrombotic therapy in atrial fibrillation.[30] During follow-up in the randomized trial, anticoagulation was used in 7.8% of patients in the VVI group and in 2.7% of the AAI group ($p = 0.16$). In patients who developed chronic atrial fibrillation during follow-up, the annual rate of thromboembolism was 14.5% per year in the VVI group and 4.2% per year in the AAI group. In the meta-analysis in nonpaced patients with atrial fibrillation, the annual risk of stroke or systemic embolism was 5% per year without anticoagulation and 1.7% per year on anticoagulation. Thus, the rate of thromboembolism in the VVI-paced group with atrial fibrillation was 3–8 times higher than expected for patients with atrial fibrillation, whereas the rate in the AAI group was similar to or slightly higher than expected.

The explanation for the very high frequency of thromboembolic events in patients treated with a VVI pacemaker is uncertain. It may be related to the abnormal depolarization pattern of the ventricular myocardium caused by ventricular stimulation. During atrial fibrillation (with or without an AAI pacemaker), the ventricular myocardium is activated through the AV-junction and the bundle branches, and a normal physiological contraction is preserved in the ventricles. In contrast, during atrial fibrillation with a VVI pacemaker (or a DDD pacemaker) the apical ventricular stimulation changes the activation and the contraction pattern of the ventricles. This change in ventricular contraction has been shown to be followed by decreased coronary artery blood flow, dilatation of the ventricles, increased end-diastolic pressure, and increased atrial pressure.[31–37] Such changes may further lead to atrial dilatation, decreased left atrial wall motion, and slow the blood flow in perimural areas of the atrium which may further predispose to development of cardiac thrombus[38] and subsequently increase the risk of thromboembolism. In the randomized trial by Andersen *et al.*,[22] echocardiography performed before implantation and at subsequent follow-up visits showed that there was significantly more dilation of the left atrium in the VVI than in the AAI group, and atrial enlargement was not a consequence of atrial fibrillation, because it occurred before atrial fibrillation developed.

Thus, based on both observational studies and one randomized trial, it seems evident that VVI pacing is associated with an increased risk of thromboembolism compared with AAI/DDD pacing. The risk seems especially high in patients with 'tachy-brady syndrome'.

Haemodynamics and Congestive Heart Failure

Normally, cardiac output increases about 200–400% during maximal exercise; the largest component is provided by an increase in heart rate, whereas increased stroke volume makes only a modest contribution. In a normal heart, AV synchrony at rest contributes about 20–30% of the cardiac output.[39] The haemodynamic importance of a properly timed atrial systole has been recognized in a large number of studies to be associated with a higher cardiac output at rest with AAI/DDD than with VVI pacing.[40,41] Repeated haemodynamic studies have shown that this difference between atrial and ventricular pacing is maintained with time.[42,43]

Many studies have demonstrated that cardiac output is greater during AAI pacing than during VVI pacing[40,41,44] and during DDD pacing.[32,33,35,36,45–47] The haemodynamic superiority of AAI pacing is partly a result of the effect of the atrial contraction upon ventricular filling. However, the abnormal contraction sequence of the ventricular myocardium induced by ventricular stimulation may obviously also play a negative role in VVI and DDD pacing (see later). Several studies have reported the long-term haemodynamic benefits of atrial compared with ventricular pacing in SSS. Rosenqvist *et al.*[15] evaluated the development of congestive heart failure after pacemaker implantation for SSS and found a statistically higher incidence with VVI than with AAI pacing, whereas Stangl *et al.*[17] demonstrated only a trend in the same direction. In contrast, other groups comparing VVI with

AAI pacing in SSS patients reported no statistically significant differences with regard to the development of congestive heart failure.[16,19] Sgarbossa *et al.*[48] compared VVI pacing with physiological pacing in a large group of patients (VVI: $n = 112$; AAI: $n = 19$; DDD: $n = 376$) and found no difference in congestive heart failure. In that study, progressive or new-onset congestive heart failure was more a consequence of the underlying cardiovascular disease, and VVI pacing was not associated with an increased incidence of heart failure compared with physiological pacing. However, preservation of the 'atrial kick' is not the only mechanism at work in this context. Impairment of the ventricular function may have occurred in both groups owing to right ventricular stimulation, because 95% of the patients in the 'physiological' group were actually stimulated in the ventricle. This may explain why Sgarbossa *et al.*[48] did not find a significant difference between VVI pacing and physiological pacing. In the randomized trial by Andersen *et al.*[22] comparing AAI with VVI pacing, there was no significant difference in congestive heart failure. However, reliable assessment of the NYHA classification during a short ambulatory visit to the outpatient clinic is difficult in these older patients (mean age in 1996 was 80 years). As a surrogate end-point on heart failure, the left atrial diameter was measured by M-mode echocardiography. Left atrial diameter in the AAI and VVI groups before implantation were 34 ± 6 mm and 34 ± 7 mm, respectively. During follow-up, there was a significant increase in the diameter to 40 ± 7 mm in the VVI group and to 36 ± 7 mm in the AAI group ($p = 0.0001$, VVI versus AAI). Compared with preoperative values, the increase was significant within both groups (VVI: $p = 0.0001$; AAI: $p = 0.006$). The larger dilatation in the VVI group may be a consequence of the compromised left ventricular function caused by the apical right ventricular stimulation.

Thus, there is evidence of a haemodynamic benefit of AV synchrony maintained by AAI and DDD pacing, and of a physiological contraction pattern of the ventricles maintained by AAI pacing. However, the lack of large randomized trials designed to prospectively study haemodynamics and heart failure in different pacing modalities (AAI versus VVI versus DDD) makes it difficult to demonstrate that these elements also translate into less congestive heart failure for patients with SSS.

Mortality

Several studies indicate that the survival rate among paced patients with SSS is approximately comparable to the survival rate of the nonpaced population. Early in the 1980s some reports of the natural history of unpaced patients with sick sinus syndrome showed survival to be similar to the normal population.[8,23] At the same time, VVI patients did not show an improvement in survival compared with unpaced patients.[49] That is, VVI pacing was useful in improving symptoms but was not useful in improving survival. The prognosis for survival is, furthermore, related to the underlying heart disease. Mortality is increased by congestive heart failure and ischaemic heart disease.[20,50,51] Several observational studies have compared mortality in AAI/DDD-paced patients with those paced in VVI (Table 5.3).

Table 5.3 Effect of mode of pacing on mortality in nonrandomized trials

	No. of patients		Mean follow-up (months)		Mortality (% per year)[a]	
	AAI/DDD	VVI	AAI/DDD	VVI	AAI/DDD	VVI
Rosenqvist et al. (1988)[15]	89/0	79	44	47	2.2	5.9
Sasaki et al. (1988)[14]	12/12	25	20	35	7.6	8.2
Bianconi et al. (1989)[11]	153	150	44	59	3.8	6.3
Santini et al. (1990)[10]	135/79	125	60	60	3.1	7.7
Stangl et al. (1990)[17]	110/0	112	40	33	5.1	9.8
Zanini et al. (1989)[16]	53/0	57	45	40	2.5	5.3
Sasaki et al. (1991)[19]	17/24	34	62	39	2.4	10.9
Nürnberg et al. (1991)[28b]	15/22	93	41		7.1	13.8
Hesselson et al. (1992)[20c]	0/336	193	42	44	6.5	12.9
Sgarbossa et al. (1993)[50b]	19/376	112	66		3.9	7.5
Tung et al. (1994)[52b]	0/36	112	44		8.3	16.4

[a] Mean for AAI/DDD: 4.8%; for VVI: 9.5%.
[b] Only one follow-up period was reported for the total group.
[c] Follow-up period was reported for a total study population of 950 patients of which 559 patients had SSS.

Rosenqvist et al.[15] reported that mortality was significantly higher in the VVI group (23%) compared with 8% among AAI-paced patients during a 4-year follow-up. This difference was significant following a Cox proportional hazards analysis which adjusted for age and sex within the two groups and used a one-sided test. The observed survival did not, however, differ significantly from the expected in any of the two groups. Hesselson et al.[20] studied 950 pacemaker patients with follow-up to 7 years, and SSS was present in 59% of the population. The mortality rates for SSS patients were higher with VVI pacing (12.9% per year) than with AAI/DDD (6.5%). In a randomized trial, Andersen et al.[22] found no significant improvement of survival in the AAI patients compared with VVI pacing. At 40-months follow-up, mortality was 21.7% in the VVI group and 19.1% in the AAI group ($p = 0.74$). Preliminary data from an ongoing randomized trial comparing VVI(R) with DDD(R) in 163 patients showed a 12% mortality in the VVI(R) group versus 6% mortality in the DDD(R) group at 1-year follow-up.[5]

Thus, there is only a weak tendency for improved survival with AAI/DDD pacing compared with VVI pacing. We cannot definitively conclude that AAI/DDD pacing is associated with better survival than VVI pacing in patients with SSS. Only large-scale randomized trials can give the answer, and it is hoped that some of the ongoing trials will resolve the question about which pacing mode has the highest survival prospects.[5,53–55]

Atrioventricular Conduction Defects

Because SSS has been regarded as part of a more generalized dysfunction of the conduction system, it is still debated whether these patients should be treated with an

AAI pacemaker, because of the risk of developing AV block during follow-up. Sutton and Kenny[9] reviewed 28 studies reporting on 1395 patients followed over an average of 34 months. Progression of the AV conduction disturbance was present in 8% of the patients with an annual incidence of 3%. These authors considered a PR interval over 0.24 seconds, complete bundle branch block, a Wenckebach point of 120 bpm or less, His–ventricular prolongation and second- and third-degree AV block as indices of progressive AV conduction disturbance. Although most of the electrocardiographic changes were asymptomatic and without the need for ventricular backup-pacing, it was concluded that permanent AAI pacing was not a safe pacing mode for SSS patients. In contrast, Rosenqvist and Obel[56] collected data from 1878 patients from 28 studies in which it was possible to assess the development of second- and third-degree AV block and only include progression in AV nodal conduction disease which required replacement of the AAI pacemaker with a system providing ventricular stimulation. Applying their criteria, the total prevalence of progression was 2.5% during a median follow-up time of 36 months. The median annual incidence was 0.65%. Thus, they found a very low risk for the development of a clinically important conduction disturbance in these patients, and claimed that 'atrial pacing is a reliable and superior method to treat patients with sinus node disease without significant AV conduction disturbances'.

Brandt[57] reviewed ten additional studies including 571 AAI-paced patients with a median follow-up of 34 months and reported a median 0.9% annual incidence of second- and third-degree AV block. Santini[24] reported an overall prevalence of 3.9% and an incidence of 0.9% per year and declared that it is possible to treat over 50% of SSS patients with AAI pacing.

In the randomized trial by Andersen et al.[22] patients were excluded from randomization if a standard electrocardiogram showed first-, second- or third-degree AV block (first-degree AV block was defined as a PQ interval >0.22 seconds in patients $\leqslant 70$ years, and a PQ interval >0.26 seconds in patients >70 years). Furthermore, patients were excluded if the electrocardiogram showed left bundle branch block or bifascicular block or if patients with 'tachy-brady syndrome' had an RR interval >3 seconds or a QRS rate <40 bpm for 1 minute during atrial tachycardia. Thus, patients with right bundle branch block or single fascicular block were included. After randomization, an atrial pacing test was performed at the time of implantation. The Wenckebach point was required to be $\geqslant 100$ bpm for an AAI implant. Medical treatment was not discontinued before implantation and neither atropine nor isoprenaline was used to enhance AV conduction during the atrial pacing test. Using these simple selection criteria for AAI pacing, only two AAI patients needed upgrading of the pacemaker system during follow-up because of second- and third-degree AV block, respectively (incidence 0.6% per year). One patient aged 79 had no bundle branch or fascicular block, a PQ interval of 0.24 seconds, a stimulus–Q interval of 0.34 seconds at 100 bpm, and a Wenckebach point between 100 and 120 bpm. The other patient was 80 years old and had right bundle branch block, a PQ interval of 0.18 seconds, a stimulus–Q interval of 0.21 seconds at 100 bpm, and a Wenckebach point >120 bpm. Thus, in these patients randomized to AAI pacing, 1 of 7 (14%) with right bundle branch block developed symptomatic AV block during follow-up.

Brandt *et al.*[58] also observed that in patients with right or left bundle branch block or bifascicular block at the time of implantation, the incidence of high-grade AV block during follow-up seemed to be higher than in patients without such intraventricular conduction defects.

Most observational studies have used a Wenckebach point $\geqslant 120$ bpm as a criteria for implantation of an AAI pacemaker. However, it has never been clearly documented in a prospective trial that measurement of the Wenckebach point or pre-implant electrophysiological assessment of the His–ventricular interval, in patients with a normal PQ interval and without bundle branch or bifascicular block, has any significant prognostic advantage above a standard electrocardiogram (ECG) to identify patients at high risk for developing symptomatic AV block after implantation of an AAI pacemaker.

Thus, based on careful clinical selection, review of Holter recordings and ECGs, and an atrial pacing test performed at implantation, more than 50% of SSS patients can be identified where the risk of subsequent AV block is under 1% per year. In the small proportion of patients where AV block develops it normally progresses slowly without clinical symptoms and is frequently produced by drug therapy.[10,59] The slow progression of impairment in the AV conduction enables the physician to adjust drug therapy or to implant an extra ventricular lead in most patients before clinical symptoms occur.

Obviously, ventricular bradycardia due to progressive deterioration of the atrioventricular conduction can be avoided by implantation of a VVI or a DDD pacemaker in all patients. However, the potential disadvantages of ventricular stimulation in SSS patients should be considered and weighted against the small risk of clinically significant AV block. Instead of treating all patients with ventricular stimulation to avoid bradycardia in fewer than 1% per year, it may be more appropriate to treat only the small fraction of patients who develop impairment of AV conduction during follow-up. It should be recognized that ventricular stimulation leads to abnormality in ventricular performance and it may create new problems for the patient. Therefore, in patients with SSS and a normal AV and intraventricular conduction, the traditional statement that 'the ventricles should not be left unprotected' may not be correct. Instead, it might appear much more appropriate to claim that 'the ventricles should remain untouched' if only the sinus node is sick.

Pacemaker Syndrome with VVI, AAI and DDD Pacing

The pacemaker syndrome was first described by Mitsui *et al.*[60] Later, Ausubel and Furman[61] defined the pacemaker syndrome as a clinical complex of signs and symptoms related to the adverse haemodynamic and electrophysiological consequences of ventricular pacing in the presence of a normally functioning implanted ventricular pacemaker. Subsequently, Schüller and Brandt[62] suggested that the pacemaker syndrome be redefined more broadly as 'symptoms and signs present in the pacemaker patient which are caused by inadequate timing of atrial and ventricular contraction'. Thus, the latter definition also includes pacemaker syndrome associated with pacing modes other than VVI.

The pathophysiology of the pacemaker syndrome is very complex and not yet fully understood. The inadequate timing of atrial and ventricular contractions causes atrial contraction against partially or completely closed mitral and tricuspid AV valves. This may lead to systemic and pulmonary venous regurgitation and congestion with atrial distension followed by activation of stretch receptors in the walls of the atria and pulmonary veins, producing a reflex vasodepressor effect.[63] The presence of atrial cannon waves appears to be essential for the development of symptoms because atrial fibrillation with ventricular pacing cannot produce the pacemaker syndrome.[64] In extreme cases, SSS patients with the pacemaker syndrome may suffer substantial hypotension, especially in the first few seconds of ventricular pacing when switching from normal sinus rhythm. Syncope or near syncope can occur. Other symptoms and signs include dyspnoea, limitation of exercise capacity, induction of congestive heart failure, pulmonary venous congestion, patient awareness of beat-to-beat variation of cardiac response (from spontaneous to pacemaker beats), cough, a lump in the throat, unpleasant pulsation in the neck or chest, headache, chest pain, apprehension, weakness, fatigue, malaise, and pressure sensation of fullness in the chest, neck or head. Physical examination may show cannon waves in the jugular veins and a marked drop in blood pressure when the rhythm changes from sinus to pacing rhythm. Reproduction of symptoms during pacing and improvement during spontaneous sinus rhythm support the diagnosis. The true incidence of pacemaker syndrome is unknown. If patients with DDD pacemakers are blindly randomized to reprogramming of their pacemaker to either VVI mode or DDD mode, 60–80% of patients will prefer the DDD mode.[65,66]

During VVI(R) pacing at rest in patients with chronotropic atrial incompetence, the ventricular stimulation may cause 1:1 retrograde VA conduction and pacemaker syndrome. During VVI(R) pacing at low activity in patients with moderate chronotropic atrial incompetence, the spontaneous sinus rate may increase above the pacemaker rate; but on more heavy exercise inadequate increase of the sinus rate gives way to ventricular pacing associated with retrograde VA conduction.[67] VA conduction is dynamic,[68] and some patients with blocked VA conduction at rest may develop improved and restored VA conduction on exercise during VVI(R) pacing under the influence of catecholamine.[69] Alternatively, the pacemaker syndrome at rest may actually disappear on exercise if an increase in the ventricular pacing rate blocks VA conduction.

During AAI pacing, a marked delay between the pacemaker stimulus and the onset of ventricular systole can produce atrial systole against closed AV valves, a situation haemodynamically identical to VVI pacing with retrograde VA conduction. This form of pacemaker syndrome can occur in the AAI(R) mode when the atrial pacing rate increases.[70] A fast activity sensor response in the AAI(R) mode with sudden increase in the atrial rate without exercise can lengthen the PR interval before the sympathetic activity has the opportunity to improve or shorten AV conduction. This is especially pronounced during sleep and in patients treated with antiarrhythmic drugs such as beta-blockers.[71] It tends to correct itself as sympathetic tone progressively increases during exercise.[58,71] In most patients, a pacing rate of 90–100 bpm during normal walking is quite satisfactory, and an AAI(R) device should be programmed accordingly.

During DDD pacing the pacemaker syndrome can occur if the AV delay is programmed either too long or too short resulting in inadequate timing of atrial and ventricular contraction.[72] Furthermore, permanent or intermittent dysfunction of the atrial lead may result in VVI pacing with retrograde VA conduction.[62] In the presence of severe atrial disease, propagation of electrical activity from the right atrium to the left atrium can be markedly delayed and provide inadequate timing of left atrial and left ventricular contraction. In extreme cases, the left atrial systole begins after the onset of left ventricular systole,[73] and therefore contracts against the closed mitral valve. Dual atrial pacing with simultaneous stimulation in the right atria and the left atria (via the coronary sinus) may restore mechanical AV synchrony.[74] Another mechanism of pacemaker syndrome in DDD pacing occurs if the pacemaker resets from DDD mode to VVI mode (automatic mode conversion) as a response to noise interference or as a response to sinus tachycardia during exercise when the sinus rate increases above the programmed upper rate limit for automatic mode conversion.

Pacing and Abnormal Ventricular Activation

More than 25 years ago, Boerth and Covell[34] showed that right ventricular stimulation produced an abnormal contraction pattern, which depressed the function and efficiency of the left ventricle. Since then, a number of animal experimental studies have demonstrated the importance of a normal contraction pattern for preservation of optimal left ventricular function.[32,35,75] Clinical studies have confirmed the importance of a normal ventricular depolarization in optimizing left ventricular function. The cardiac pumping efficiency is higher with AAI pacing than with VVI pacing, whereas DDD pacing occupies an intermediate position, even when the atrial and the ventricular stimulation is properly synchronized.[33,36,76,77] Many studies have also demonstrated that cardiac output is greater during AAI pacing when the ventricles are activated through the normal ventricular conduction system than during VVI pacing[40,41,44] and during DDD pacing.[32,33,35,36,45–47,77] Thus, stimulation in the ventricles (VVI and DDD) always alters the physiological contraction of the ventricular myocardium and may potentially compromise cardiac function.

Programming a long AV interval in DDD pacemakers to promote spontaneous AV conduction so that the pacing mode becomes functionally equivalent to AAI mode has been proposed as a method to avoid ventricular stimulation.[36] On the other hand, an excessively long PR interval can restrict the programming of a sufficiently high upper rate limit and an appropriate atrial refractory period. Furthermore, DDD pacemakers programmed with a long AV interval do not prevent ventricular stimulation. Sgarbossa *et al.*[78] reported that programming the AV delay approximately 20% longer than the spontaneous PR interval still resulted in 80% ventricular stimulation, and it was concluded that 'since no clear advantage derives from programming a long AV interval, a "normal" AV delay is preferable; pts unlikely to develop AV block may benefit from pacing in AAI mode'.

Another alternative to avoid the detrimental effect of stimulation in the right ventricular apex would be to change the site of ventricular pacing to the His bundle.

Experimental and clinical studies with pacing in the proximal septum have so far revealed promising results.[75,79,80]

How Should Patients with SSS be Paced?

It is evident that the atrium should be sensed and paced (AAI or DDD) in patients with SSS to maintain AV synchrony and to reduce atrial fibrillation and thromboembolism. The presence of paroxysmal supraventricular tachyarrhythmias in SSS, previously considered a contraindication to AAI and DDD pacing as it was believed that progression to chronic atrial fibrillation was common, now constitutes an important indication for physiological pacing.[81] Thus, only in patients with chronic atrial fibrillation should VVI pacing be considered as a first-choice pacing modality. The crucial question is, therefore, whether patients with SSS and a normal AV conduction fare better with AAI than with DDD pacing. No prospective study has yet reported such results, but it is hoped that an ongoing randomized trial may answer the question in the future.[55] Obviously, for SSS patients with impairment of the AV conduction or with concomitant bundle branch block or bifascicular block, DDD pacing should be chosen.

If a DDD pacemaker is implanted, approximately 15–20% of SSS patients will be paced VVI after 2–4 years because of chronic atrial fibrillation.[82–86] In SSS patients where chronic atrial fibrillation develops, the risk of thromboembolism seems much higher if the patient is paced VVI than AAI. The explanation is probably that during atrial fibrillation with a VVI pacemaker, the apical ventricular stimulation changes the activation and the contraction of the ventricles which is followed by ventricular dilation, increased end-diastolic pressure, increased atrial pressure and subsequent atrial dilatation, which may further predispose to development of thrombus in the heart. Therefore, when chronic atrial fibrillation develops while ventricular function is simultaneously compromised because of apical ventricular stimulation, the ventricular pacing can further increase the risk of thromboembolism. By contrast, during atrial fibrillation with an AAI pacemaker, the ventricular myocardium is activated through the AV junction and the bundle branches. Thus a normal physiological ventricular contraction is preserved. In the event of development of permanent atrial fibrillation in a patient with SSS with AAI/DDD pacing, DC-conversion and antiarrhythmic drug therapy should be contemplated.

One argument for DDD pacing has been that in the 15–20% of patients who develop chronic atrial fibrillation there may be a need for bradycardia pacing. However, if the SSS disease progresses to chronic atrial fibrillation, the ventricular rate can be adequately controlled in nearly all patients by drugs modulating the AV conduction. Only very few SSS patients who develop chronic atrial fibrillation need bradycardia pacing.[10,22,58,87–89]

In the future, another technical solution may be available with modern DDD units; i.e. automatic mode switching from AAI to DDD if the ventricular rate drops significantly. Such a DDD pacemaker should be programmed to work as an AAI pacemaker with the ventricular channel continuously sensing the QRS activity but inactivated from stimulation until significant ventricular bradycardia appears (for example RR interval $\geqslant 3$ seconds). Then, automatic mode conversion from AAI to DDD should appear and DDD pacing should continue at a normal rate until spontaneous ventricular activity is sensed again through the ventricular channel which triggers reversion to AAI mode at the same rate (hysteresis in mode switching). Such a feature will allow normal ventricular contraction most of the time and nearly eliminate the inappropriate ventricular stimulation in patients with normal AV conduction.

Until then, AAI pacing, preserving both AV synchrony and a normal ventricular activation pattern, should be used when possible. In SSS patients already implanted with a DDD pacemaker, reprogramming to AAI mode must be considered.

Selection of Patients for AAI Pacing

Most patients with SSS are candidates for AAI pacing. Consequently, implantation of an AAI pacemaker should be considered in all patients with SSS unless there are contraindications (Table 5.4).

Preimplant evaluation of SSS patients must be based on careful clinical examination and review of the ECG and Holter recordings which may also be useful in determining the presence of atrial chronotropic incompetence. Alternatively, a preimplant stress test may be helpful. Approximately 40–60% of patients with SSS exhibit an inadequate increase in heart rate during exercise and are, therefore, candidates for rate-adaptive pacemakers.[58,90] At implantation, an atrial pacing test should be performed, and the final decision to implant an AAI or a DDD pacemaker is made based on the test. A preimplant invasive electrophysiological study can be helpful in a few selected cases, but in most cases it is not needed.[91]

Obviously, SSS patients with concomitant second- or third-degree AV block and patients with bundle branch block or bifascicular block should be treated with DDD pacing. A PQ interval between 0.22 and 0.26 seconds diagnosed on preimplant ECG or Holter recording does not exclude implantation of an AAI pacemaker. Andersen *et al.*[22] used different exclusion criteria for PQ intervals in patients aged under or over 70 years: those 70 or under were excluded from randomization if the PQ interval was >0.22 seconds and patients older than 70 were excluded if the PQ interval was >0.26 seconds.

Table 5.4 Contraindications for AAI(R) pacemaker implantation in SSS

First-, second- or third-degree AV block[a]
Chronic atrial fibrillation
Bundle branch block and bifascicular block
'Tachy-brady syndrome' with RR interval >3 seconds during atrial tachycardia
Atrial tachycardia with a ventricular rate <40 bpm for more than 1 min
Wenckebach point <100 bpm
Carotid sinus syndrome

[a] First degree AV block: Patients $\leqslant 70$ years; PQ > 0.22 s.
Patients >70 years; PQ > 0.26 s. (reference 22)

Assessment of the Wenckebach point by an atrial pacing test performed during implantation may be helpful in making the final decision as to which patients should be implanted with an AAI or DDD pacemaker. It has been suggested that a Wenckebach point above 120–130 bpm was predictive for a low risk of late AV conduction abnormalities, whereas those with a lower Wenckebach point would have a higher risk. Andersen et al.[22] used a Wenckebach point ⩾100 bpm as a selection criterion, and observed only a very low incidence of AV block during follow-up (0.6% per year). In their study, 11% of patients would have been excluded as candidates for AAI pacing if a Wenckebach point ⩾120 bpm had been applied as a selection criterion, whereas only 1% of patients were excluded because of a Wenckebach point <100 bpm. However, no prospective study has so far proved that the Wenckebach point has predictive value in assessing the risk for AV block.[56,92] Therefore, the value of an atrial pacing test can still be questioned. However, the atrial pacing test may be useful in disclosing a very long stimulus–Q interval at a low pacing rate (⩽100 bpm), which may be helpful in identifying patients at risk of pacemaker syndrome with AAI pacing, especially if rate-adaptive mode is applied.[71,93] In addition, the presence of carotid sinus syndrome constitutes a contraindication for AAI pacing.[81]

In patients with 'tachy-brady syndrome', the ventricular rate must not be too low during attacks of atrial tachycardia if an AAI pacemaker is to be implanted. Andersen et al.[22] excluded patients if the RR interval was >3 seconds and if the ventricular rate was <40 bpm for more than 1 min during atrial tachycardia. Patients with 'tachy-brady syndrome' were considered candidates for AAI pacing if atrial tachycardia was present for ⩽50% of the time before implantation.[22] The time before implantation was 'defined' as the preimplant period (days, weeks, months) where ECG or Holter documentation had been obtained. Mostly, the time period was only a few days and seldom longer than 1 week. Based on the excellent results obtained with AAI pacing in patients with 'tachy-brady syndrome' in the randomized trial,[22] we now implant atrial leads also in patients with atrial tachycardia >50% of the time.

References

1. Silverman LF, Mankin HT, McGoon DC. Surgical treatment of an inadequate sinus mechanism by implantation of a right atrial pacemaker electrode. *J Thorac Cardiovasc Surg* 1968; **55**: 264–70.
2. Smith NPD, Vasarhelyi L, McNamara W, Kakascik GE. A permanent transvenous atrial electrode catheter. *J Thorac Cardiovasc Surg* 1969; **58**: 773–82.
3. Parsonnet V, Bernstein AD. The 1989 world survey of cardiac pacing. *Pacing Clin Electrophysiol* 1991; **69**: 331–8.
4. Feruglio GA. Cardiac pacing in Europe in 1992: a new survey. In: Aubert AE, Ector H, Stroobandt R (eds), *Cardiac Pacing and Electrophysiology: A Bridge to the 21st Century.* AA Dordrecht, The Netherlands: Kluwer Academic, 1994: 157–68.
5. Lamas GA, Pashos CL, Normand SLT, McNeil B. Permanent pacemaker selection and subsequent survival in elderly Medicare pacemaker recipients. *Circulation* 1995; **91**: 1063–9.
6. Kusumoto FM, Goldschlager N. Cardiac pacing. *N Engl J Med* 1996; **334**: 89–98.
7. Sutton R, Bourgeois I. Cost benefit analysis of single and dual chamber pacing for sick sinus syndrome and atrioventricular block. *Eur Heart J* 1996; **17**: 574–82.

8. Shaw DB, Holman RR, Gowers JI. Survival in sinoatrial disorder (sick sinus syndrome). *Br Med J* 1980; **280**: 139–41.
9. Sutton R, Kenny RA. The natural history of sick sinus syndrome. *Pacing Clin Electrophysiol* 1986; **9**: 1110–14.
10. Santini M, Alexidou G, Ansalone G, Cacciatore G, Cine R, Turitto G. Relation of prognosis in sick sinus syndrome to age, conduction defects and modes of permanent cardiac pacing. *Am J Cardiol* 1990; **65**: 729–35.
11. Bianconi I, Boccadamo R, Di Florio A, *et al.* Atrial versus ventricular stimulation in sick sinus syndrome (abstract). *Pacing Clin Electrophysiol* 1989; **12**: 1236.
12. Markewitz A, Schad N, Hemmer W, Bernheim C, Ciavolella M, Weinhold C. What is the most appropriate stimulation mode in patients with sinus node dysfunction? *Pacing Clin Electrophysiol* 1986; **9**: 1115–20.
13. Feuer JM, Shandling AH, Messenger JC, Castellanet CD, Thomas LA. Influence of cardiac pacing mode on the long-term development of atrial fibrillation. *Am J Cardiol* 1989; **64**: 1376–9.
14. Sasaki Y, Shimotori M, Akahane K, *et al.* Long-term follow-up of patients with sick sinus syndrome: a comparison of clinical aspects among unpaced, ventricular inhibited paced, and physiologically paced groups. *Pacing Clin Electrophysiol* 1988; **11**: 1575–83.
15. Rosenqvist M, Brandt J, Schüller H. Long-term pacing in sinus node disease: effects of stimulation mode on cardiovascular morbidity and mortality. *Am Heart J* 1988; **116**: 16–22.
16. Zanini R. Facchinetti AI, Gallo G, *et al.* Survival rates after pacemaker implantation: a study of patients paced for sick sinus syndrome and atrioventricular block. *Pacing Clin Electrophysiol* 1989; **12**: 1065–9.
17. Stangl K, Seitz K, Wirtzfeld A, Alt E, Blömer H. Differences between atrial single chamber pacing (AAI) and ventricular single chamber pacing (VVI) with respect to prognosis and antiarrhythmic effect in patients with sick sinus syndrome. *Pacing Clin Electrophysiol* 1990; **13**: 2080–5.
18. Grimm W, Langenfeld H, Maisch B, Kochsiek K. Symptoms, cardiovascular profile and spontaneous ECG in paced patients: a five-year follow-up study. *Pacing Clin Electrophysiol* 1990; **13**: 2086–90.
19. Sasaki Y, Furihata A, Suyama K, *et al.* Comparison between ventricular inhibited pacing and physiologic pacing in sick sinus syndrome. *Am J Cardiol* 1991; **67**: 771–4.
20. Hesselson AB, Parsonnet V, Bernstein AD, Bonavita GJ. Deleterious effects of long-term single-chamber ventricular pacing in patients with sick sinus syndrome: the hidden benefits of dual-chamber pacing. *JACC* 1992; **19**: 1542–9.
21. Sgarbossa EB, Pinski SL, Maloney JD, *et al.* Chronic atrial fibrillation and stroke in paced patients with sick sinus syndrome: relevance of clinical characteristics and pacing modalities. *Circulation* 1993; **88**: 1045–53.
22. Andersen HR, Thuesen L, Bagger JP, Vesterlund T, Thomsen PEB. Prospective randomized trial of atrial versus ventricular pacing in sick-sinus syndrome. *Lancet* 1994; **344**: 1523–8.
23. Rasmussen K. Chronic sinus node disease: natural course and indications for pacing. *Eur Heart J* 1981; **2**: 455–60.
24. Santini M, Ansalone G, Auriti A. Sick sinus syndrome: natural history before and after pacing. *Eur J Cardiac Pacing Electrophysiol* 1993; **3**: 220–31.
25. Curzi GF, Mocchegiani R, Ciampani N, Pasetti L, Berrettini U, Purcaro A. Thromboembolism during VVI permanent pacing. In: Gomez FR (ed.), *Cardiac Pacing: Electrophysiology, Tachyarrhythmias.* Madrid: Editorial Grouz, 1985: 1203–6.
26. Sasaki Y, Takeuchi A, Shzeki M, *et al.* Long-term follow-up of paced patients with sick sinus syndrome. In: Steinbach K, Glogar D, Laszkovics A, Scheibelhofer W, Weber H (eds), *Proceedings of the Seventh World Symposium on Cardiac Pacing.* Darmstadt: Steinkopff Verlag, 1983, 85–90.
27. Sethi KK, Bajaj V, Mohan JC, Arora R, Khalilullah M. Comparison of atrial and VVI pacing modes in symptomatic sinus node dysfunction without associated tachyarrhythmias. *Ind Heart J* 1990; **42**: 143–7.
28. Nürnberg M, Frohner K, Podczeck A, Steinbach K, Boltzmann L. Is VVI pacing more

dangerous than AV-sequential pacing in patients with sick sinus node syndrome? (abstract). *Pacing Clin Electrophysiol* 1991; **14**: 674.

29. Lamas GA, Stambler B, Mittelman R, *et al.* Clinical events following DDDR versus VVIR pacing: results of a prospective trial (abstract). *Pacing Clin Electrophysiol* 1996; **19**: 619.

30. Atrial Fibrillation Investigators. Risk factor for stroke and efficacy of antithrombotic therapy in atrial fibrillation. *Arch Intern Med* 1994; **154**: 1449–57.

31. Amitzur G, Manor D, Pressman A, *et al.* Modulation of the arterial coronary blood flow by asynchronous activation with ventricular pacing. *Pacing Clin Electrophysiol* 1995; **18**: 697–710.

32. Askenazi J, Alexander JH, Koenigsberg DI, Belic N, Lesch M. Alteration of left ventricular performance by left bundle branch block simulated with atrioventricular sequential pacing. *Am J Cardiol* 1984; **53**: 99–104.

33. Bedotto JB, Grayburn PA, Black WH, *et al.* Alteration in left ventricular relaxation during atrioventricular pacing in humans. *JACC* 1990; **15**: 658–64.

34. Boerth RC, Covell JW. Mechanical performance and efficiency of the left ventricle during ventricular stimulation. *Am J Physiol* 1971; **221**: 1686–91.

35. Lee MA, Dae MW, Langberg JJ, *et al.* Effects of long-term right ventricular apical pacing on left ventricular perfusion, innervation, function and histology. *JACC* 1994; **24**: 225–32.

36. Rosenqvist M, Isaaz K, Botvinick EH, *et al.* Relative importance of activation sequence compared to atrioventricular synchrony in left ventricular function. *Am J Cardiol* 1991; **67**: 148–56.

37. Zile MR, Blaustein AS, Shimizu G, Gaasch WH. Right ventricular pacing reduces the rate of ventricular relaxation and filling. *JACC* 1987; **10**: 702–9.

38. Kubica J, Stolarczyk L, Krzyminska E, *et al.* Left atrial size and wall motion in patients with permanent ventricular and atrial pacing. *Pacing Clin Electrophysiol* 1990; **13**: 1737–41.

39. Goldreyer BN. Physiologic pacing: the role of AV synchrony. *Pacing Clin Electrophysiol* 1982; **5**: 613–15.

40. Sutton R, Perrins J, Citron P. Physiological cardiac pacing. *Pacing Clin Electrophysiol* 1980; **3**: 207–19.

41. Wirtzfeld A, Schmidt G, Himmler FC, Stangl K. Physiological pacing: present status and future developments. *Pacing Clin Electrophysiol* 1987; **10**: 41–57.

42. Wirtzfeld A, Himmler FC, Klein G, *et al.* Atrial pacing in patients with sick sinus syndrome: acute and long-term hemodynamic effects. In: Feruglio GA (ed.), *Cardiac Pacing: Electrophysiology and Pacemaker Technology*. Padova: Piccin Medical Books, 1982: 651–4.

43. El Gamal MIH, van Gelder LM. Preliminary experience with the Helifix electrode for transvenous atrial implantation. *Pacing Clin Electrophysiol* 1981; **4**: 100–5.

44. Rydén L, Kruse I. Haemodynamic aspects of physiologic pacing. In: Barold SS (ed.), *Modern Cardiac Pacing*. New York: Futura, 1985: 19–32.

45. Samet P, Castillo C, Bernstein WH. Hemodynamic consequences of sequential atrioventricular pacing: subjects with normal hearts. *Am J Cardiol* 1968; **21**: 207–12.

46. Samet P, Castillo C, Bernstein WH. Hemodynamic sequelae of atrial, ventricular and sequential atrio-ventricular pacing in cardiac patients. *Am Heart J* 1966; **72**: 725–9.

47. Shefer A, Rozenman Y, Ben-David Y, Flugelman MY, Gotsman MS, Lewis BS. Left ventricular function during physiological cardiac pacing: relation to rate, pacing mode, and underlying myocardial disease. *Pacing Clin Electrophysiol* 1987; **10**: 315–25.

48. Sgarbossa EB, Pinski SL, Trohman RG, Castle LW, Maloney JD. Single-chamber ventricular pacing is not associated with worsening heart failure in sick sinus syndrome. *Am J Cardiol* 1994; **73**: 693–7.

49. Simon AB, Janz N. Symptomatic bradyarrhythmias in the adult: natural history following ventricular pacemaker implantation. *Pacing Clin Electrophysiol* 1982; **5**: 372–83.

50. Sgarbossa EB, Pinski SL, Maloney JD. The role of pacing modality in determining long-term survival in the sick sinus syndrome. *Ann Intern Med* 1993; **119**: 359–65.

51. Zehender M, Büchner C, Meinertz T, Just H. Prevalence, circumstances, mechanisms, and risk stratification of sudden cardiac death in unipolar single chamber ventricular pacing. *Circulation* 1992; **85**: 596–605.

52. Tung RT, Shen WK, Hayes DL, *et al.* Long term survival after permanent pacemaker implantation for sick sinus syndrome. *Am J Cardiol* 1994; **344**: 1523–8.
53. Lamas GA, Estes NM, Schneller S, Flaker GC. Does dual chamber or atrial pacing prevent atrial fibrillation? The need for a randomized controlled trial. *Pacing Clin Electrophysiol* 1992; **15**: 1109–13.
54. Connolly SJ, Kerr C, Gent M, Yusuf S. Dual-chamber versus ventricular pacing: critical appraisal of current data. *Circulation* 1996; **94**: 578–83.
55. Andersen HR, Vesterlund T, Thuesen L, Bagger JP, Thomsen PEB. Atrial versus ventricular pacing (letter). *Lancet* 1995; **345**: 733–4.
56. Rosenqvist M, Obel IWP. Atrial pacing and the risk for AV block: is there a time for change in attitude? *Pacing Clin Electrophysiol* 1989; **12**: 97–101.
57. Brandt J. *Permanent Atrial Pacing: Clinical Studies.* Thesis, University of Lund, Sweden, 1991.
58. Brandt J, Anderson H, Fåhraeus T, Schüller H. Natural history of sinus node disease treated with atrial pacing in 213 patients: implications for selection of stimulation mode. *JACC* 1992; **20**: 633–9.
59. van Mechelen R, Segers A, Hagemeijer, *et al.* Serial electrophysiologic studies after single chamber atrial pacemaker implantation in patients with symptomatic sinus node dysfunction. *Eur Heart J* 1984; **6**: 628–36.
60. Mitsui T, Hori M, Suma K, Wanibuchi Y, Saigusa M. The 'pacemaking syndrome' (abstract). In: Jacobs JE (ed.), *Proceedings of the Eighth Annual International Conference on Medical and Biological Engineering.* Chicago: Association for the Advancement of Medical Instrumentation, 1969: 29/3.
61. Ausubel K, Furman S. The pacemaker syndrome. *Ann Intern Med* 1985; **103**: 420–9.
62. Schüller H, Brandt J. The pacemaker syndrome: old and new causes. *Clin Cardiol* 1991; **14**: 336–40.
63. Ellenbogen KA, Thames MD, Mohanty PK, Rogers R, Brands D. New insights into pacemaker syndrome gained from hemodynamic, humoral and vascular responses during ventriculo-atrial pacing. *Am J Cardiol* 1990; **65**: 53–9.
64. McCormick DJ, Shuck JW, Ansinelli RA. Intermittent pacemaker syndrome: revision of VVI pacemaker to a new cardiac pacing mode for tachy-brady syndrome. *Pacing Clin Electrophysiol* 1987; **10**: 372–7.
65. Heldman D, Mulvihill D, Nguyen H, *et al.* True incidence of pacemaker syndrome. *Pacing Clinical Electrophysiol* 1990; **13**: 1742–50.
66. Mitsuoka T, Kenny RA, Yeung TA, Chan SL, Perrins JE, Sutton R. Benefits of dual chamber pacing in sick sinus syndrome. *Br Heart J* 1988; **60**: 338–47.
67. Liebert HP, O'Donoghue S, Tullner WF, Platia EV. Pacemaker syndrome in activity-responsive VVI pacing. *Am J Cardiol* 1989; **64**: 124–6.
68. Klementowicz P, Ausubel K, Furman S. The dynamic nature of ventriculoatrial conduction. *Pacing Clin Electrophysiol* 1986; **9**: 1050–4.
69. Cazeau S, Daubert C, Mabo P, *et al.* Dynamic electrophysiology of ventriculoatrial conduction: implications for DDD and DDDR pacing. *Pacing Clin Electrophysiol* 1990; **13**: 1646–55.
70. Mabo P, Pouillot C, Kermarrec A. Lack of physiological adaptation of the atrioventricular interval to heart rate in patients chronically paced in the AAIR mode. *Pacing Clin Electrophysiology* 1991; **14**: 2133–42.
71. Linde C, Nordlander R, Rosenqvist M. Atrial rate adaptive pacing: what happens to AV conduction? *Pacing Clin Electrophysiol* 1994; **17**: 1581–9.
72. Torresani J, Ebagosti A, Allard-Latour G. Pacemaker syndrome with DDD pacing. *Pacing Clin Electrophysiol* 1984; **7**: 1148–51.
73. Wish M, Fletcher RD, Gottdiener JS, Cohen AI. Importance of left atrial timing in the programming of dual-chamber pacemakers. *Am J Cardiol* 1987; **60**: 566–71.
74. Daubert C, Ritter P, Mabo P, *et al.* AV delay optimization in DDD and DDDR pacing. In: Barold SS, Mugica J (eds), *New Perspectives in Cardiac Pacing.* Mount Kisco, NY: Futura, 1993: 259–87.

75. Karpawich PP, Justice CD, Chang CH, Gause CY, Kuhns LR. Septal ventricular pacing in the immature canine heart: a new perspective. *Am Heart J* 1991; **121**: 827–33.
76. Gallik DM, Guidry GW, Mahmarian JJ, Verani MS, Spencer WH. Comparison of ventricular function in atrial rate adaptive versus dual chamber rate adaptive pacing during exercise. *Pacing Clin Electrophysiol* 1994; **17**: 179–85.
77. Leclercq C, Gras D, Helloco AI, Nicol L, Mabo P, Daubert C. Hemodynamic importance of preserving the normal sequence of ventricular activation in permanent cardiac pacing. *Am Heart J* 1995; **129**: 1133–41.
78. Sgarbossa EB, Pinski SL, Wilkoff BL, *et al.* Is programming a long AV delay effective in permitting spontaneous ventricular activation? (abstract). *Pacing Clin Electrophysiol* 1993; **16**: 872.
79. Barin ES, Jones SM, Ward DE, Camm AJ, Nathan AW. The right ventricular outflow tract as an alternative permanent pacing site: long-term follow-up. *Pacing Clin Electrophysiol* 1991; **14**: 3–5.
80. Giudici MC, Thornburg GA, Buck DL, Alldredge SG. Permanent right ventricular outflow tract pacing improves cardiac output: comparison with apical lead placement (abstract). *JACC* 1993; **21** (suppl A): 382.
81. Clarke M, Sutton R, Ward D, *et al.* Recommendations for pacemaker prescription for symptomatic bradycardia: report of the working party of the British Pacing and Electrophysiology Group. *Br Heart J* 1991; **66**: 185–91.
82. Chamberlain-Webber R, Petersen MEV, Ingram A, Briers L, Sutton R. Reasons for reprogramming dual chamber pacemakers to VVI mode: a retrospective review using a computer database. *Pacing Clin Electrophysiol* 1994; **17**: 1730–6.
83. Gross JN, Moser S, Benedek ZM, Andrews C, Furman S. DDD pacing mode survival in patients with a dual-chamber pacemaker. *JACC* 1992; **19**: 1536–41.
84. Ibrahim B, Sanderson JE, Wright B, Palmer R. Dual chamber pacing: how many patients remain in DDD mode over the long term? *Br Heart J* 1995; **74**: 76–9.
85. Sgarbossa EB, Pinski SL, Castle LW, Trohman RG, Maloney JD. Incidence and predictors of loss of pacing in the atrium in patients with sick sinus syndrome. *Pacing Clin Electrophysiol* 1992; **15**: 2050–4.
86. Hummel J, Fazio G, Lawrence J, Midel M, Walford GD, Brinker JA. The natural history of dual chamber pacing. *Pacing Clin Electrophysiol* 1991; **14**: 1745–7.
87. Elshot SRE, Mamdouh IH, Gamal E, Tielen KHJ, van Gelder BM. Incidence of atrioventricular block and chronic atrial flutter/fibrillation after implantation of atrial pacemakers: follow-up of more than ten years. *Int J Cardiol* 1993; **38**: 303–8.
88. Kolettis TM, Miller HC, Boon NA. Atrial pacing: who do we pace and what do we expect? Experiences with 100 atrial pacemakers. *Pacing Clin Electrophysiol* 1990; **13**: 625–30.
89. Pollak A, Falk RH. Pacemaker therapy in patients with atrial fibrillation. *Am Heart J* 1993; **125**: 824–30.
90. Rosenqvist M, Arén C, Kristensson BE, Nordlander R, Schüller H. Atrial rate-responsive pacing in sinus node disease. *Eur Heart J* 1990; **11**: 537–42.
91. Simonsen E. *Sinus Node Dysfunction: A Prospective Clinical Study with Special Reference to the Diagnostic Value of Ambulatory Electrocardiography, Electrophysiologic Study and Exercise Testing.* Thesis, University of Odense, Denmark, 1987.
92. Haywood GA, Ward J, Ward DE, Camm AJ. Atrioventricular Wenckebach point and progression to atrioventricular block in sinoatrial disease. *Pacing Clin Electrophysiol* 1990; **13**: 2054–8.
93. Lau CP, Tai YT, Leung WH, Wong CK, Lee P, Chung FLW. Rate adaptive pacing in sick sinus syndrome: effects of pacing modes and intrinsic conduction on physiological responses, arrhythmias, symptomatology and quality of life. *Eur Heart J* 1994; **15**: 1445–55.

6

Stroke in Sinus Node Disease

M. Santini, G. Ansalone, A. Auriti and B. Magris

Atrial fibrillation (AF), which is common in patients with sinus node disease (SND), is an important and well-known risk factor for stroke. The incidence of stroke in SND varies in different series, according to the length of the follow-up, from 3% at 1 year[1] to 11% at 5 years[2]. In one series, this cerebrovascular event significantly worsened the prognosis, causing death in up to 15% of patients over a period of 5 years.[3] The main pathogenetic factor involved in these cerebrovascular accidents seems to be the thomboembolism that is fast bound to the atrial fibrillation. However, it should be recognized that, although atrial tachyarrhythmias occur in the major proportion of SND patients, only a minority of them experience cerebrovascular accidents during the clinical course. So, other clinical variables such as age, hypertension, diabetes, history of cerebrovascular disease and concomitant coronary artery or valvular heart disease could be involved. Moreover, it is well accepted that ventricular pacing (VVI) increases the incidence of chronic atrial fibrillation and stroke in SND,[4–11] but it should be also underlined that these complications are strongly determined by other clinical variables such as the presence before implantation of paroxysmal atrial fibrillation and by the pacing modality.[1] This chapter reviews the main physiopathological, clinical and therapeutic aspects of stroke in SND.

Epidemiology

Thromboembolism and Stroke in Unpaced Patients

In 1976, Fairfax et al.[12] demonstrated a higher thromboembolic risk in SND patients. This has been confirmed by others.[11,13–21] The risk of thromboembolism is higher in elderly people, in the presence of atrial tachyarrhythmias, and especially in those patients with both fast and slow components of atrial arrhythmia.[3] There are few published data concerning the incidence of embolic cerebrovascular accidents in unpaced patients because of the tendency to implant the pacemaker in an early stage of the disease. Moreover, the embolic stroke is usually included in all thromboembolic events. In a meta-analysis of five studies on 475 patients, the rate of all systemic embolic events approached about 15.2% in unpaced patients,[19] whereas the incidence of systemic embolism was significantly less (1.3%) in a group of 712 age-matched

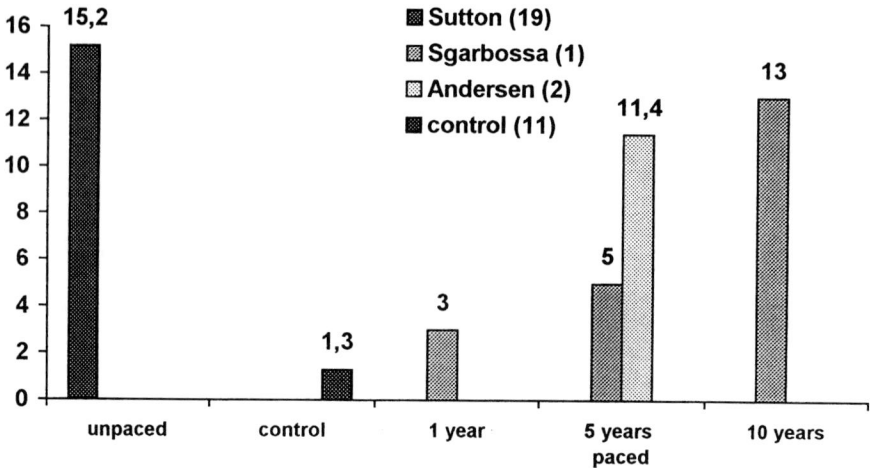

Figure 6.1 Percentages of thromboembolisms and strokes in unpaced and paced patients with SND in three studies.

controls[11] (Figure 6.1). The risk seems to be higher in women, in older patients (>60 years), in patients with left atrial enlargement[11,17] and in those with atrial tachy-arrhythmia before they are treated with pacing (20% before vs 7.1% after pacing, $p < 0.05$).[11,22] It seems higher in stable than in paroxysmal atrial fibrillation although many events can appear close to the onset or to the end of the arrhythmia episodes.[23,24]

Thromboembolism and Stroke in Paced Patients

Several studies have reported the annual incidence of stroke in SND paced patients ranging from 6% to 10%, while the incidence of stroke in patients with atrial fibrillation is about 2–4% and about 0.1% in the normal population.[3] Sgarbossa et al.[1] found an incidence of stroke of 6.3% in 507 paced patients over a follow-up of 65 ± 37 months, whereas in the same series the actuarial incidence of stroke was 3% at 1 year, 5% at 5 years and 13% at 10 years[1] (Figure 6.1). Considering a global incidence of stroke or peripheral arterial embolus, Andersen et al.[2] in a prospective randomized trial on 225 patients found an overall incidence of thromboembolic events of 11.4% over 5 years (Figure 6.1): 8.8% were in the ventricular group and 2.6% in the atrial group ($P = 0.0083$) (Figure 6.2). Other authors in a meta-analysis of retrospective studies reported a greater incidence of thromboembolic events in VVI (13%) than in AAI (1.6%) paced patients for SND ($p < 0.001$)[19] (Figure 6.2). This rate was also significantly higher than that observed in VVI-paced patients (1.3%) for atrioventricular block.[11] Thus, in patients with SND there is a basic tendency to embolisms that seems to be favoured by pacing modality *per se*. Indeed, in 507 patients referred by Sgarbossa et al.,[1] multivariate analysis showed that a history of cerebrovascular disease was the strongest predictor for stroke after pacemaker implantation

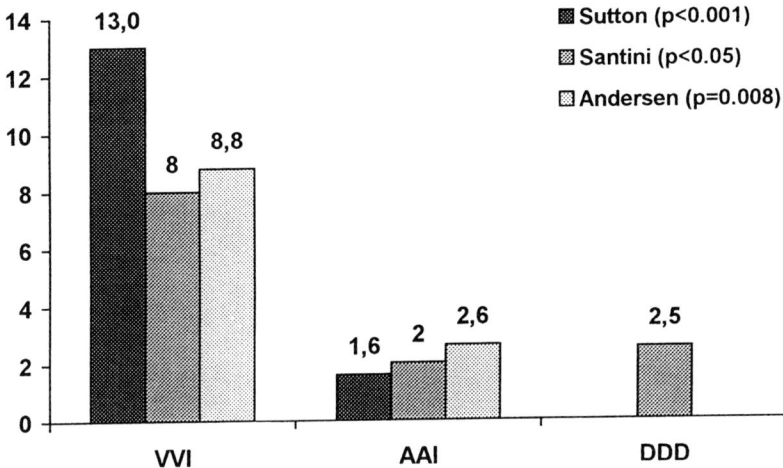

Figure 6.2 Percentages of thromboembolisms and strokes in patients with SND according to pacing modality.

($p < 0.001$) with a risk ratio of 5.22. Other independent predictors were ventricular pacing mode ($p = 0.008$) with a risk ratio of 2.61 and history of paroxysmal atrial fibrillation ($p < 0.037$) with a risk ratio of 2.81.[1] It is noteworthy that ventricular pacing mode remained an independent predictor for stroke even after adjusting for paroxysmal atrial fibrillation.[1] Otherwise, stroke was predicted by VVI pacing as an independent factor of atrial fibrillation development. Therefore, mechanisms other than atrial tachyarrhythmias could be involved in the VVI pacing mode with an embolic stroke link. Table 6.1 shows the results of the main studies on the incidence of embolism in patients with physiological compared with nonphysiological VVI pacing. The average incidence of embolic events was $1.3 \pm 1.2\%$ per year in 1033 patients followed-up for an average period of 38 ± 19 months.[5,19,25–28,32–35] Systemic embolisms and stroke strongly worsen the prognosis in patients with SND. Like others, we have found a higher mortality for embolism in patients with VVI pacing (8%) than in patients with AAI (2%) or DDD (2.5%) pacing[15] (Figure 6.2), with a high rate of fatal events (from 41% to 65%).[25,26,28–31] For this reason, it has been proposed by the majority of authors to establish oral anticoagulant therapy in VVI patients, considering the reduction of embolic events observed with this therapy compared with controls (8% *vs* 31%).[7]

Atrial Fibrillation and Thromboembolic Stroke

The incidence of stroke in patients free from SND and with isolated atrial fibrillation ranges from 1.8% or less to 8.8% per year. The risk of embolic stroke in permanent atrial fibrillation is up to eightfold when compared with normal sinus rhythm, and rises to 35% if one considers the whole lifespan.[36–41] Likewise, in patients with SND, a history of paroxysmal atrial fibrillation was an independent predictor of stroke

Table 6.1   Incidence of thromboembolic events and stroke in physiologically paced patients

Author	Patients	Pacing mode	Follow-up (months)	Events (%)
Ihara et al. (1979)[26]	25	AAI	13	0.0
Curzi et al. (1985)[25]	44	AAI	46	0.0
Sutton and Kenny (1986)[19]	321	AAI	30	1.6
Bianconi et al. (1989)[32]	153	AAI	44	2.3
Rosenqvist et al. (1988)[35]	40	AAIR	12	0.0
Bana et al. (1990)[33]	30	DDI	23	0.0
Santini et al. (1990)[5]	135	AAI	60	2.2
Kolettis et al. (1990)[34]	100	AAI	33	3.0
Kosakai et al. (1991)[27]	144	AAI/DDD	60	2.0
Sasaki et al. (1991)[28]	41	AAI/DDD	62	2.0
Totals	1033		38 ± 19	1.3 ± 1.2

together with history of cerebrovascular disease.[1] On this matter, it should be considered that multivariate analysis in such retrospective reports could be influenced by basal clinical characteristics of the selected population, so that in the Sgarbossa *et al.* series[1] a statistically significant higher prevalence of cerebrovascular disease in the VVI group could explain why atrial fibrillation was found to be an independent but weak predictor of stroke with an increased risk of about threefold. On the basis of the published data, it can be suggested that atrial fibrillation and a ventricular pacing mode are two independent risk factors for stroke, with the same statistical power but weaker than a history of previous cerebrovascular disease.

Pathophysiology

The main pathogenetic factors of stroke in SND are paroxysmal and chronic atrial fibrillation, systemic thromboembolism, peripheral artery and cerebrovascular disease and, in paced patients, ventricular pacing mode. The physiopathological mechanisms of transient ischaemic attacks related to haemodynamic changes during sinus bradycardia or supraventricular tachycardia are investigated below.

Atrial Fibrillation

Chronic atrial fibrillation marks the natural history of SND.[42–44] The loss of functioning pacemaker cells and the inability to maintain sinus rhythm causing the escape of subsidiary atrial pacemaker cells are the natural consequence of an age-related process of sinus node fibrosis.[45–48] Atrial re-entry may be favoured by concomitant ultrastructural and electrophysiological alterations of the atrial myocardial cells and is not strictly dependent on the associated bradycardia.[49] The fact of these alterations may mark the transition from 'paroxysmal' to 'chronic' atrial fibrillation, the latter reflecting a prevalence of sick atrial myocardial cells on the remaining healthy sinus cells. As this process develops, progressive loss of stability of automatic control of the atrium occurs, refractory periods of cells become scattered, conduction slows down, and atrial re-entry takes place. It has been suggested that a prior history of paroxysmal atrial fibrillation is the strongest independent predictor of postimplant chronic atrial fibrillation, with an increased risk of almost 17-fold.[1] Furthermore, other important risk factors for postimplant chronic atrial fibrillation are the preimplant characteristics of paroxysmal atrial fibrillation (number and duration of previous episodes),[1] VVI pacing mode,[1,2,5] the use of antiarrhythmic drugs before implant[1] and age.[1]

Systemic Thromboembolism

The association of systemic emboli with atrial fibrillation is well established, depending primarily on the formation of intracavitary thrombi in the left atrium and particularly in its left appendage. However, the exact mechanism for thrombi formation in the left atrial appendage during atrial fibrillation has not yet been defined. It is believed that attenuation of left atrial appendage contractile activity and stasis of blood flow within the appendage are important factors. Echocardiographic correlates of thromboembolic risk in atrial fibrillation are enlargement of the left atrium, mitigated by mitral regurgitation, and impairment of left ventricular systolic function,[18,50–52] which may promote stasis of blood within the left atrium in the presence of atrial fibrillation.[19,36,51] Transoesophageal echocardiography offers better visualization of the left atrium and its appendage than transthoracic echocardiography and identifies atrial thrombi and spontaneous echogenic contrast ('smoke effect'). They are probably indicative of stasis more often in patients with atrial fibrillation and thromboembolism than in those without.[51,53]

In a series of 80 patients with SND, after adjusting for age (> 65 years) and history of cerebral ischaemia, a multivariate analysis underlined the role of low atrial ejection force and spontaneous echo-contrast in the development of embolic episodes.[54] Many authors found that the appendage ejection fraction during atrial fibrillation was markedly lower than during sinus rhythm.[55,56] It was also observed that during atrial fibrillation the appendage seems to display only passive filling and emptying owing to mechanical compression by the adjacent left ventricle.[57] According to this hypothesis, in the presence of a high ventricular rate response due to atrial fibrillation, left atrial appendage emptying is markedly reduced because of the reduction of the diastolic volume of the left ventricle which is determined by the ventricular rate response. On the other hand, lower ventricular rate response prolongs ventricular diastolic filling duration and leads to greater distension of the left ventricular chamber. Consequently, because the cardiac chambers share the pericardial space, the increased left ventricular diastolic volume may cause a greater compression of the left atrial appendage during atrial systole. Thus, a higher ventricular rate response in atrial fibrillation may be an important predisposing factor for blood flow stasis and thrombus formation in the left atrial appendage.[57]

The increase in left atrial appendage emptying immediately after DC cardioversion to sinus rhythm is due to a change in the intrinsic emptying or in contractile capability of the appendage, but does not seem to depend on heart rate.[57] However, further studies are needed to define the influence of ventricular rate response control during atrial fibrillation on the incidence of left atrial appendage thrombus formation. It has been suggested that the incidence of embolic complications in patients with chronic atrial fibrillation is higher at the onset of the arrhythmia or shortly after conversion to sinus rhythm.[58,59] Selzer[60] hypothesized that transient intermittent bouts of atrial fibrillation could be a risk for systemic embolism. Nevertheless, the incidence of embolic complications in patients with paroxysmal atrial fibrillation appears to be lower than that reported for chronic arrhythmia. Therefore, the syndrome of 'brady-tachy' atrial arrhythmias could be a mechanism less important than sustained or chronic atrial fibrillation in the pathophysiology of thromboembolism.

Peripheral Artery and Cerebrovascular Disease

In patients with SND, it is likely that perhaps 15% (25% in AF) of strokes associated with atrial arrhythmias are due to intrinsic cerebrovascular diseases, other cardiac sources of embolism, or atheromatous pathology in the proximal aorta.[61,62] Approximately 25–30% (50% in AF) of elderly patients with SND have chronic hypertension (a major risk for cerebrovascular disease) and 5–10% of these harbour cervical carotid stenosis.[63] However, the frequency of carotid stenosis is not substantially greater in these patients with stroke, and carotid stenosis is a minor contributing factor to the increased stroke risk associated with atrial tachyarrhythmias.[63] Although atherosclerotic carotid lesions may contribute to stroke risk through a thromboembolic mechanism unrelated to the severity of luminal stenosis, this kind of pathogenetic event is relatively uncommon.

Sinus Bradycardia and Cerebral Ischaemia

It has been demonstrated[64] that a mechanism of cerebral ischaemia in bradycardic patients besides thromboembolism can be a reduction of global or regional cerebral flow. A cerebral ischaemia caused by thromboembolism is not a common event in bradycardic patients because bradycardia *per se* is not likely to cause thrombus formation in the atria, apart from in some rare cases of great atrial enlargement with inner slowed flow.

Conversely, cerebral ischaemia during marked bradycardia or sinus arrest can be ascribed to a reduction of cerebral flow in the presence of atherosclerotic narrowing of brain vessels. In this field much is still unknown about the role of such mechanisms in the genesis of symptoms in the elderly, usually attributed to the cerebral involution. Actually, it has been suggested that minor cerebral symptoms like lack of memory, somnolence, minimal speech troubles and dizziness, in the presence of sinus bradycardia, could be a consequence of a chronic reduction of cerebral flow and of an excessive rise of cerebral vessel resistance, more than just the result of atherosclerotic involutive brain disease. A sudden reduction of cardiac output caused by an atrioventricular block, an atrial standstill or a very severe bradycardia (<20 bpm) can cause the so-called Adam–Stokes syndrome with syncope and seizures resulting from the reduction of cerebral blood flow.

While the effects of an acute reduction of cerebral blood flow are quite well known, this is not the case for a chronic reduction of the flow as in the presence of marked stable sinus bradycardia.[64–68] The distinction between a physiological and a pathological bradycardia, as an expression of sinus node disease, is still controversial and often represents a practical problem. Bradycardia of marked degree is a common finding in trained healthy athletes and is usually considered almost a normal finding in elderly patients. Whether or not a severe bradycardia, even in the absence of any specific symptoms, has to be considered deleterious for the brain is still a debated topic. It is known that during a stable marked heart rate reduction the cerebral perfusion is maintained at a sufficient level by a regulatory mechanism of the cerebral circulation which increases the cerebral vascular resistance and the stroke volume.[67] This mechanism is sometimes not working adequately in elderly patients with atherosclerotic lesions of brain vessels and a reduction of cardiac performance especially under effort. Solti *et al.*[65] found, in 10 bradycardic patients compared with controls, a reduction of cerebral blood flow beside a rise of vessel resistance. After relief of the bradycardia by pacing, they observed in the same subjects a rise of cerebral blood flow, of brain oxygen uptake and a resetting of cerebral vascular resistance to the physiological level, together with complete regression of the related symptoms. In patients with chronotropic incompetence, especially when they are elderly, symptoms of cerebral hypoperfusion such as dizziness, fainting or syncope can appear only under effort. This is probably due to the association between the lack of heart rate increase and the fall in the muscular vessel resistance. Both factors lead to a reduction of cerebral blood flow and to a rise of brain vessel resistance. As a consequence, a further reduction of cerebral flow can ensue. In some other instances the impairment of cerebral flow can be limited to a restricted region of the brain and causes events like transient ischaemic attacks or stroke. This is particularly frequent in the vertebrobasilar region, which has fewer collateral vessels, when in the presence of critical narrowing of a main cerebral artery.[64,69,70] Further studies are needed to verify the real role of long-standing severe sinus bradycardia in the pathogenesis of minor neurological and psychiatric disturbances in the elderly.

Supraventricular Tachycardia and Cerebral Ischaemia

Like marked sinus bradycardia, supraventricular tachyarrhythmias (atrial or nodal re-entrant or focal supraventricular tachycardia) also can compromise cerebral flow, leading to a significant reduction of the stroke volume and of cardiac output, particularly in patients with SND with left ventricular dysfunction. In these patients, although the atrial mechanical activity is still working, the high rate can unmask systolic and/or diastolic ventricular failure, critically reducing the cerebral circulation. Similarly, a global reduction of the cerebral flow could induce a regional ischaemia because of atheromatous narrowing of some brain vessels. This selective reduction of regional flow could be another mechanism working in the genesis of transient ischaemic attacks, and the global reduction of cerebral output could be responsible for lipothimic or syncopal attacks.

Clinical Evaluation

Subgroups with High and Low Incidence of Strokes

The identification of subgroups of patients with relatively high or low incidence of strokes is important in establishing who gains the greatest benefit from long-term anticoagulation with warfarin, counterbalancing its risk, expense and inconvenience. Because the clinical classification of ischaemic strokes according to aetiologic subtypes is imperfect and not adequately validated,[61] risk stratification is presently based on combined analysis of all ischaemic strokes. In patients with SND, clinical variables of risk frequently overlap. Heart failure, hypertension and diabetes are more frequent in older patients. Chronic, and probably also intermittent, atrial fibrillation seems to correlate with an independent risk of thromboembolism, but it should be noted that stroke in patients with SND is also directly related to coexistent heart disease, hypertension, age and perhaps female sex. Whether the alternation of bradycardia and tachycardia in the 'brady-tachy syndrome' lies in the increasing risk of embolic events is not yet well established. On the other hand, it is likely that in patients with SND there is an intrinsic tendency to embolic events that could be explained by multiple pathogenetic factors.

Techniques to Aid the Diagnosis of a Cerebral Accident

Computed tomography and magnetic resonance

Animal studies have shown that the course of brain infarctions is over several hours, during which time the core lesion appears and enlarges to its final size.[71] Computed tomography (CT) can reveal changes related to the stroke symptoms just a few hours from onset. In one study on 36 patients with middle cerebral artery infarctions, 70% of CT scans performed within 4 hours of the stroke were positive.[72] With regard to the magnetic resonance (MR) technique, recent studies in animal models using contrast-enhanced and diffusion-weighted techniques demonstrated changes as early as 10 minutes after middle cerebral ligation.[73] The enhanced MR signals are due to the increased brain water as documented in histochemical studies.[74] One large recent study (based on early technology) compared patients with symptoms of cerebral ischaemia lasting more or less than 24 hours, studied with both CT and MR scan.[75] This did not find a difference in the diagnostic efficacy between the two methods at 24 hours analysis; the number of positive scans was high in patients with long-lasting or worsening symptoms, and was low for patients with brief symptomatology with both techniques. With reference to symptomatology, the difference was significant both for CT ($p < 0.01$) and for MR ($p < 0.01$). The conclusion was that there was not a notable difference between CT and MR scans in the early detection of ischaemic lesions, and by 24 hours the lesions were equally evident with both techniques.

However, other investigations have yielded different results. Bryan *et al.*[76] found that by 24 hours the sensitivity of CT was remarkably less (58%) than that of MR. Smaller lesions, particularly in the basal ganglia and in the posterior fossa, can be seen by MR and not by CT.[77] However, the use of contrast agents may shorten the time to imaging in both CT and MR.

Concerning transient ischaemic attacks (TIAs), Salgado *et al.*[78] found that 86% of patients displayed a positive MR scan versus 42% on CT, and Awad *et al.*[79] found focal changes in 17 (77%) using MR and only in 7 (32%) using CT. In a series of 62 patients[80] the type of lesions found on MR were as reported in Table 6.2 with an overall positivity of 81%. However, acute infarcts related to the TIA symptomatology were detected only in 19 of these patients (31%), old infarcts in 63% of patients with previous cerebrovascular attacks, and in 45% of previously asymptomatic individuals.[80] The lesion characteristics of the 19 TIA patients with acute infarction are listed in Table 6.3. Thus, TIA-related infarcts tend to be small and limited to the cortex and formed by multiple lesions. In conclusion, it seems that after 24 hours there is no evident difference between the two techniques, but MR seems more sensitive in the early detection of small and fading areas of ischaemia.

In order to distinguish CT features presumed to be due to a cardioembolic mechanism from those suspected to be due to an atherosclerotic narrowing of brain artery, and consequently an attempt to characterize CT patterns that could be more specific of SND, the result of a large study[81] will be reported. In a comparison between baseline CT patterns from two cohorts of patients with TIA and minor stroke having nonrheumatic AF ($n = 985$) and in sinus rhythm ($n = 2987$), patients with AF more often had multiple infarcts not related to the current symptomatology. Considering symptomatic infarcts, patients with AF more often had cortical end-zone infarcts and cortical border-zone infarcts. However, the CT characteristics of the two groups

Table 6.2 Magnetic resonance findings in 62 TIA patients

MR findings	Number of lesions	95% confidence interval
Acute infarcts	19	20–44
Old infarcts	14	13–44
Lacunes	27	31–57
White-matter hyperintensities	37	46–72
Punctate	22	24–49
Early confluent	9	7–26
Confluent	6	4–22
Any focal lesion	50	68–90

Source: Reference 80 (modified).

Table 6.3 Lesion characteristics in 19 TIA patients with acute infarction

Infarct characteristics	Number of lesions	95% confidence interval
Cortical	14	49–91
Cortical/subcortical	3	3–40
Subcortical	5	9–51
Size < 1.5 cm	13	44–87
Multiple	7	16–62
Contrast enhancement	5	14–68

Source: Reference 80 (modified).

overlapped at statistical analysis and did not allow a reliable distinction between cardioembolic and atherosclerotic causes of the stroke. The small deep infarcts (lacunae) were more often seen in sinus rhythm patients, confirming the current opinion that this feature is typical of atherosclerotic small vessel narrowing. On the other hand, it cannot be excluded that in a small percentage of lacunar infarct patients, AF can be the direct cause of the lesion.

Echocardiography

Stroke registries report that 22–39% of strokes are caused by emboli from various cardiac sources.[82,83] Concerning SND, paroxysmal atrial fibrillation (PAF) is the arrhythmia which is likely to cause cerebral embolism in nonpaced patients. On the other hand, unphysiological pacing *per se* can represent an adjunctive risk factor for embolism in patients with SND. The prevalence of PAF is difficult to assess because of its transient and often asymptomatic characteristics. In the Framingham Study, atrial fibrillation was classified as intermittent in 25% of those initially free from the arrhythmia who subsequently developed a documented AF.[84] In a study of 341 patients with intermittent AF,[85] the echocardiographic predictors of PAF recurrence were the mean left atrial dimensions and left ventricular function. On a multivariate analysis a left atrial diameter of 4.1–5 cm carried a 1.6-fold increased risk of recurrent AF than diameters $\leqslant 4.0$ cm, and a size >5 cm had a 4.5 times increased risk of recurrent AF than diameters $\leqslant 4.0$ cm. In addition, patients who developed constant AF had more heart failure and larger ventricular size. For each 1 cm increase in left ventricular systolic dimension there was a 1.8-fold increased risk of constant AF.

Left atrial spontaneous echo contrast ('smoke') and left atrial appendage thrombi are high-risk factors for subsequent thromboembolism,[86] and their formation is greatly favoured by AF. Transthoracic echocardiography (TTE) is not a sensitive tool for the detection of intrathoracic sources of embolism.[87] However, in one study[88] an abnormal TTE was a strong predictor of transoesophageal echocardiographic (TEE) findings of left atrial thrombus and spontaneous echo contrast ($p < 0.0001$) in patients with stroke. In contrast, in the same study TEE had a low yield (1% for the smoke effect, 0% for left atrial thrombi) in patients with normal TTE (no detection of septal defects, valvular abnormalities, ventricular enlargement etc.) and sinus rhythm, but 95% of patients with the smoke effect or left atrial thrombus had an abnormal TTE and/or atrial fibrillation. However, in general we share the opinion that TEE should be performed in cases of stroke of unknown origin.[89]

In patients with stable AF the prevalence of left atrial appendage thrombi is quite high, approaching 36%.[90] The pathophysiological mechanism of thrombi formation during AF is the absence of a regular flow pattern in the appendage[90] and/or left ventricular dysfunction leading to an increase in the inner atrial pressure and slower flow. The same mechanism operates during PAF, and thrombus formation then depends on the duration of the PAF, the frequency of recurrences together with the coagulability state. This can explain the finding of a higher prevalence of left atrial appendage thrombi in patients with stroke and a history of PAF.[88]

Recently, TEE has been used for guiding AF cardioversion without the need for prolonged oral anticoagulation. In a study[91] of 94 eligible consecutive patients with

AF of more than 2 days' duration, 12 had atrial thrombi visible on TEE and were given prolonged oral anticoagulation before cardioversion; 78 of the remainder were admitted to cardioversion under a heparin regimen and without a preceding prolonged oral anticoagulation, and with no subsequent embolic events and a safe outcome.[91] Oral anticoagulation, however, is strongly warranted after cardioversion owing to the risk of embolization due to *de novo* thrombi formation or the smoke effect.[91,92]

Holter monitoring

In SND, the alternating bradycardia and tachycardia has been considered a potential mechanism for cerebral hypoperfusion and consequent neurological symptoms.[64] However, the presence of paroxysmal atrial fibrillation alone can be considered a real risk factor for developing cerebral ischaemia.

In a general population the variability of the arrhythmia makes Holter monitoring of limited value in the diagnosis of paroxysmal atrial fibrillation.[92] On the other hand, the Holter technique has been shown also to have a low sensitivity for the detection of significant arrhythmias in patients with stroke.[94] The relationship between detected arrhythmias and the neurological symptomatology remains uncertain after this costly examination.[95] In one study,[96] atrial fibrillation was found in 12% of patients after a cerebral ischaemic event and was unsuspected before the exams in 5%; and in a second trial on 100 patients, Holter findings did not lead to a change in clinical management of patients with stroke.[97] However, because the incidence of atrial fibrillation is high in SND, when a sign of cerebral ischaemia ensues in this cohort of patients, Holter monitoring can yield useful information and be cost-efficient for the management of the patient, especially for the evaluation of antiarrhythmic therapy.

The relatively new application of Holter monitoring in studying variability of the RR interval opens new fields for the classification of patients. The finding of altered sympathovagal balancement before the arrhythmia ensues[98] could be extrapolated in patients without documented atrial fibrillation in the evaluation of the risk of arrhythmia. Prospective studies are necessary to evaluate the use of information about heart period variability in classifying patients regarding the risk of PAF.

Reducing the Incidence of Strokes in SND

Electrical Therapy

Before the era of pacing the treatment of AF, as a predisposing factor for stroke development, was a difficult task. All drugs worsened the bradycardic component of the syndrome. Many authors have now reported the benefits of associated anti-arrhythmic and electrical therapy.[5,10,14,42] In the early days of electrical therapy of SND, the ability of VVI pacing to relieve tachyarrhythmias was pointed out. In fact, VVI pacing has been shown to have a proarrhythmic effect in SND, especially in those having backward ventriculoatrial conduction, and to increase the risk of AF and thromboembolism.[69,99-101] Because the risk of developing atrioventricular block is less than 2% per year in patients with SND without bundle branch block and good preoperative atrioventricular conduction (Wenckebach point >120 bpm), atrial pacing is generally indicated in SND. Atrial pacing or dual-chamber pacing can have an intrinsic antiarrhythmic therapeutic efficacy. By raising heart rate at rest and during effort (rate-responsive pacing) these pacing modalities can provide an anti-arrhythmic effect by resynchronizing atrial cells.[19,102–104]

A randomized prospective trial comparing AAI with VVI packing was undertaken to assess the matter.[2] In 225 patients randomized to VVI pacing ($n = 115$) or AAI pacing ($n = 110$) and followed for 5 years, the frequency of atrial fibrillation was higher in the ventricular group than in the atrial group, although without significance at one or more visits (23% vs 14%, $p = 0.12$). As already reported above, the incidence of thromboembolism was significantly higher in the ventricular than in atrial groups (20 cases vs 6 cases, $p = 0.0083$); multivariate analysis identified randomization to ventricular pacing as the only variable significantly associated with an increased risk of a thromboembolic event during follow-up ($p = 0.039$). The left atrial dimensions increased in the VVI group to a larger extent than in the AAI group ($p = 0.0001$), predisposing to the development of AF probably because of the increase of the atrial pressure due to a disorganized ventricular function provoked by apical ventricular activation. A second randomized trial is ongoing to assess the efficacy of DDD pacing in reducing the incidence of AF in SND.[105]

Anticoagulation and Antiplatelet Therapy

Several trials[106–110] have compared the efficacy of long-term anticoagulation and/or antiplatelet therapy in stroke primary prevention in patients with nonvalvular AF (Table 6.4). They have mainly related to the chronic form of AF. The SPAF trial excluded patients with lone AF, randomizing them to aspirin or placebo because of the low risk for stroke ($<0.5\%$ per year). The AFASAK trial excluded patients with PAF. All the studies reported a relative risk for stroke <1 for patients receiving anticoagulation, with an overall reduction rate of events of about two-thirds. Moreover, the rate of complications was not adversely affected by oral anticoagulation,

Table 6.4 Trials for the prevention of stroke in atrial fibrillation

Comparison	Study	Dose[a]	No. of patients
Warfarin/controls	AFASAK	INR 2.8–4.2	825
Warfarin/controls	SPAF	INR ≈ 2.0–4.5	504
Warfarin/controls	CAFA	INR 2–3	479
Warfarin/controls [b]	BAATAF	INR ≈ 1.5–2.7	822
Warfarin/controls	SPINAF	INR ≈ 1.4–2.8	896
Aspirin/placebo	AFASAK	75 mg/d	826
Aspirin/placebo	SPAF	325 mg/d	1451
Warfarin/aspirin	AFASAK	INR 2.8–4.2/75 mg/d	825
Warfarin/indobufen	SIFA	INR 2–3.5/200 mg bid	916
Anticoagulants/aspirin	EAFT	INR 2.5–4.0/300 mg/d	1007

[a] INR = International Normalized Ratio.
[b] Primary prevention

being 1% per year for intracerebral bleeding. Aspirin given 325 mg/d in the SPAF trial yielded a relative risk for stroke of 0.56 and a risk reduction of 42%, whereas no benefit was reported in the AFASAK study which tested an older population at a dose of 75 mg/d and yielded a risk reduction of 16%. Combination of the data suggests a modest reduction of the relative risk (0.68, $p < 0.001$).[111,112] One-thousand and seven patients with nonrheumatic AF having had a TIA or a minor stroke were randomized to oral anticoagulant (INR 2.5–4.0) or aspirin (300 mg/d) or placebo in a large European trial (EAFT).[113] The efficacy of aspirin was low, with an annual incidence of vascular events of 15% (placebo 19%) and a risk ratio of 0.83; whereas anti-coagulants were more effective than aspirin, with a risk ratio of 0.60.

In summary, warfarin is the drug of choice (target INR 2–3) in patients with nonrheumatic chronic AF, except for younger patients (<65 years) without adjunctive risk factors for stroke (previous thromboembolism, hypertension, diabetes, impaired ventricular function, atrial enlargement) who do not strictly need oral anticoagula-tion.[112] In such patients, or in patients in whom anticoagulation is in some way contraindicated, aspirin given at 325 mg/d is a good alternative but the efficacy is poor in patients >75 years. Results from SPAF-III and a Dutch PATAF ongoing trial will help in a better identification of patients candidated to oral anticoagulation or aspirin for a risk reduction of stroke in nonrheumatic AF.

Concerning paroxysmal AF, one of the hallmarks of SND, stroke is less common than for patients with chronic AF (about 2% per year). Therefore anticoagulant therapy is not indicated for primary prevention, unless perhaps attacks are very frequent, and treatment with aspirin may be taken into consideration.

The preliminary results have been reported of an Italian trial (SIFA) comparing warfarin (INR 2–3.5) and indobufen (200 mg bid) in the prevention of stroke in 916 patients with nonvalvular AF and recent stroke or TIA.[114] The efficacy of indobufen has been comparable to that of warfarin. These results should be considered when choosing the drug for antithrombotic therapy. It is, however, important to emphasize that there is no study evaluating, in a prospective manner, anticoagulation therapy in patients with SND.

Summary

Stroke occurs in a limited number of patients with SND (6–10%) and rarely is a fatal event. It is mainly related to cardioembolism due to atrial fibrillation (either paroxysmal or chronic) in unpaced patients. In paced patients, the VVI pacing modality can itself represent an adjunctive risk factor for developing a thromboem-bolic stroke. Conversely, physiological pacing (AAI/DDD) can significantly reduce the rate of embolic events, probably preventing the occurrence of atrial fibrillation. Other risk factors for stroke in SND are previous cerebrovascular disease, hyper-tension, diabetes, age >65 years, associated coronary artery disease or other cardio-pathy. CT scan and MR imaging are equally useful techniques in the first 24 hours for the diagnosis of stroke, whereas TTE is useful for the detection of intracardiac thrombi or the smoke effect. Holter monitoring can be a useful tool for the assessment of a therapeutic strategy. Oral anticoagulation has been effective in reducing the rate of stroke in AF patients. In younger patients (<65 years), and in those without associated cardiopathy or other risk factors or having a contraindication to oral anticoagulation, antithrombotic therapy with aspirin or indobufen can be considered as an alternative.

References

1. Sgarbossa EB, Pinski SL, Maloney JD, Simmons TW, Wilkoff BL, Castle LW, Trohman RG. Chronic atrial fibrillation and stroke in paced patients with sick sinus syndrome: relevance of clinical characteristics and pacing modalities. *Circulation* 1993; **88**: 1045–53.
2. Andersen HR, Thuesen L, Bagger JP, Vesterlund T, Thomsen PE. Prospective randomised trial of atrial versus ventricular pacing in sick sinus syndrome. *Lancet* 1994; **344**(8936): 1523–8.
3. Mattioli AV, Rossi R, Annichiarico E, Mattioli G. Causes of death in patients with unipolar single chamber ventricular pacing: prevalence and circumstances in dependence on arrhythmias leading to pacemaker implantation. *PACE* 1995; **18**: 11–17.
4. Rosenqvist M, Brandt J, Schuller H. Long-term pacing in sinus node dysfunction: effects of stimulation mode on cardiovascular morbidity and mortality. *Am Heart J* 1988; **116**: 16–22.
5. Santini M, Alexidou G, Ansalone G, Cacciatore G, Cini R, Turitto G. Relation of prognosis in sick sinus syndrome to age, conduction defects and modes of permanent cardiac pacing. *Am J Cardiol* 1990; **65**: 729–35.
6. Hesselson AB, Parsonnet V, Bernstein AD, Bonavita G. Deleterious effects of long-term single-chamber ventricular pacing in patients with sick sinus syndrome: the hidden benefits of dual-chamber pacing. *JACC* 1992; **19**: 1542–9.
7. Sasaki Y, Shimotori M, Akahane K, Yonekura H, Hirano K, Endoh R, Koike S, Furuta S, Homma RT. Long-term follow-up of patients with sick sinus syndrome: a comparison of clinical aspects among unpaced, ventricular inhibited paced, and physiologically paced groups. *PACE* 1988; **11**: 1575–83.
8. Lagenfeld H, Grimm W, Maisch B, Kochsiek K. Atrial fibrillation and embolic complications in paced patients. *PACE* 1988; **11**: 1667–72.
9. Stone JM, Bhakta RD, Lutgen J. Dual chamber sequential pacing management of sinus node dysfunction: advantages over single chamber pacing. *Am Heart J* 1982; **104**: 1319–27.
10. Brandt J, Anderson H, Fahraeus T, Schuller H. Natural history of sinus node disease treated with atrial pacing in 213 patients: implications for selection of stimulation mode. *JACC* 1992; **20**: 633–9.
11. Stangl K, Seitz K, Wirtzfeld A, Alt E, Blomer H. Differences between atrial single chamber pacing (AAI) and ventricular single chamber pacing (VVI) with respect to prognosis and antiarrhythmic effect in patients with sick sinus syndrome. *PACE* 1990; **13**: 2080–5.
12. Fairfax AJ, Lambert CD, Leatham A. Systemic embolism in chronic sinoatrial disorder. *N Engl J Med* 1976; **295**: 190–2.
13. Eraut D, Shaw DB. Sinus bradycardia. *Br Heart J* 1971; **33**: 742–9.
14. Aroesty JM, Cohen SI, Morkin E. Bradycardia–tachycardia syndrome: results in twenty-eight patients treated by combined pharmacologic therapy and pacemaker implantation. *Chest* 1974; **66**: 257–63.
15. Kaul TK, Kumar EB, Thomson RM, Bain WH. Sino-atrial disorders, the sick sinus syndrome: experience with implanted cardiac pacemakers. *J Cardiovasc Surg* (Torino) 1978; **19**: 261–6.
16. Altamura G, Boccadamo R, Antonini L, Toscano S, Roncella A. Pistolese M. Treatment of the brady–tachy syndrome: comparative analysis between atrial and ventricular pacing. In: Feruglio GA (ed.), *Cardiac Pacing: Electrophysiology and Pacemaker Technology*. Padova: Piccin Medical Books, 1982; 511–14.
17. Santini M, Messina G, Porto MP. Sick sinus syndrome: single chamber packing. In: Gomez

FP (ed), *Cardiac Pacing: Electrophysiology, Tachyarrhythmias*. Madrid: Editorial Grouz, 1985; 144–52.

18. Koudstaal PJ, van Gijn J, Klootwijk APJ, van der Meche FGA, Kapelle LJ. Holter monitoring in patients with transient and focal ischemic attacks of the brain. *Stroke* 1986; 17: 192–5.

19. Sutton R, Kenny RA, The natural history of sick sinus syndrome. *PACE* 1986; 9: 1110–14.

20. Kopecky SL, Gersh BJ, McGoon MD, Whisnant JP, Holmes DR, Ilstrup DM, Frye RL. The natural history of lone atrial fibrillation: a population-based study over three decades. *N Engl J Med* 1987, 317: 669–74.

21. Cabin HS, Clubb KS, Hall C, Perlmutter RA, Feinstein AR. Risk for systemic embolization of atrial fibrillation without mitral stenosis. *Am J Cardiol* 1990; 65: 1112–16.

22. Bathen J, Sparr S, Rokseth R. Embolism in sinoatrial disease. *Acta Med Scand* 1978; 203: 7–11.

23. Petersen P, Godtfredsen J. Embolic complications in paroxysmal atrial fibrillation. *Stroke* 1986; 17: 622–6.

24. Wolf PA, Kannel WB, McGee DL, Meeks SL, Bharucha NE, McNamara PM. Duration of atrial fibrillation and imminence of stroke: the Framingham study. *Stroke* 1983; 14: 664–7.

25. Curzi GF, Moccheggiani R, Ciampani N, Pasetti L, Berrettini U, Purcaro A. Thromboembolism during VVI permanent pacing. In: Gomez FP (ed.), *Cardiac Pacing: Electrophysiology, Tachyarrhythmias*. Madrid: Editorial Grouz, 1985: 1203–6.

26. Ihara K, Sato S, Ogitani N, Minamino T, Morisaki H, Onishi K, Kosakai Y, Hirose H, Kitamura S, Mori T, Kawashima Y. Evaluation of atrial pacing therapy for sick sinus syndrome: a comparison with ventricular pacing therapy. In: Meere C (ed.), *Proceedings of the Sixth World Symposium on Cardiac Pacing*. Montreal: Pacesymp, 1979: 17-3.

27. Kosakai Y, Ohe T, Kamakura S, Aihara N, Kurita T, Takaki H, Isobe F, Shimomura K, Kawashima Y. Long-term follow-up of incidence of embolism in sick sinus syndrome after pacing (abstract). *PACE* 1991; 14: 680.

28. Sasaki Y, Furihata A, Suyama K, Furihata Y, Koike S, Kobayashi T, Shimotori M, Akahane K, Furuta S. Comparison between ventricular inhibited pacing and physiologic pacing in sick sinus syndrome. *Am J Cardiol* 1991; 67: 771–4.

29. Krishnaswami V, Geraci AR. Permanent pacing in disorders of sinus node function. *Am Heart J* 1975; 89: 579–85.

30. Simonsen E, Straede Nielsen J, Lyager Nielsen B. Sinus mode dysfunction in 128 patients. *Acta Med Scand* 1980; 208: 343–8.

31. Rosenqvist M, Vallin H, Edhag O. Clinical and electro-physiologic course of sinus node disease: five-year follow-up study. *Am Heart J* 1985; 109: 513–22.

32. Bianconi L, Boccadamo R, Di Florio A, Carpino A, Catalano F, Stella C, Pistolese M. Atrial versus ventricular stimulation in sick sinus syndrome: effects on morbidity and mortality (abstract). *PACE* 1989; 12: 1236.

33. Bana G, Locatelli V, Piatti L, Gerosa C, Knippel M. DDI pacing in the bradycardia–tachycardia syndrome. *PACE* 1990; 13: 264–70.

34. Kolettis TM, Miller HC, Boon NA. Atrial pacing: who do we pace and what do we expect? Experiences with 100 atrial pacemakers. *PACE* 1990; 13: 625–30.

35. Rosenqvist M, Aren C, Kristensson BE, Nordlander R, Schuller H. Atrial rate-responsive pacing in sinus node disease. *Eur Heart J* 1990; 11: 537–42.

36. Sherman DG, Dyken ML, Fisher M, Harrison MJG, Hart RG. Cerebral embolism. *Chest* 1986; 89: 82S–98S.

37. Brand FN, Abbott RD, Kannel WB, Wolf PA. Characteristics and prognosis of lone atrial fibrillation. 30-year follow-up in the Framingham study. *JAMA* 1985; 254: 3449–53.

38. Flegel KM, Shipley MJ, Rose G. Risk of stroke in non-rheumatic atrial fibrillation. *Lancet* 1987; 1: 526–9.

39. Halperin JL, Hart RG. Atrial fibrillation and stroke: new ideas, persisting dilemmas (editorial). *Stroke* 1988; 19: 937–41.

40. Hinton RC, Kistler JP, Fallon JT, Friedlich AL, Fisher CM. Influence of etiology of atrial fibrillation on incidence of systemic embolism. *Am J Cardiol* 1977; 40: 509–13.

41. Wolf PA, Dawber TR, Thomas Jr. HE, Kannel WB. Epidemiologic assessment of chronic atrial fibrillation and risk of stroke: the Framingham study. *Neurology* 1978; **28**: 973–7.
42. Rubenstein JJ, Schulmann CL, Yurchak PM, DeSantis R. Clinical spectrum of the sick sinus syndrome. *Circulation* 1972; **46**: 5–13.
43. Ferrer I. The sick sinus syndrome. *Circulation* 1973; **67**: 635–41.
44. Vera Z, Mason DT, Awan NA, Miller RR, Janzen D, Tonkon MJ, Vismara LA. Improvement of symptoms in patients with sick sinus syndrome by spontaneous development of stable atrial fibrillation. *Br Heart J* 1977; **39**: 160–5.
45. Davies MJ, Pomerance A. Pathology of atrial fibrillation in man. *Br Heart J* 1972; **34**: 520–5.
46. Thery C, Grosselin B, Lekieffre J, Warembourg H. Pathology of sinoatrial node: correlations with echocardiographic findings in 111 patients. *Am Heart J* 1977; **93**: 735–40.
47. Bharati S, Nordenberg A, Bauernfiend R, Varghese JP, Carvalho AG, Rosen K, Lev M. The anatomic substrate for the sick sinus syndrome in adolescence. *Am J Cardiol* 1980; **46**: 163–72.
48. Inoue S, Shinohara F, Niitani H, Gotoh K. A new method for the histological study of aging changes in the sinoatrial node. *Jpn Heart J* 1986; **27**: 653–60.
49. Luck JC, Engel TR. Dispersion of atrial refractoriness in patients with sinus node dysfunction. *Circulation* 1979; **60**: 404–12.
50. Smith NPD, Citron P, Keshishian JM, Garcia JM, Kelly LC. Permanent pervenous atrial sensing and pacing with a new J-shaped lead. *J Thorac Cardiovasc Surg* 1976; **72**: 565–70.
51. Hart RG, Halperin JL. Atrial fibrillation and stroke: revisiting the dilemmas. *Stroke* 1994; **25**: 1337–41.
52. Corbalàn R, Arriagada D, Braun S, Tapia J, Huete I, Kramer A, Chavez A. Risk fractors for systemic embolism in patients with paroxysmal atrial fibrillation. *Am Heart J* 1992; **124**: 149–53.
53. Feruglio GA, Rickards AF, Steinbach K, Feldman S, Parsonnet V. Cardiac pacing in the world: a survey of the state of the art in 1986. *PACE* 1987; **10**: 768–77.
54. Mattioli AV, Castellani ET, Paolillo C, Fusco A, Molinari R, Palladini G, Mattioli G. Stroke in pacemaker users for sinus node disease: relevance of atrial function and clinical characteristics. *Cardiologia* 1995; **40**(2): 123–8.
55. Pollick C, Taylor D. Assessment of left atrial appendage function by transesophageal echocardiography: implications for the development of thrombus. *Circulation* 1991; **84**: 223–31.
56. Garcia-Fernandez MA, Torrecilla EG, San Roman D. Left atrial appendage Doppler flow patterns: implications on thrombus formation. *Am Heart J* 1992; **124**: 955–61.
57. Kwame OA, Funai JT, Porter TR, Jesse RL, Mohanty PK. Left atrial appendage contractile function in atrial fibrillation: influence of heart rate and cardioversion to sinus rhythm. *Chest* 1995; **107**: 690–6.
58. Sherman DG, Goldman L, Whiting R, Jurgensen K, Kaste M, Easton D. Thromboembolism in patients with atrial fibrillation. *Arch Neurol* 1984; **41**: 708–10.
59. Moss AJ. Atrial fibrillation and cerebral embolism. *Arch Neurol* 1984; **41**: 707–14.
60. Selzer A. Atrial fibrillation revisited. *N Engl J Med* 1982; **306**: 1044–5.
61. Miller VT, Tothrock JF, Pearce LA, Feinberg WM, Hart RG, Anderson DC. Ischemic stroke in patients with atrial fibrillation: effect of aspirin according to stroke mechanism. *Neurology* 1993; **43**: 32–6.
62. Bogousslavsky J, Van Melle G, Regli F, Kappenberger L. Pathogenesis of anterior circulation stroke in patients with nonvalvular atrial fibrillation: the Lausanne Stroke Registry. *Neurology* 1990; **40**: 1046–50.
63. Kanter MC, Tegeler CH, Pearce LA, Weinberg J, Feinberg WM, Anderson DC, Gomez CR, Rothrock JF, Helgason CM, Hart RG, on behalf of the SPAF Investigators. Carotid stenosis in patients with atrial fibrillation: prevalence, risk factors and relationship to stroke. *Arch Intern Med* 1994; **154**: 1372–7.
64. Di Pasquale G, Ruffini M, Andreoli A, Limoni P, Urbinati S, Pinelli G. Bradicardia sinusale persistente: quali effetti sulla funzione cerebrale? Aritmie Cardiache, International Workshop, Venice 24–26 Oct. 1991: 187–95.

65. Solti F, Iskum M, Varadi A. The regulation of the cerebral circulation in long-lasting bradycardia. *Acta Physiol Hung* 1987; **69**(1): 15–19.
66. Wilcox BR, Coulter NA, Rackley ChE, Croom RD. The effect of changing heart rate on blood flow: power dissipation and resistance in the control carotid artery of man. *Ann Surg* 1970; **171**: 24–80.
67. Sulg IA, Cronqvist S, Schuller H, Ingvar DH. The effect of intracardial pacemaker therapy on cerebral blood flow and electroencephalogram in patients with complete atrioventricular block. *Circulation* 1969; **39**: 487–94.
68. Agruss NS, Rosin EY, Adolph RJ, Fowler NO. Significance of chronic sinus bradycardia in elderly people. *Circulation* 1972; **46**: 924–30.
69. Kendall RE, Marshall J. Role of hypotension in the genesis of transient focal cerebral ischemic attacks. *Br Med J* 1963; **2**: 344–8.
70. Denny-Brown D, Meyer JS. The cerebral collateral circulation. *Neurology* 1957; **7**: 657–62.
71. Garcia JH, Yoshida Y, Chen H, Li Y, Zhang ZG, Lian J, Chen S, Chopp M. Progression from ischemic injury to infarct following middle cerebral artery occlusion in the rat. *Am J Pathol* 1993; **142**: 623–5.
72. Bozzao L, Bastianello S, Fantozzi LM, Angeloni U, Argentino C, Fieschi C. Correlation of angiographic and sequential CT findings in patients with evolving cerebral infarction. *Am J Neuroradiol* 1989; **10**: 1215–22.
73. Kucharczyk J, Mintorovitch J, Asgary HS, Moseley M. Diffusion/perfusion MR imaging of acute cerebral ischemia. *Magn Reson Med* 1991; **19**: 311–15.
74. De La Paz RL, Shibata D, Steinberg GK, Zarnegar R, George C. Acute cerebral ischemia in rabbits: correlation between MR and histopathology. *Am J Neuroradiol* 1991; **12**: 89–95.
75. Mohr JP, Biller J, Hilal SK, Yuh WTC, Tatemichi TK, Hedges S, Tali E, Nguyen H, Mun I, Adams HP, Grimsman K, Marler JR. Magnetic resonance versus computed tomographic imaging in acute stroke. *Stroke* 1995; **26**: 807–12.
76. Bryan RN, Levy LM, Whitlow WD, Killian JM, Preziosi TJ, Rosario JA. Diagnosis of acute cerebral infarction: comparison of CT and MR imaging. *Am J Neuroradiol* 1991, **12**: 611–20.
77. Biller J, Sand JJ, Corbett JJ. Syndrome of the paramedian thalamic arteries: clinical and neuroimaging correlation. *J Clin Neuroophthalmol* 1985; **5**: 217–23.
78. Salgado ED, Weinstein M, Furlan AJ. Proton magnetic resonance imaging in ischemic cerebrovascular disease. *Ann Neurol* 1986; **20**: 502–7.
79. Awad IA, Modic M, Little JR, Furlan AJ, Weinstein M. Focal parenchymal lesions in transient ischemic attacks: correlation of computed tomography and magnetic resonance imaging. *Stroke* 1986; **17**: 399–403.
80. Fazekas F, Fazekas G, Schmidt R, Kapeller P, Offenbacher H. Magnetic resonance imaging correlates of transient cerebral ischemic attacks. *Stroke* 1996; **27**: 607–11.
81. Van Latum JC, Kodstaal PJ, Kappelle LJ, Van Kooten F, Algra A, van Gijn J, for the European Atrial Fibrillation Trial and Dutch TIA Trial Study Groups. Comparison of CT in patients with cerebral ischaemia with or without non-rheumatic atrial fibrillation. *J Neurol Neurosurg Psychiat* 1995; **59**: 132–7.
82. Olsen TS, Skriver EB, Herning M. Cause of cerebral infarction in the carotid territory: its relation to the size and the location of the infarct and the underlying vascular lesion. *Stroke* 1985; **16**: 459–66.
83. Bogousslavsky J, Melle GV, Regli F. The Lausanne Stroke Study: analysis of 1000 consecutive patients with first stroke. *Stroke* 1988; **19**: 1083–92.
84. Kannel WB, Abbott RD, Savage DD, McNamara PM. Coronary artery disease and atrial fibrillation: the Framingham Study. *Am Heart J* 1983; **106**: 389–96.
85. Flaker GC, Fletcher KA, Rothbart RM, Halperin JL, Hart RG, for the Stroke Prevention in Atrial Fibrillation (SPAF) Investigators. Clinical and echocardiographic features of intermittent atrial fibrillation that predict recurrent atrial fibrillation. *Am J Cardiol* 1995; **76**: 355–8.
86. Leung DY, Black IW, Cranney GB, Hopkins AP, Walsh WF. Prognostic implications of

left atrial spontaneous echo contrast in nonvalvular atrial fibrillation. *JACC* 1994; **24**: 755–62.

87. Sansoy V, Abbott RD, Jayaweera AR, Kaul S. Low yield of transthoracic echocardiography for cardiac source of embolism. *Am J Cardiol* **75**: 166–9.
88. Leung DY, Black IW, Cranney GB, Walsh WF, Grimm RA, Stewart WJ, Thomas JD. Selection of patients for transesophageal echocardiography after stroke and systemic embolic events: role of transthoracic echocardiography. *Stroke* 1995; **26**: 1820–4.
89. Rauh G, Fischereder M, Spengel FA. Transesophageal echocardiography in patients with focal cerebral ischemia of unknown cause. *Stroke* 1996; **27**: 691–4.
90. Santiago D, Warshofsky M, Mandri G, Di Tullio M, Coromilas J, Reiffel J, Homma S. Left atrial appendage function and thrombus formation in atrial fibrillation-flutter: a transesophageal echocardiographic study. *JACC* 1994; **24**: 159–64.
91. Manning WJ, Silverman DI, Gordon SPF, Krumholz HM, Douglas PS. Cardioversion from atrial fibrillation without a prolonged anticoagulation with use of transesophageal echocardiography to exclude the presence of atrial thrombi. *N Engl J Med* 1993; **328**: 750–5.
92. Black IW, Fatkin D, Sagar KB, *et al.* Exclusion of atrial thrombus by transesophageal echocardiography does not preclude embolism after cardioversion of atrial fibrillation: a multicenter study. *Circulation* 1994; **89**: 2509–13.
93. Di Marco JP, Philbrick JT. Use of ambulatory electrocardiographic (Holter) monitoring. *Ann Intern Med* 1990; **113**: 53–68.
94. Kessler DK, Kessler KM, Myerburg RJ. Ambulatory electrocardiography: a cost per management decision analysis. *Arch Intern Med* 1995; **155**: 165–9.
95. Clark PI, Glasser SP, Spoto E. Arrhythmias detected by ambulatory monitoring. *Chest* 1980; **77**: 722–5.
96. Richardt G, Ensle G, Swarz F. Diagnostik kardialer ursachen zerebraler embolien: beitrag von 2D-echokardiographie und lagzeit-EKG. *Z Kardiol* 1989; **78**: 598–601.
97. Kessler DK, Kessler KM. Is ambulatory electrocardiography useful in the evaluation of patients with recent stroke? *Chest* 1995; **107**: 916–18.
98. Coumel P. Paroxysmal atrial fibrillation: a disorder of autonomic tone? *Eur Heart J* 1994; **15** (suppl A): 9–16.
99. Camm AJ, Katritsis D. Ventricular pacing for sick sinus syndrome: a risky business? *PACE* 1990; **13**: 695–9.
100. Zanni R, Facchinetti AI, Gallo G, Cazzamalli L, Bonandi L, Cas LD. Morbidity and mortality of patients with sinus node disease: comparative effects of atrial and ventricular pacing. *PACE* 1990; **13**: 2076–9.
101. Santini M, Ansalone G, Auriti A. Sick sinus syndrome: natural history before and after pacing. *Eur J CPE* 1993; **3**: 220–31.
102. Gilette PC, Wampler DG, Shannon C, Ott D. Use of atrial pacing in a young population. *PACE* 1985; **8**: 94–100.
103. Pouillot C, Daubert C, Mabo P, Paillard F, Kermarrec A, Le Breton H. Is AAIR pacing the gold standard to treat sinus node disease with atrial chronotropic incompetence? (abstract). *PACE* 1991; **14**: 690.
104. Hayes DL, Neubauer SA. Incidence of atrial fibrillation after DDD pacing (abstract). *PACE* 1990; **13**: 501.
105. Lamas GA, Estes NM, Schneller S, Flaker GC. Does dual chamber or atrial pacing prevent atrial fibrillation? The need for a randomised controlled trial. *PACE* 1992; **15**: 1109–13.
106. Stroke Prevention in Atrial Fibrillation Investigators. Stroke prevention in atrial fibrillation study: final results. *Circulation* 1991; **84**: 527–39.
107. Petersen P, Boysen G, Gotdfredsen J, Anderson ED, Andersen B. Placebo-controlled, randomised trial of warfarin and aspirin for prevention of thromboembolic complication in chronic atrial fibrillation: the Copenhagen AFASAK study. *Lancet* 1989; **1**: 175–9.
108. Connolly SJ, Laupacis A, Gent M, Roberts RS, Cairns JA, Joyner C. Canadian Atrial Fibrillation Anticoagulation (CAFA) Study. *JACC* 1991; **18**: 394–55.
109. The Boston Area Anticoagulation Trial for Atrial Fibrillation Investigators. The effect of

low-dose warfarin on the risk of stroke in patients with nonrheumatic atrial fibrillation. *N Engl J Med* 1990; **323**: 1505–11.

110. Ezekovitz MD, Bridgers SL, James KE, Carliner NH, Colling CL, Gornick CC: Veterans Affairs Stroke Prevention in Nonrheumatic Atrial Fibrillation Investigators. Warfarin in the prevention of stroke associated with nonrheumatic atrial fibrillation. *N Engl J Med* 1992; **327**: 1406–12.

111. Matchar DB, McCrory DC, Barnett HJM, Feussner JR. Medical treatment for stroke prevention. *Ann Intern Med* 1994; **121**: 41–53.

112. Prystowsky EN, Benson W, Fuster W, Hart R, Kay N, Myerburg RJ, Baccarelli GV, Wyse G. Management of patients with atrial fibrillation: a statement for healthcare professionals from the subcommittee on electrocardiography and electrophysiology, American Heart Association. *Circulation* 1996; **93**: 1262–77.

113. EAFT Study Group: European Atrial Fibrillation Trial. Secondary prevention in nonrheumatic atrial fibrillation after transient ischemic attack or minor stroke. *Lancet* 1993; **342**: 1255–62.

114. Cataldo G, on behalf of the SIFA Study Group. Warfarin vs indobufen for secondary prevention of thromboembolism in non-valvular atrial fibrillation: the SIFA (Studio Italiano Fibrillazione Atriale) Trial. *Circulation* 1995; **92**: I-485.

7

Pacing in Carotid Sinus Syndrome

R. Sutton

Carotid sinus syndrome is a syncopal disease of older people which is of unknown aetiology. The syndrome has been recognized for over 60 years,[1,2] but it was not devoted great attention at the outset because it was considered to be rare. It has, more recently, been subjected to an increased level of interest since an effective method of therapy was introduced.[3] Pacing was first employed by means of a single-chamber VVI system[4] in 1970 with some success; this was more easily and less traumatically applied than the earlier methods of surgical[5,6] or radiotherapeutic[7,8] denervation of the carotid sinus. The work of the Westminster Hospital group[3] demonstrated that dual-chamber pacing in the DVI mode was more effective than single-chamber VVI. This prompted many centres to study the syndrome in relation to its aetiology, clinical presentation, natural history as well as therapy. Much has been learnt but its cause still remains obscure.

Diagnosis

Carotid sinus syndrome is diagnosed by performance of carotid sinus massage, preferably today, on a tilt table in the erect position with the patient supported by straps for protection in the event of syncope. The carotid artery is palpated just above the thyroid cartilage and in front of the sterno-cleido-mastoid muscle, the site of the carotid sinus (Figure 7.1). Massage is strongly recommended to be massage rather than aggressive occlusion of the vessel, and this is best done by the ball of the thumb. Massage is a sustained to and fro rubbing movement, over a limited distance of about 2 cm, exerting moderate pressure which is maintained for 5–10 seconds,[9,10] sufficient time to cover a full respiratory cycle with its intrinsic autonomic changes. At the same time it is wise to monitor the ipsilateral temporal artery with the other hand to be certain that the massage is not occluding the artery. The right carotid sinus is usually massaged first; the two arteries must not be massaged simultaneously for fear of prejudicing the cerebral circulation. After a brief interval of perhaps 30 seconds the left artery is massaged. Positive results tend to occur on only one side. During the massage the electrocardiogram is monitored and, preferably, the arterial pressure is also monitored by means of digital plethysmography (Finapres system); intermittent cuff arterial pressures are not adequate for the appreciation of the rapid changes

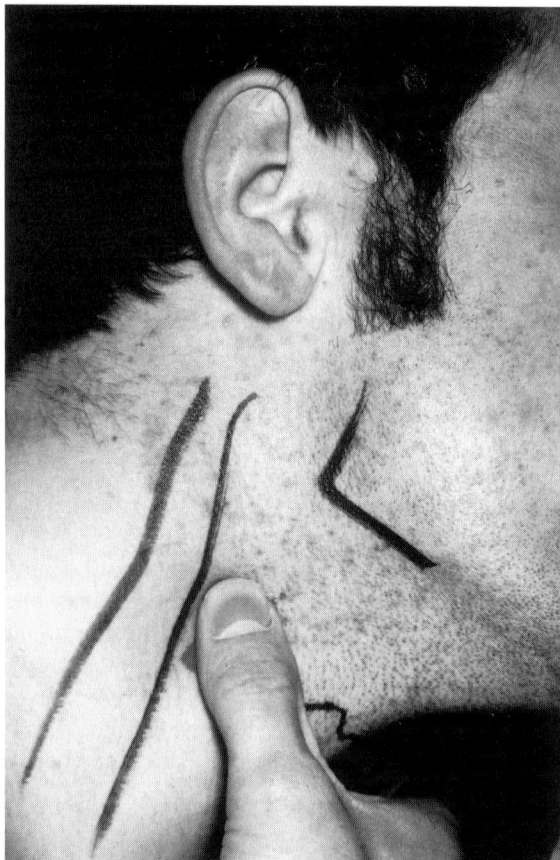

Figure 7.1 The right side of the neck with the anterior border of the sterno-cleido-mastoid muscle and the angle of the mandible clearly outlined. The site of the carotid sinus is exactly where massage is being performed.

which take place in a positive test. Digital plethysmography has been shown to reflect, very closely, changes in arterial pressure but not to give great accuracy in absolute terms.[11]

A positive result is induction of syncope which, in the patient's estimation, reproduces the symptoms experienced. Electrocardiographically this is asystole for a period of at least 3 seconds. There will, of course, be hypotension which can be expected to persist for as much as 20 seconds (Figure 7.2).[12,13] The reason to perform the test in the upright posture is that 3–4 seconds asystole can be asymptomatic in the supine position and it is now considered most important to reproduce the patient's symptoms for a definitive diagnosis. Thus, the diagnosis of carotid sinus syndrome is reproduction of symptoms by means of carotid sinus massage in a syncopal patient in whom there is considered to be no other cause of syncope after extensive investigation.

Carotid sinus massage may result in more than 3 seconds asystole in subjects who

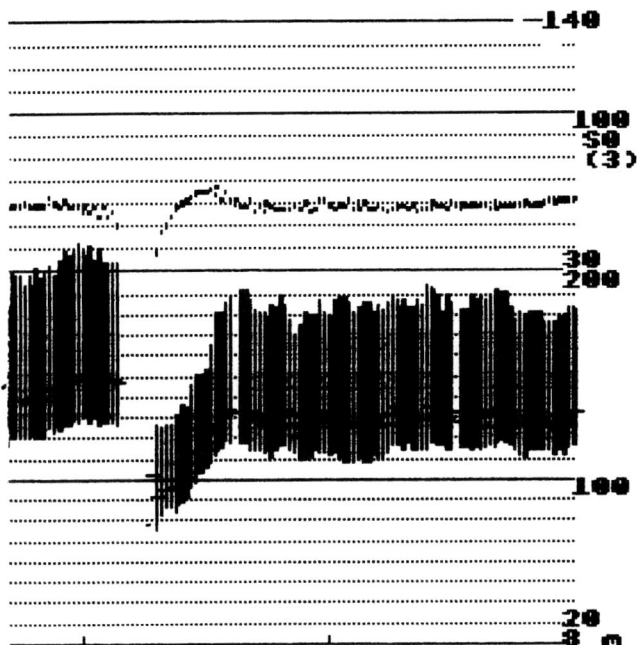

Figure 7.2 Carotid sinus massage. The upper panel depicts heart rate (30–140 bpm) and the lower panel blood pressure by digital plethysmography (20–200 mmHg). Massage (duration 6 s) of the right carotid commenced immediately after the first time bar on the lower line of the recording (time bars at 60 s intervals). The heart rate falls precipitously to be followed by 8.5 s asystole. Blood pressure recovers more slowly than heart rate after massage has ceased.

have not experienced syncope. This is described as a hypersensitive carotid sinus reflex, which must be distinguished from carotid sinus syndrome as it may carry a benign prognosis. Hyperreflexia was thought to be common[14] and associated with the ageing process, but more recent studies have denied this.[15] When a positive response has been found in an unselected population there proved to be a high incidence of unreported syncope amongst responders.[16]

It is important to be aware that carotid sinus massage is a test not without morbidity or mortality. Both cerebrovascular accidents and serious ventricular arrhythmias have been reported.[17] The former occurs presumably by dislodgement of plaque material during the act of massage: this has an incidence of 0.14% in 5000 massages.[18] Its evolution is typically that of cerebral embolism, usually with no permanent sequelae. Arrhythmias have occurred as escape tachyarrhythmias due to the bradycardia engendered by the massage. Complications can be minimized by withholding massage from patients who have carotid bruits. However, this policy is not entirely logical as it is well known that carotid bruits do not offer a good index of degree of carotid artery disease, and in the series of Dehn *et al.*[19] extensive carotid disease was seen in patients without bruits and in whom multiple massages were safely performed. With respect to arrhythmias it is essential to have full resuscitation equipment available when massage is undertaken.

Carotid sinus massage is essentially a very crude and entirely uncontrolled diagnostic tool. Attempts have been made to standardize it by use of a neck chamber to apply known negative pressures to achieve reproducible amounts of distortion of the carotid sinus that mimic digital pressure during clinical massage.[19] These methods have not been widely adopted because they compare unfavourably with the ease of carotid sinus massage.

It is possible for the diagnostic criteria for carotid sinus syndrome to coexist with those of vasovagal syndrome where a tilt test is positive with syncope and, in the patient's estimation, symptoms are reproduced. The final diagnosis will be made on clinical grounds: younger patients who have some warning of impending syncope will be likely to be termed vasovagal; in contrast, older patients without a significant prodrome will be pronounced to have carotid sinus syndrome. This picture of overlap of the neurally mediated syncopes has been further blurred by the findings of Brignole et al.[20] who demonstrated that the syncope of sinoatrial node disease is also largely neurally mediated. In these cases separation is easier as it is essential to have evidence of sinoatrial node dysfunction in terms of sinoatrial block, sinus arrest, intense sinus bradycardia or escape atrial tachyarrhythmias to make this diagnosis.

New information on the diagnosis of carotid sinus syndrome has been reported by Dey et al.[21] Patients presenting with falls which are unexplained are often carotid sinus syncopal events with amnesia for the syncope. Syncope for which there is amnesia has recently been witnessed during both carotid sinus massage (R. A. Kenny, personal communication) and during tilt testing (R. Sutton and M. E. V. Petersen, personal observations). Right carotid sinus massage is more often positive than massage on the left. The effects are also different, with right massage tending to cause sinus arrest and left causing atrioventricular block. This is explained by a degree of lateralization of the reflex; the right side influencing the sinoatrial node, probably by imposing exit block rather than suppression of impulse formation,[22] and the left having its effect on atrioventricular conduction at the atrioventricular node.

The reproducibility of carotid sinus massage is somewhat controversial, but there is, at least, some agreement on the long-term reproducibility which has been found to be good in two studies.[23,24] There are circumstances in which carotid sinus massage may give misleading results. The most notable of these is in the first 6 months after myocardial infarction,[25] where baroreceptor function is known to be altered. Furthermore, it is important, as implied above, to distinguish between carotid sinus syndrome as it has been defined involving both symptoms and laboratory findings, from carotid sinus hypersensitivity which has the same laboratory findings but is not associated with symptoms in everyday life.

Graux et al.[26] have drawn attention to secondary types of carotid sinus syndrome: these can be due to local causes such as tumours, local radiotherapy, lymphadenopathy or arterial aneurysms, or to drug therapy which may act by enhancement of an insignificant hypersensitive carotid sinus reflex to become a symptomatic problem.

Clinical Presentation

Carotid sinus syndrome presents with syncope without a significant warning phase, with significant injury occurring in up to 25%,[3] and in this respect it mimics Stokes–

Adams attacks of AV block. Attacks may be precipitated by neck movements as described by Weiss and Baker,[2] but other triggers for attacks exist such as abdominal pain or nausea noted by Morley and Sutton.[9] Carotid sinus syndrome is a misnomer for this disease as it is a form of neurally mediated syncope for which carotid sinus massage is an access point to permit a diagnosis, but other autonomic access points are known although much less available for clinical assessment.

An important new finding is the amnesia for syncope which can occur in older people.[21,27] This distorts the clinical history and may obscure diagnosis or lead the clinician toward another investigative route. Additionally attacks may be associated with neurological sequelae due possibly to embolic phenomena or simply to a greater duration of attack than typically seen in Stokes–Adams syncope because of the persistent nature of vasodepression. This vasodilatation is not a feature of syncope in AV block. The implication of these features of the presentation is that patients can be misdiagnosed as suffering from epilepsy or other neurological conditions.

In descriptions by observers a carotid sinus syncope has pallor throughout, including after recovery of consciousness; while, by way of comparison, a Stokes–Adams attack is followed by a brief flushing of the skin and a return to normal colour. Very prolonged attacks can occur in carotid sinus syndrome, lasting minutes or even hours, the explanation for which is probably a restoration of cardiac activity paralleled by a persistence of vasodilatation and insufficient blood pressure to procure full consciousness; these situations have led to erroneous assumptions by lay people that the patient is dead.

Patients with carotid sinus syndrome are predominantly male (2:1) and aged over 70 years. Recorded cases under the age of 40 are very rare. In view of this, incidental findings of hypertension and coronary artery disease are common.

Aetiology and Pathophysiology

The precise aetiology of carotid sinus syndrome is not known. The most plausible theories involve a malfunction at or around the vasomotor centre in the medulla. Excessive gain in the central part of the reflex loop[28] involving a chemical neurotransmitter such as GABA[29] seems possible.

The efferent arm of the loop uses the vagus nerve to achieve bradycardia. It is thought that the vasodilatation is under sympathetic control and the splanchnic bed is the major site at which venular dilatation occurs. The time course of the reflex depends to some extent on the duration of the trigger, beyond this the limiting factors are unknown. Bradycardia tends to be brief while vasodilatation lasts much longer. In contrast, the limiting factor in vasovagal syncope is usually adoption of the supine position, by fainting and falling, which offers an autotransfusion of blood from the legs serving to reverse the abnormal reaction. Perhaps this is also an important limiting factor in carotid sinus syncope.

Carotid sinus syncope has been divided by some workers into three types: cardioinhibitory, vasodepressor, and mixed. This is an unhelpful division because there is now clear evidence that pure vasodepressive attacks are rare and all cardioinhibitory episodes are associated with at least some vasodepression.[9] Thus, the vast majority of carotid sinus syncope is mixed with, in some, cardioinhibition dominating over vasodepression and in a lesser number of cases the opposite. The degree of vasodepression is best appreciated by using the technique described by Morley et al.,[3] whereby bradycardia is controlled by dual-chamber pacing at a rate just above the spontaneous sinus rate, and carotid sinus massage is performed during arterial pressure monitoring. This revealed that hypotension occurs in all independently of the bradycardia or asystole. When it is <30 mmHg it is considered clinically insignificant. These assessments were later repeated more appropriately by Madigan et al.[30] using the upright posture and they reached identical conclusions.

Incidence and Natural History

Two estimates of the incidence of symptomatic carotid sinus syndrome have been made, and they are strikingly similar despite their origination at different times and from different countries.[9,31] They drew their data from the south-east coast of England and the west coast and central Italy, arriving at figures of, respectively, 35 and 40 per million new cases per year. Both of these centres could be described as enthusiasts for testing in order to make this diagnosis. These numbers would seem to constitute approximately 10% of the average implant rate in North America and Europe. It is therefore surprising that a world survey on cardiac pacing[32] indicates numbers of implants for carotid sinus syndrome that fall far short of 10%, being, in the main, barely 1%. The reasons for this huge discrepancy require analysis. At this point underdiagnosis and classification in another diagnostic category can be advanced as explanations.

A large contribution of underdiagnosis implies that a great many patients are not receiving pacemakers from which they would undoubtedly benefit. Recent work from the group of Kenny[33] suggests that this is the case. Their approach has been to examine older patients in a syncope and falls clinic who have earlier presented at the emergency room with a fall. There is a high incidence of hypersensitive carotid sinus reflexes amongst them. A prospective study of these patients is now in hand (R. A. Kenny 1996, personal communication) designed to demonstrate the value of pacing in this population. If a benefit can be shown in terms of elimination of unexplained falls and reduction in costs of emergency room and subsequent treatment (e.g. hip surgery) a vast increase in the numbers of pacemaker implants can be expected.

Insufficient is known about natural history of carotid sinus syndrome. Few longitudinal studies have been reported. In their review of a series of 202 patients over 12 years, Sutton and coworkers[34,35] found a 5-year survival of 64%, supported by Brignole et al.[36] (66%), which suggests no excess mortality in paced patients with this condition. Similar conclusions have been drawn in a later study from the same group[37] and by Graux et al.[38] The causes of death in these patients are those expected at this age: cerebrovascular accident, myocardial infarction, heart failure, and cancer. The influence of pacing on mortality is unknown, but Blanc et al.[39] and Brignole et al.[36,40] have shown that syncope recurs much more frequently in patients who have not been paced. This strongly implies that morbidity is reduced by pacing.

Therapy

Early treatment of carotid sinus syndrome was surgical[5,6] or radiotherapeutic.[7,8] These were small series and they were quickly outmoded by the facility and results of cardiac pacing,[3,4] which remains the mainstay of therapy. The mode of pacing, however, is still somewhat controversial. The first patients were necessarily paced VVI and it was not until the report of Morley *et al.*[3] in 1982 that dual-chamber pacing was seriously applied. The results were good and dual-chamber systems, then DVI, offered better control of the vasodepressor element by their ability to pace physiologically during the bradycardia of an attack. At the same time the Westminster group drew attention to what they called the 'pacemaker effect'. This was evident in patients who did not experience retrograde atrioventricular conduction during VVI pacing but a fall in systolic arterial pressure occurred sufficient to cause symptoms as VVI pacing phased in and out of sinus rhythm, the two rates being similar. Where retrograde AV conduction was present, even supine arterial pressures could fall by as much as 70 mmHg. Madigan *et al.*[30] confirmed the results of Morley and coworkers in another large series. The report of Morley *et al.*[3] also showed that the AAI mode was unsuitable for pacing carotid sinus syndrome. In spite of laboratory confirmation in the supine position that the AAI mode was adequate, there was a high recurrence rate of symptoms and all patients later showed AV block during carotid sinus massage.

In the early 1980s pacemaker technology evolved rapidly, permitting Morley and Sutton[9] to recommend the DDI mode of pacing with rate hysteresis (Figures 7.3 and 7.4). The DDI mode was chosen both to avoid competitive pacing in the atrium as may occur in the DVI mode, and the problem of pacemaker-mediated tachycardia,[41] especially as a persistence of retrograde AV conduction during a carotid sinus attack had been observed by Morley and Sutton.

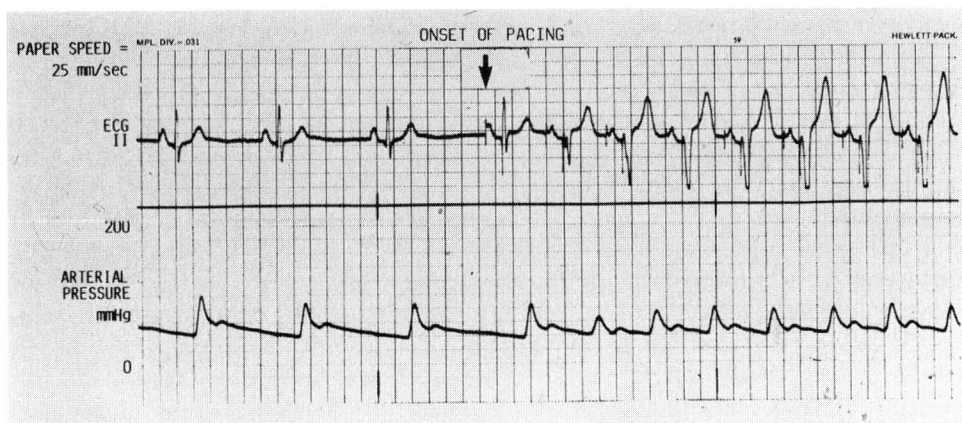

Figure 7.3 Polygraph showing a single-lead electrocardiogram combined with direct brachial artery pressure monitoring. The patient has a dual-chamber pacemaker programmed in the DDI mode with rate hysteresis 45/85 ppm. Sinus rhythm slows during the recording to allow the pacemaker to commence pacing in an AV sequential manner. Note that the arterial pressure falls only slightly.

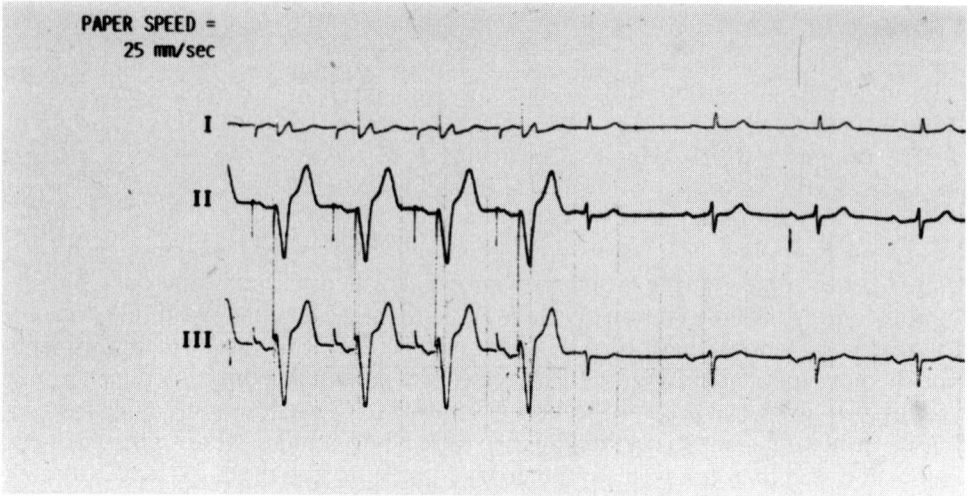

Figure 7.4 Three-lead electrocardiogram showing how pacing is inhibited when a carotid sinus attack is over and sinus rhythm increases in rate. The DDI pacemaker is programmed in the same way as that in Figure 7.3.

Subsequently, pacemakers have become able to recognize this arrhythmia and apply algorithms in order to terminate it. Thus, today, it is probably unnecessary to burden pacemaker physicians and technicians with this ill-understood mode, and the DDD mode can be considered adequate for all normal purposes. The rate hysteresis in the original concept of Morley and Sutton was to attempt to provide effective dual-chamber pacing at a stimulation rate above that which is usually delivered, and well above the patient's heart rate at the time of the carotid sinus crisis, with a view to overcoming the vasodepression as well as the cardioinhibition (Figure 7.3). This pacing approach remains the method of choice today, although further modifications have been made. Some of these are described in Chapter 9 on vasovagal syncope as they are more pertinent in that context. However, the vasovagal modifications to pacemaker algorithms have been enthusiastically adopted by the Newcastle group.[27]

Another problem with conventional dual-chamber pacing and rate hysteresis, either DDI or DDD, is the setting of the AV delay. For optimal function during the pacing of an attack it should be quite short (e.g. <150 ms), but this may result in permanent ventricular stimulation which might be negatively inotropic. In order to overcome this, a type of mode-switching has been introduced.[42,43] The dual-chamber pacemaker runs in the AAI mode but maintains sensing in the ventricles until an unexpected degree of AV block develops, when ventricular pacing supervenes with the AV delay at that memorized from previous normal rhythm. To this can be added an option to accelerate the pacing rate. This function is known as 'automatic mode conversion' (AMC) and is a programmable feature of some ELA dual-chamber pacemakers. An acute study performed on 41 patients to compare DDI, DDD with AMC and DDD with AMC with the rate acceleration option indicated that the third of these modes was the superior in haemodynamic terms.[42] A double-blind randomized controlled crossover comparison of DDI and VVI pacing modes, each with and without rate hysteresis, showed a clear patient preference for the DDI mode with rate hysteresis.[44]

The advice of Morley and Sutton in 1984 has been sustained to the present time, which is to choose dual-chamber pacing for all (except those in chronic atrial fibrillation). This view is not accepted by Brignole *et al.*[20] as they believe it possible to separate patients who will do well with VVI pacing by means of what they call the 'method of symptoms'. They perform carotid sinus massage for 10 seconds before and after intravenous atropine 0.02 mg/kg, and conclude that patients with important sinus bradycardia <50 bpm, retrograde atrioventricular conduction, a symptomatic pacemaker effect in the erect position, an important vasodepressor component of the reflex, and orthostatic hypotension, are unsuitable for VVI pacing; while the remainder will safely respond to this mode (approximately 57%).

The question of medical therapy need not be considered in a newly presenting patient with several syncopal episodes, over a short period such as 6 months, and carotid sinus syndrome diagnosed as described above. There may be a case for withholding pacing in very mildly affected patients,[45] but any possible benefit of medication is unproven. Kenny *et al.*[46] attempted the use of aminophylline, as an antagonist to naturally occurring adenosine, without success. In an exhaustive effort to find a drug capable of rapidly resolving the vasodepressor component of this syndrome, Morley *et al.*[47] noted that clonidine had a reversing effect with the arterial pressure rising on carotid sinus massage, but the background hypotension precluded its use for all but those significantly hypertensive. Dihydroergotamine abolished vasodepression (Figure 7.5), but clinical use was associated with overwhelming side-effects. The other drugs studied, including beta-blockers (pindolol, prenalterol), atropine, methoxamine and ephedrine, showed no benefit. More recently, Kenny's group have had some success with fludrocortisone[48] and midodrine (Ward *et al.* 1997, unpublished data), an alpha-agonist. Selective serotonin reuptake inhibitors may also favourably influence the central processing of the reflex.[49] The context in which medication most often requires consideration is as an addition to pacing to combat vasodepression incompletely treated by a sophisticated mode of dual-chamber pacing. The choice of drug remains unresolved and weak alpha- and beta-agonists such as etilefrine or midodrine offer some promise, possibly combined with fludrocortisone.

The results of pacing by dual-chamber pacing systems are quite good,[35,45] but they fail to achieve complete abolition of syncope as is expected when symptomatic AV block is paced. Sutton *et al.*[35] in their 5-year review of the effect of treatment found that syncope recurred in 18% of patients paced VVI and in 9% of those paced dual-chamber. These figures have been confirmed by Brignole *et al*;[20] using their selection methods for mode of pacing they found similar rates of recurrence between the modes of 15% VVI and 12% dual-chamber. Brignole's group maintain that recurrence of syncope can be predicted in patients who have a positive head-up tilt test.[50] Appropriate medication may add some improvement to these figures but it is unlikely that they will reach zero syncopal recurrences. An approach which might yield this is to combine a dual-chamber pacing system with an intravenous drug dispenser. Using this method it may be possible to deliver a drug such as dihydroergotamine in effective doses without engendering side-effects that

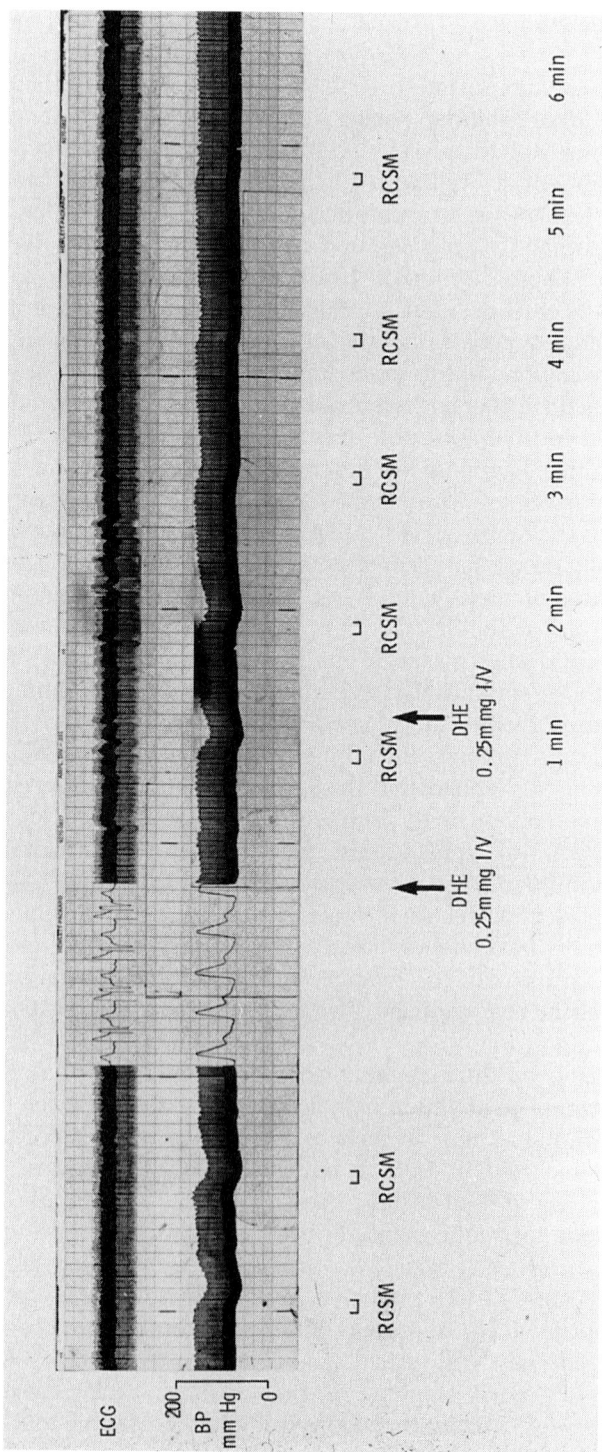

Figure 7.5 Polygraph showing the effect of bolus doses of dihydroergotamine (DHE). There is an elimination of the normally reproducible vasodepressor effect of carotid sinus massage during dual-chamber pacing.

inevitably complicate oral administration. The question of variable bioavailability is also overcome.

Conclusion

Carotid sinus syndrome is an important cause of syncope and mortality in the elderly. It remains insufficiently recognized mainly because it is not considered as a diagnosis and no appropriate investigations are performed. It is a treatable condition and the results of pacing are very good, although some further progress is required in amelioration of the vasodepressor component.

References

1. Roskam J. Un syndrome nouveau; syncopes cardiaques graves et syncopes repetees par hypereflectivite sinocarotidienne. *Press Medical* 1930; **28**: 590–1.
2. Weiss H, Baker JP. The carotid sinus reflex in health and disease: its role in the causation of fainting and convulsions. *Medicine* 1933; **12**: 297–354.
3. Morley CA, Perrins EJ, Grant P, *et al*. Carotid sinus syncope treated by pacing: analysis of persistent symptoms and role of atrioventricular sequential pacing. *Br Heart J* 1982; **47**: 411–18.
4. Voss DM, Magnin GE. Demand pacing and carotid sinus syncope. *Am Heart J* 1970; **79**: 544–7.
5. Craig WMK, Smith HI. The surgical treatment of hypersensitive carotid sinus reflex: a report of thirteen cases. *Yale J Biol Med* 1939; **11**: 415–22.
6. Trout HH, Brown LL, Thompson JE. Carotid sinus syndrome: treatment by denervation. *Ann Surg* 1979; **89**: 575–80.
7. Stevenson CA. The role of roentgen therapy in the carotid sinus syndrome. *Radiology* 1939; **32**: 209.
8. Greeley HP, Smedal MI, Morset W. The treatment of the carotid sinus syndrome by irradiation. *N Eng J Med* 1955; **252**: 91–4.
9. Morley CA, Sutton R. Carotid sinus syncope. *Int J Cardiol* 1984; **6**: 287–93.
10. Brignole M, Menozzi C, Gianfranchi L, *et al*. Neurally mediated syncope detected by carotid sinus massage and head-up tilt test in sick sinus syndrome. *Am J Cardiol* 1991; **68**: 1032–6.
11. Petersen MEV, Williams TR, Sutton R. A comparison of non-invasive continuous finger blood pressure measurement (Finapres) with intra-arterial pressure during prolonged head-up tilt. *Eur Heart J* 1995; **16**: 1647–54.
12. McIntosh SJ, Lawson J, Kenny RA. Clinical characteristics of vasodepressor, cardioinhibitory and mixed carotid sinus syndrome in the elderly. *Am J Med* 1993; **95**: 203–8.
13. Gaggioli G, Brignole M, Menozzi C, *et al*. Re-appraisal of the vasodepressor reflex in carotid sinus syndrome. *Am J Cardiol* 1995; **75**: 518.
14. Heidorn GH, McNamara AP. Effect of carotid sinus stimulation on the electrocardiograms of clinically normal individuals. *Circulation* 1956; **14**: 1104–13.
15. McIntosh SJ, da Costa D, Lawson J, *et al*. Heart rate and blood pressure responses to carotid sinus massage in healthy elderly subjects. *Age Ageing* 1994; **23**: 57–61.
16. Hudson WM, Morley CA, Perrins EJ, *et al*. Is a hypersensitive carotid sinus reflex relevant? *Clin Prog Electrophysiol Pacing* 1985; **3**: 155–9.
17. Friedberg AS. Carotid sinus and angina pectoris. *N Engl J Med* 1969; **281**: 330–1.
18. Munro NC, McIntosh S, Lawson J, *et al*. Incidence of complications after carotid sinus massage in older patients with syncope. *J Am Ger Soc* 1994; **42**: 1242–51.

19. Dehn TCB, Morley CA, Sutton R. The use of the neck chamber test in the evaluation of the carotid sinus baroreceptor control of heart interval in patients with carotid sinus syndrome. *Cardiovasc Res* 1984; **18**: 746–51.
20. Brignole M, Menozzi C, Lolli G. *et al*. Validation of a new method for the choice of pacing mode in carotid sinus syndrome with or without sinus bradycardia. *PACE* 1991; **14**: 196–203.
21. Dey AB, Bexton RS, Tyman MM, *et al*. The impact of a dedicated 'syncope and falls' clinic on pacing practice in northeastern England. *PACE* 1997; **20**: in press.
22. Reiffel JA, Bigger JT. Current status of direct recordings of the sinus node in man. *PACE* 1983; **6**: 1143–50.
23. Brignole M, Gigli G, Altomonte, *et al*. Il riflesso cardioinibitore provocato dalla stimulazione del seno carotideo nei soggetti normali e con malatti cardiovascolari. *G Ital Cardiol* 1985; **15**: 514–19.
24. Morley CA, Perrins EJ, Sutton R. Is there a difference between carotid sinus syndrome and sick sinus syndrome? *Eur J Cardiac Pacing Electrophysiol* 1991; **1**: 62–70.
25. Brown KA, Maloney JD, Smith HC. Carotid sinus reflex in patients undergoing coronary angiography: relationship of degree and location of coronary artery disease to response to carotid sinus massage. *Circulation* 1980; **62**: 697–703.
26. Graux P, Guyomar Y, Carliez R, *et al*. Secondary carotid sinus syndrome. In: Blanc JJ, Benditt D, Sutton R (eds), *Neurally Mediated Syncope: Pathophysiology, Investigations, and Treatment*. Armonk, NY: 1996; Futura, 145–51.
27. Richardson DA, Bexton R, Shaw FE. Prevalence of cardioinhibitory carotid sinus hypersensitivity in patients 50 years or over presenting to the accident and emergency department with 'unexplained' or 'recurrent' falls. *PACE* 1997; **20**: in press.
28. Kenny RA, Lyon CC, Ingram AM, *et al*. Enhanced vagal activity and normal arginine vasopressin response in carotid sinus syndrome: implications for a central abnormality in carotid sinus hypersensitivity. *Cardiovasc Res* 1987; **21**: 545–50.
29. Wahba MMAE, Morley CA, AL-Shamma YMH, *et al*. Cardiovascular reflex responses in patients with unexplained syncope. *Clin Sci* 1989; **77**: 547–53.
30. Madigan NP, Flaker GC, Curtiss JJ, *et al*. Carotid sinus hypersensitivity: beneficial effects of dual chamber pacing. *Am J Cardiol* 1984; **53**: 1034–40.
31. Brignole M, Menozzi C, Lolli G, *et al*. Pacing for carotid sinus syndrome and sick sinus syndrome. *PACE* 1990; **13**: 2071–5.
32. Parsonnet V, Bernstein D. The 1989 world survey of cardiac pacing, *PACE* 1991; **14**: 2073–6.
33. Dey AB, Stout NR, Kenny RA. Cardiovascular syncope is the most common cause of drop attacks in the elderly. *PACE* 1997; **20**: in press.
34. Sutton R. Pacing in patients with carotid sinus and vasovagal syndromes. *PACE* 1989; **12**: 1260–3.
35. Sutton R, Ahmed R, Ingram A. 12-year pacing experience in carotid sinus syndrome (abstract). *PACE* 1989; 1253.
36. Brignole M, Menozzi C, Lolli G, *et al*. Long-term outcome of paced and non-paced patients with severe carotid sinus syndrome. *Am J Cardiol* 1992; **69**: 1039–43.
37. Ahmed R, Ingram A, Sutton R. 16 years' experience of pacing in carotid sinus syndrome (abstract). *PACE* 1993; **16**: 284.
38. Graux P, Cardioz R, Guyoma Y. A prospective study of the background and follow-up in carotid sinus syndrome. *Eur J Cardiac Pacing Electrophysiol* 1994; **4**: 161–9.
39. Blanc JJ, Boschat J, Penther PH. Hypersensibilite sino-carotidienne: evolution a moyen terme en fonction du traitement et des symptomes. *Arch Mal Coeur* 1984; **77**: 330–6.
40. Brignole M, Oddone D, Cogorno S, *et al*. Long-term outcome in symptomatic carotid sinus hypersensitivity. *Am Heart J* 1992; **123**: 687–92.
41. den Dulk K, Lindemans FW, Bar FW, *et al*. Pacemaker related tachycardias. *PACE* 1982; **5**: 476–85.
42. Cazeau S, for the CSS Cooperative Study Group. Improved hemodynamics provided by automatic mode conversion from AAI to DDD in carotid sinus syndrome (abstract). *PACE* 1993; **7**: 1589.

43. Blanc J, Cazeau S, Ritter P, *et al*. Carotid sinus syndrome: acute hemodynamic evaluation of a new dual chamber pacing mode. *PACE* 1995; **18**: 1902–8.
44. Ahmed R, Guneri S, Hills W, *et al*. Double blind comparison of DDI, DDI with rate hysteresis, VVI and VVI with rate hysteresis in symptom control in carotid sinus syndrome (abstract). *PACE* 1991; **14**: 623.
45. Brignole M, Menozzi C. Why and when to treat a patient with carotid sinus syndrome. In: Blanc JJ, Benditt D, Sutton R (eds), *Neurally Mediated Syncope: Pathophysiology, Investigations, and Treatment*. Armonk, NY: Futura, 1996: 153–9.
46. Kenny RA, Siddique S, Mitsuoka T, *et al*. The influence of methylxanthine on the vasodepressor response of carotid sinus syndrome (abstract). *PACE* 1985; **8**: 315.
47. Morley CA, Perrins EJ, Sutton R. Pharmacological intervention in the carotid sinus syndrome (abstract). *PACE* 1983; **6**: A16.
48. da Costa D, McIntosh S, Kenny RA. Benefits of fludrocortisone in the treatment of symptomatic vasodepressor carotid sinus syndrome. *Br Heart J* 1993; **69**: 308–10.
49. Grubb BP, Samoil D, Kosinski D, *et al*. The use of serotonin reuptake inhibitors for the treatment of recurrent syncope due to carotid sinus hypersensitivity unresponsive to dual chamber cardiac pacing. *PACE* 1994; **17**: 1434–6.
50. Gaggioli G, Brignole M, Menozzi C, *et al*. A positive response to head-up tilt testing predicts syncopal recurrence in carotid sinus syndrome patients with permanent pacemakers. *Am J Cardiol* 1995; **76**: 720–2.

8

Pacing in Bifascicular Block

A. Englund

A bifascicular block (BFB) is usually defined as left bundle branch block or right bundle branch block with left anterior or left posterior fascicular block. This definition is based on the trifascicular concept.[1] Although the anatomical basis for this definition is less clearly defined,[2] the trifascicular concept has been useful in explaining electrocardiographic patterns and functional abnormalities associated with intraventricular conduction disturbances.

An increased prevalence of BFB with increasing age has been reported in an unselected population.[3] A prevalence of approximately 1% was found in a population >35 years.[4,5] It is uncommon at younger age and was found in only 0.1% of a large group of air-force personnel.[6] It seems to be more common among patients with a history of syncopal attacks, and an ECG showing BFB was found in 7% of a large population of patients with syncope admitted to emergency wards.[7]

Patients with BFB have a high prevalence of associated heart disease, mainly coronary artery disease and hypertensive heart disease.[8–10] It is therefore not surprising that the mortality is high at 2–14% per year.[11] The incidence of sudden death is also increased and occurs in 3–5% of patients per year.[8,9,12,13] In a large population of patients undergoing chronic pacemaker treatment, BFB proved to be an independent risk factor for sudden death.[14] In patients without associated heart disease, cardiac mortality is increased in patients with left bundle branch block but not in patients with right bundle branch block, compared with age- and sex-matched controls.[3]

The symptom of greatest concern is syncope, which is reported in up to 25% of patients first seen with BFB.[11] This symptom is the only clinical feature that has been shown to be predictive of impending high-grade AV block. Other symptoms are mainly related to the underlying heart disease.

Bifascicular Block and High-Grade AV-Block Development

The trifascicular concept implies that AV conduction in patients with BFB is dependent on normal functioning of the third remaining fascicle. A dysfunction may result in chronic or intermittent high-grade AV block. The overall yearly incidence of this progression in an unselected population of patients with BFB seems to be, however, only 1–4%.[8,11,15–17]

As mentioned above, the only symptom or noninvasive test that has been found to be useful in predicting subsequent high-grade AV block is a history of syncopal attacks. With a follow-up of 42 months, McAnulty et al.[9] reported that patients with a history of syncope had a 17% incidence of this arrhythmia, compared with only 2% in the group of patients without this symptom; this corresponds to an annual incidence of 5% in the syncope group and 0.6% in the other group.

The most common way of including patients in earlier studies was by screening routinely performed ECGs, selecting those patients with more remote syncopal attacks and possible lower likelihood for progression to AV block. Patients with intermittent high-grade AV block as the mechanism behind their syncope might develop a high-grade AV block early and could therefore not be included by ECG screening. This hypothesis was supported by our group in a study of 101 patients with BFB.[18] Forty-one patients had a history of unexplained syncope and 60 were asymptomatic. The annual progression rate to high-grade AV block was higher (11%) in the syncope group compared with previous studies, but was similar (0.8%) in the non-syncope group. The majority of the syncope patients were included after they had been admitted to an emergency room for a syncopal attack. A median time of only 14 days elapsed between the syncope and the inclusion. It can therefore be speculated that the true progression rate to high-grade AV block in patients with BFB and syncope is higher than what has been shown in studies based on ECG screening.

Identifying Patients with an Increased Risk for High-Grade AV Block

The only way to eliminate the risk of bradyarrhythmias in patients with BFB is to implant a pacemaker. According to the Framingham study, the incidence of BFB is approximately 130 cases per 100 000 inhabitants per year.[4,5] The high costs involved, and the potential risks involved in pacemaker treatment, prohibits the idea of including all patients with BFB in such treatment. Moreover, since the rate of progression to high-grade AV block is low, a strategy of identifying the high-risk patients is essential.

Noninvasive Evaluation

The diagnostic value of long-term ECG recording in patients with BFB and syncope is not well studied. Most studies of patients with BFB have been based on an invasive electrophysiological investigation and have included only patients with 'unexplained syncope' (i.e. those with no documented arrhythmias on long-term ECG monitoring and other noninvasive testing). Since the number of patients excluded owing to a positive finding on a long-term ECG recording has not been stated in most studies, the diagnostic value of this investigation is unknown. Previous studies of 24-hour ambulatory ECG-recording in unselected patients with syncopal attacks have, however, shown that the sensitivity of this investigation is limited.[19–21] A significantly longer recording time is needed to reach a diagnosis in most cases owing to the often intermittent nature of arrhythmias in patients with syncopal attacks.

In the last few years, new methods of long-term ECG-recording have become available. Small ECG recorders which continuously store significant arrhythmias or patient-activated events offer possibilities to monitor a patient for more than a week.[22] Another method of monitoring patients with syncope which remains unexplained despite a complete invasive and noninvasive investigation is to use an implantable device.[23,24] In this way it is possible to monitor the heart rhythm for several months, and when a diagnosis is established the device is explanted.

An exercise test can serve several purposes in the evaluation of a patient with syncope:

(1) First, it can provoke the arrhythmia, bradycardia or tachycardia responsible for the patient's symptoms. Some case reports have been reported in which high-grade AV block was induced by an exercise test,[25] but a systematic evaluation is not available. In our study of 41 patients with BFB and unexplained syncope,[7] all patients underwent a symptom-limited bicycle exercise test according to a modified Bruce protocol; in no patient could a high-grade AV block be induced.
(2) Secondly, an exercise test can be helpful in deciding whether the patient has a chronotropic incompetence and would benefit from a rate-response pacemaker.
(3) Thirdly, the test can sometimes detect signs of myocardial ischaemia, although this is often difficult to determine in the presence of bundle branch block.

Invasive Electrophysiological Investigations

Studies performed in the basal state

The evaluation of patients with BFB was one of the first applications of the invasive electrophysiological technique reported in 1971 by Berkowitz *et al.*[26] Theoretically, slow conduction in the remaining third fascicle, reflected as a prolonged HV interval, would suggest a trifascicular disease. Measurement of this interval would thereby allow the identification of a subgroup of patients at high risk for high-grade AV block or sudden death. In the mid-1970s and early 1980s this hypothesis was studied extensively in a large number of patients,[8,9,16,17,27–29] but the result was somewhat disappointing since no or only a weak correlation between the HV interval and subsequent high-grade AV block was found. Only a severely prolonged HV interval (>100 ms) had a high specificity, but owing to the low prevalence of this finding the sensitivity was very low.[17] Another condition studied was His–Purkinje block induced by incremental atrial pacing.[30,31] The normal response to this procedure is the development of block in the AV node (i.e. proximal to the bundle of His). A block within or distal to the bundle of His suggests conduction abnormality in the remaining third fascicle. However, as with a severely prolonged HV interval, this was found in only 3–4% of all recordings. It was, however, found to be highly predictive for the development of high-grade AV block. This has been confirmed recently by Petrac *et al.*[32]

In summary, these reports indicate that an invasive electrophysiological study is often of limited value in patients with BFB, when performed in the basal state.

Studies performed with pharmacological provocation

In order to increase the diagnostic and prognostic value of an invasive electrophysiological study, pharmacological stress tests have been proposed. Ajmaline, procainamide and disopyramide have been used for this purpose.

Ajmaline. This is a Class 1A antiarrhythmic agent with a complicated pharmaco-
kinetic profile.[33,34] It has been shown to unmask latent bundle branch block as well as
induce high-grade AV block.[35] Several investigators have studied the utility of
intravenous provocation with ajmaline for the evaluation of patients with intraventricular conduction disorders in whom symptomatic transient high-grade AV block
was suspected.[35–46] Only a few of these have been reported in the English language.
    Kaul *et al.*[42] reported on 35 patients with bundle branch block and unexplained
syncope who underwent an invasive electrophysiological study including provocation by ajmaline at 1 mg/kg. Eleven patients had only right bundle branch block
whereas the remainder had BFB. A positive test was defined as a post-ajmaline
second-degree or third-degree AV block occurring spontaneously. This was found in
twelve patients (34%) and appeared only in patients with BFB. All patients with a
positive test received a pacemaker and were asymptomatic during a mean follow-up
period of 18.5 months. A progression to complete AV block was seen in one patient on
inhibiting the pacemaker. In the group with a negative ajmaline test, six patients had
recurrence of symptoms but in none was a high-grade AV block documented. Since
only one patient had a documented high-grade AV block and no controls were
included, the diagnostic value of the ajmaline test cannot be certain from this study.
    Wunderlich and Hetze[40] reported the results of the ajmaline test in 259 patients
with intraventricular conduction disorders of whom 235 patients had a BFB. They
used a protocol which did not include His bundle recordings or atrial pacing. Instead,
only a ventricular lead was used for rapid ventricular pacing for up to 2 min after
intravenous administration of 50 or 100 mg of ajmaline. A positive test was defined as
second- or third-degree AV block after abrupt termination of ventricular pacing. In
the group of 109 patients with previously documented high-grade AV block the test
was positive in 93%; this is a sensitivity of 85%. The specificity was assessed in a group
of 38 patients without syncope or documented bradyarrhythmias: only three had a
positive test which corresponds to a specificity of 92%. This study did not present any
follow-up data.

Procainamide. This drug has been shown to decrease the conduction velocity and
increase the refractoriness of the His–Purkinje system.[47] This occurs both in normal
individuals and in patients with prolonged HV intervals, and a 10–20% increase in the
HV interval has been reported.[47,48] A more prolonged increase or the induction of
high-grade AV block indicates a defective His–Purkinje conduction reserve.
    The use of procainamide as a provocative agent of the His–Purkinje system in
patients with BFB was first proposed in 1978 by Tonkin *et al.*[49] The same group later
presented a larger study with the use of procainamide 10 mg/kg in 42 patients with
BFB and unexplained syncope;[50] a control group of five asymptomatic patients with
BFB was included. A positive test was defined as a His–Purkinje block during sinus

rhythm or an HV prolongation >15 ms. Eleven patients (26%) in the syncope group had a positive test, whereas three patients (60%) had this in the control group. After a mean follow-up of 38 months, two patients in the syncope group, both with a positive test, had a documented high-grade AV block, while all patients in the control group were in sinus rhythm. Since the follow-up did not always include an evaluation of the underlying heart rhythm, the sensitivity of the test is not possible to define. Although only a few control patients were included, the high percentage of patients with a false-positive test in this group raises concerns regarding the specificity of the test.

Other studies on patients with BFB and unexplained syncope have included provocation with procainamide.[51,52] These were, however, not designed to study the predictive value of the test.

Disopyramide. This is a Class 1A antiarrhythmic drug with anticholinergic properties.[53] The anticholinergic influence on the AV node reduces the refractory period and theoretically allows exposure of the His–Purkinje system to higher stimulation rates during atrial pacing. This would limit the risk of masking a His–Purkinje block by a slow AV nodal conduction. The Class 1 effect results in an increased refractoriness of the His–Purkinje system and an increased conduction time which may reveal a reduced conduction reserve.

The electrophysiological effects of disopyramide in patients with bundle branch block was studied by Desai *et al.*,[54] and the drug appeared to be safe in patients with intraventricular conduction defects. However, later reports indicated that disopyramide could induce high-grade AV block in vulnerable patients.[55,56]

Bergfeldt *et al.*,[57] were the first to report a study of the use of disopyramide as a pharmacological stress test in patients with BFB. This was a retrospective study, generating criteria for a positive test: second- or third-degree His–Purkinje block during (1) sinus rhythm or (2) atrial pacing (Figure 8.1), or (3) after abruptly terminated ventricular pacing, or (4) HV prolongation $\geqslant 50\%$. An extension of that study proved the usefulness of the bradycardia-detecting pacemaker in detecting intermittent high-grade AV block during follow-up.[58] The sensitivity of the disopyramide test was 75%, and the positive predictive value of a positive test was 80% for an impending high-grade AV block or pacemaker-detected bradycardia. Only the first study included asymptomatic controls, but this group was too small to allow assessment of the specificity of the test.

In order to study the specificity of the disopyramide test and to prospectively evaluate the proposed criteria for a positive test, we studied 73 patients with BFB.[59] Twenty-five patients had a history of syncope whereas 48 were asymptomatic in this respect and served as a control group. After completion of the basal electrophysiological study, disopyramide was given intravenously, 2 mg/kg body weight over a period of 5 min. Owing to the negative inotropic effects of disopyramide, exclusion criteria for the stress test were uncompensated congestive heart failure, and/or an ejection fraction (EF) <35%.

Twelve patients, 8 (32%) in the syncope group and 4 (8%) in the control group, had a positive disopyramide test ($p < 0.02$). Of these, 5 had a positive test from all aspects, 5 had His–Purkinje block during atrial pacing, and 2 had a His–Purkinje block after ventricular pacing which was combined with an HV prolongation $\geqslant 50\%$ in 1.

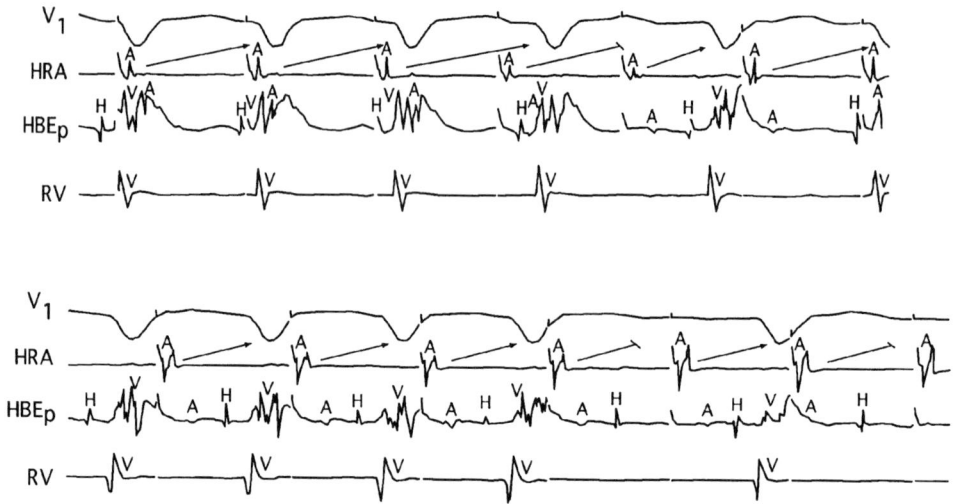

Figure 8.1 Response to incremental atrial pacing before and after disopyramide infusion in a patient with left bundle branch block and a history of syncopal attacks. In the basal state the site of block is within the AV node (the upper traces). After 150 mg of disopyramide a block in the His–Purkinje system (i.e. distal to the bundle of His) is induced. This is a positive test. V_1 = chest lead V_1; HRA = high right atrium registration; HBE_p = proximal His-potential registration; RV = right ventricular registration; A = atrial potential; H = His potential; V = ventricular potential.

The disopyramide test was positive in all seven patients in whom a high-grade AV block was documented during a median follow-up of 23 months, a sensitivity of 100%. Four of the 66 patients without a bradyarrhythmic event during follow-up had a positive disopyramide test; a specificity of 94%. This is in contrast to the poor diagnostic value of the electrophysiological study performed without pharmacological provocation, in which an HV interval >70 ms and/or a His–Purkinje block at atrial pacing had a sensitivity of 30% and a specificity of 90% for the prediction of a high-grade AV block. A life-table analysis showed a highly significant difference between patients with negative and positive disopyramide tests, as regards bradyarrhythmic events during follow-up ($p < 0.001$) (Figure 8.2).

Ventricular Arrhythmias in Patients with BFB

Most studies of patients with BFB have focused on the BFB as a substrate for bradyarrhythmias. As pointed out above, the results of these studies have been somewhat disappointing since the prognostic and diagnostic value of the various bradyarrhythmic findings were limited. Moreover, pacemaker treatment had no beneficial effect on survival. It has been suggested that this could relate to a higher prevalence of ventricular arrhythmias, but to date only a few studies have added programmed ventricular stimulation to their protocols.[10,32,42,52,60,61] Depending on the stimulation protocol, the definition of ventricular arrhythmia and the population studied, the inducibility of sustained ventricular arrhythmia ranged from 3% to 44%.

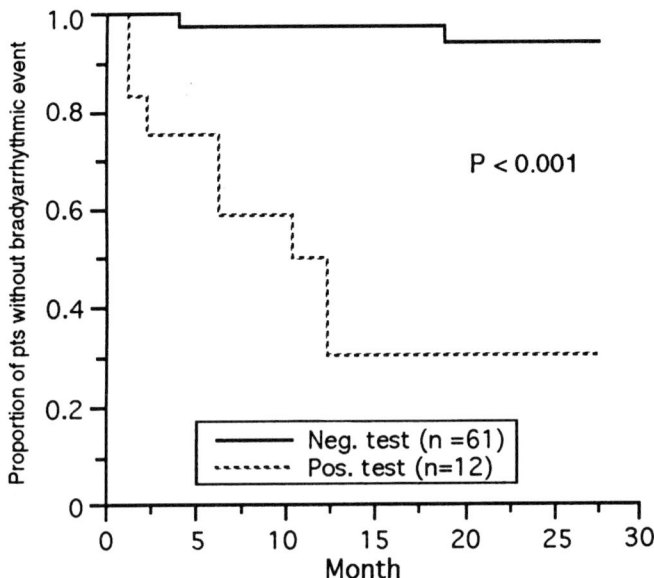

Figure 8.2 Kaplan–Meier plot, showing the progression to high-grade AV block or pacemaker-detected bradycardia in patients with positive and negative disopyramide tests. Reproduced from reference 59.

These studies included only symptomatic patients and did not address the issue of the specificity of programmed ventricular stimulation in patients with BFB.

We performed ventricular stimulation in 101 patients with BFB.[7] Forty-one patients had a history of syncope whereas the remaining 60 patients were asymptomatic in this respect and served as controls. Eight patients (20%) in the syncope group and 10 (17%) in the control group had an inducible sustained ventricular arrhythmia (p = NS). The results of the programmed ventricular stimulation were not correlated to any clinical events during a 21-month follow-up. These findings raise concerns regarding the clinical significance of inducible ventricular arrhythmias in patients with BFB. Three patients from each group had sustained monomorphic ventricular tachycardia (VT). All six patients with sustained monomorphic VT had a history of previous myocardial infarction. Of the 19 patients with a previous myocardial infarction, 32% had this arrhythmia induced.

Only two patients had findings of a dysfunctioning third remaining fascicle together with inducible ventricular arrhythmias (Figure 8.3). None of these had inducible sustained monomorphic VT. This result is similar to that of Petrac et al.[32] who found no coexistence of inducible ventricular arrhythmias and pacing-induced infranodal AV block.

Evaluation for Treatment of Patients with BFB

In the 1989 ACC/AHA Task Force Report,[62] the indications for electrophysiological studies in patients with chronic intraventricular conduction delay are stated (see

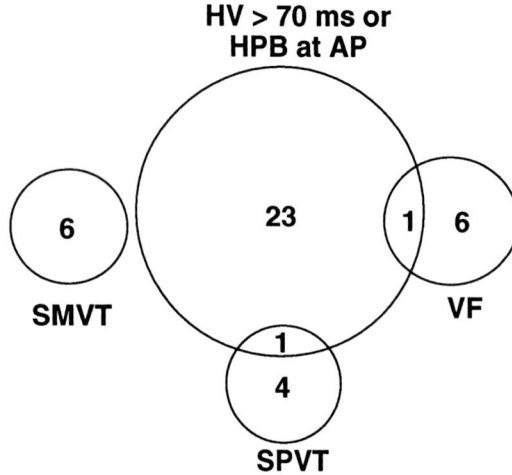

Figure 8.3 Distribution of patients with inducible ventricular arrhythmias and/or His–Purkinje block (HPB) at atrial pacing or an HV interval ⩾70 ms. SMVT = sustained monomorphic ventricular tachycardia; SPVT = sustained polymorphic ventricular tachycardia; VF = ventricular fibrillation.

Table 8.1). In summary, a Class I indication (general agreement about the usefulness of an invasive electrophysiological study) is given only for those in whom a ventricular arrhythmia is suspected to cause the patient's symptoms. A Class II indication is present in patients in whom the knowledge of the site, severity of conduction delay or response to drugs may help to direct therapy or assess prognosis. In asymptomatic patients and in patients with documented arrhythmias there is a general agreement not to perform an invasive electrophysiological study (Class III indication).

Table 8.1 ACC/AHA 1989 guidelines regarding indications for electrophysiological study in patients with chronic intraventricular conduction delay

---

Class I
(Conditions for which there is general agreement that the electrophysiological study provides information that is very useful and important for patient management)
 Symptomatic (with syncope or near syncope) patients with bundle branch block whose ventricular arrhythmia is suspected to cause the symptoms; not for study of intraventricular conduction delay itself

Class II
(Conditions for which electrophysiological studies are frequently used but there is less certainty regarding the usefulness of the information obtained)
 Symptomatic patients with bundle branch block in whom the knowledge of the site, severity of conduction delay or response to drugs may help to direct therapy or assess prognosis

Class III
(Conditions for which there is general agreement that electrophysiological studies do not provide useful information)
 (1) Asymptomatic patients with intraventricular conduction delay
 (2) Symptomatic patients with intraventricular conduction delay whose symptoms can be causally related to ECG events

---

Source: reference 62.

Table 8.2   ACC/AHA 1991 guidelines regarding indications for permanent pacing in bifascicular block and trifascicular block

---

Class I
(Conditions for which there is general agreement that permanent pacemakers should be implanted)
    A. Bifascicular block with intermittent complete heart block associated with symptomatic bradycardia
    B. Bifascicular or trifascicular block with intermittent Type II second-degree AV block without
        symptoms attributable to the heart block

Class II
(Conditions for which permanent pacemakers are frequently used but there is a divergence of opinion with respect to the necessity of their insertion)
    A. Bifascicular block with syncope that is not proved to be due to complete heart block, but other possible
        causes for syncope are not identifiable
    B. Markedly prolonged HV (>100 ms)
    C. Pacing-induced infra-His block

Class III
(Conditions for which there is general agreement that pacemakers are unnecessary)
    A. Fascicular block without AV block or symptoms
    B. Fascicular block with first-degree AV block without symptoms

---

Source: reference 63.

Similar guidelines for the indications of permanent cardiac pacing in patients with BFB were presented in 1991 (see Table 8.2).[63] According to these, only documented high-grade AV block, with or without symptoms, represent a Class I indication.

Asymptomatic patients

The risk of developing high-grade AV blocks in asymptomatic individuals with BFB is very low.[7,11,64] Since no simple, noninvasive test with a high predictive value is available as a screening method, a strategy of pacemaker treatment and/or invasive electrophysiological testing cannot be motivated. In exceptional cases, such as for insurance purposes, legal matters etc., a risk evaluation might be performed. In this situation it is of particular interest to use a method of investigating the His–Purkinje system which has a high negative predictive value. This can be performed by using the disopyramide stress test which has been found to have a high negative predictive value in asymptomatic individuals with BFB.[59]

    With regard to clinically relevant ventricular tachycardia, this has been shown to be inducible in only 5% of patients without syncope and exclusively in patients with a history of myocardial infarction.[7] However, in patients with a history of myocardial infarction *and* BFB, the inducibility of sustained monomorphic VT was high (32%). In several previous studies, this arrhythmia has been shown to indicate a poor prognosis.[65,66] This should be considered in the management of patients with BFB and myocardial infarction even in the absence of syncopal attacks.

Patients with syncope

In patients with syncopal or presyncopal attacks, there is a need for diagnostic and/or therapeutic procedures, although consensus has not been reached on how these should be performed. In some textbooks the authors advocate permanent pacemaker treatment in all symptomatic patients, whereas others recommend an invasive electrophysiological study, unless a significant bradycardia is documented.[67–70] The first policy is supported by the fact that the risk of symptomatic bradycardia is eliminated without the cost of an invasive electrophysiological study. Several arguments, however, favour the second strategy. The annual progression rate to high-grade AV block is relatively low, implying that a large number of patients will not need their pacemaker. Although modern pacemaker therapy is safe, it is certainly not free from complications and the patients are bound to a lifelong treatment. Moreover, pacemaker treatment has not been shown to influence the mortality;[9,17] and, by not performing an electrophysiological study, other arrhythmias, such as VT, might go undiagnosed.

In a cost-effectiveness study based on a computerized Markov decision analysis, empirical pacemaker treatment was compared with invasive electrophysiological testing in symptomatic patients with BFB.[71] Treatment guided by an invasive electrophysiological study was found to be substantially more cost-effective than empirical pacemaker treatment.

A tentative flow-chart of the management of patients with BFB is shown in Figure 8.4. This strategy implies that only patients with a history of myocardial infarction

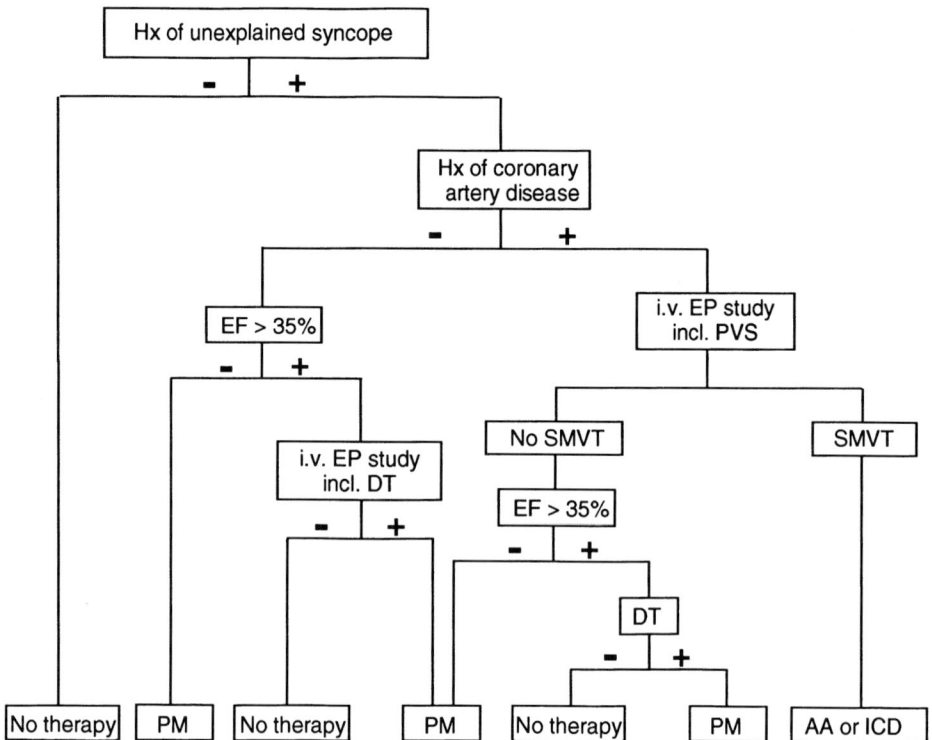

Figure 8.4 A tentative approach to the management of patients with BFB, utilizing patient history (Hx), programmed ventricular stimulation (PVS) and the disopyramide test (DT). See text for further explanations. AA = antiarrhythmic therapy found by serial drug testing; EF = ejection fraction; ICD = implantable cardioverter–defibrillator; PM = pacemaker; SMVT = sustained monomorphic ventricular tachycardia.

will undergo programmed ventricular stimulation. Owing to the low predictive value of an invasive electrophysiological study in the basal state, patients with left ventricular dysfunction, without previous myocardial infarction, will be treated with a pacemaker without further investigations. In patients with normal LV function the outcome of an invasive electrophysiological study using pharmacological stress testing decides which patients should be selected for pacemaker treatment.

Pacing in Patients with BFB and Acute Myocardial Infarction

Since patients with intraventricular conduction disorders often have an associated ischaemic heart disease, treatment of patients with BFB and an acute myocardial infarction (MI) represents a significant clinical problem. It has been recognized for more than 50 years that the prognosis of patients with an acute MI is affected adversely by the presence of bundle branch block (BBB).[72] Several studies have shown that an intraventricular conduction disorder complicates an acute MI in 5–15% of cases and is associated with an up to threefold increase in mortality.[73–82] Moreover, patients with pre-existing intraventricular conduction disorders (i.e. occurring prior to the acute MI) are a group in which the diagnosis and treatment of the myocardial infarction is complicated.

There are two major issues that have to be considered in patients with BFB and acute MI with regard to the risk of high-grade AV block development. First, is a temporary pacemaker needed as a *prophylactic* treatment for high-grade AV block during the acute phase of the infarction? Secondly, should the patient who has survived the acute phase of a myocardial infarction receive a permanent pacemaker in order to minimize the risk of sudden death from later high-grade AV block?

Temporary Pacemaker Treatment During an Acute MI

A large number of studies, performed in the prethrombolytic era, have assessed the risk of high-grade AV block development during the acute phase of a myocardial infarction in the presence of a BBB.[74,76,83–91] These studies have been excellently summarized in several review articles.[92–94] The incidence of high-grade AV block during the acute phase of MI ranged between 20% and 42%. The risk was found to be particularly high in patients with newly acquired BBB, in right BBB + left anterior fascicular block (AFB) or right BBB + left posterior fascicular block (PFB), and in anterior infarctions. The majority of high-grade AV blocks appeared suddenly; that is, they were not preceded by first- or second-degree AV block. In most studies, temporary pacemaker treatment was applied, prophylactically or at the appearance of high-grade AV block. Despite temporary right ventricular pacing, the in-hospital mortality was high (approximately 50%) and was mainly related to the development of pump failure.

Only a few studies have addressed this issue during the last decade.[77,80–82,95] These confirm the findings of previous authors and approximately 20% of the patients with acute myocardial infarction and BFB developed high-grade AV block during the acute phase of the infarction. Although these studies were mainly performed after the introduction of thrombolytic therapy, it is not clear how often thrombolytic therapy was given. A preliminary report from the GUSTO trial, however, shows that the use of thrombolytic agents has not reduced the overall incidence of high-grade AV block and that patients with BBB still have an increased risk of this arrhythmia.[96]

The issue of complications with temporary pacing was addressed in a study by Roth *et al.*[97] They studied the prognosis and complication rate of prophylactic temporary pacemaker treatment in 99 patients with right BBB. Prophylactic temporary pacing was performed in more than 50% of all patients but this did not reduce the mortality rates. Complications which were related to the temporary pacemaker treatment were found in 22% of the temporarily paced patients.

Based on these data a general recommendation to insert a prophylactic temporary pacemaker in patients with BFB and an acute myocardial infarction cannot be given, especially not if a thrombolytic agent is given. An attractive alternative approach to prophylactic transvenous pacing is the use of emergency transcutaneous cardiac pacing. This method has been shown to be reliable and safe and can be initiated within seconds.[98] It is often uncomfortable for the conscious patient but is usually tolerated until temporary transvenous pacing is initiated.

Permanent Pacing After an Acute MI

A new intraventricular conduction disturbance in conjunction with an acute myocardial infarction indicates a larger infarction, especially if a pattern of BFB occurs.[77,99] Also, patients with an old BBB or one of an undetermined duration have a poor prognosis compared with patients with normal conduction. An important question is whether the prognosis can be improved by the insertion of a permanent pacemaker. Assessment of the value of such treatment is complicated by the increased likelihood of death after discharge from hospital, from ventricular arrhythmias, ischaemic events or pump failure.[75,83,90] Results from earlier studies addressing this issue have been conflicting and, hence, the recommendations vary.

The largest of these studies[74,91] was a retrospective, multicentre study, in which patients with bundle branch block and acute myocardial infarction without cardiogenic shock preceding the BBB were included. The incidence of sudden death or high-grade AV block in the 259 patients without high-grade AV block during the acute phase of their acute MI was 13%, compared with 28% in the group of 50 patients with transient high-grade AV block ($p < 0.025$). Thirty of these 50 patients received a permanent pacemaker whereas 20 did not. Of the 14 sudden deaths or recurrent high-grade AV block during follow-up, 3 occurred in the paced group (10%) whereas 11 occurred in the 20 patients (55%) discharged without a permanent pacemaker ($p < 0.001$). Similar results have been presented by several other investigators.[83,87,100–102]

Edhag *et al.*[103] studied the incidence of severe bradycardia in patients with BFB after a myocardial infarction using a bradycardia-indicating pacemaker. They found that severe bradycardia is common, suggesting that a permanent pacemaker might reduce the morbidity after a myocardial infarction in patients with BFB. Pacemaker treatment did not, however, have an influence on the mortality rates.

In summary, most of the studies cited above indicate a beneficial effect of permanent pacemaker treatment after an acute myocardial infarction complicated with a transient high-grade AV block in patients with BBB. The interpretation of these studies is, however, difficult since most were retrospective and nonrandomized and sometimes involves a limited number of patients.

To overcome some of these limitations, Watson *et al.*[104] performed a prospective, randomized study of permanent pacing in patients with intraventricular conduction defects who survived the first 14 days after a myocardial infarction. Twenty-seven patients were randomized to permanent VVI pacing and 23 patients were discharged without a permanent pacemaker. At 5-year follow-up, 41% of the nonpaced and 61% of the paced patients had died. This difference was not statistically significant and there were no differences between the two groups regarding incidence of sudden death. Five of the seven patients who died suddenly in the paced group had a ventricular fibrillation or tachycardia documented at the time of death. An important difference compared with other earlier studies was that only a minority of the patients in the study by Watson *et al.* had a documented transient high-grade AV block during the acute phase of the MI. In most of the previously cited studies the proportion of patients with a transient AV block was much higher.

In conclusion, the occurrence of intraventricular conduction disorders, especially of the BFB type, indicate an increased mortality after an acute myocardial infarction. The major reason behind this seems to be an extensive loss of myocardial tissue, and most deaths are consequently related to left ventricular dysfunction. A substantial risk of ventricular arrhythmias is probably present which explains some of the increased risk for sudden death. The risk of sudden death due to high-grade AV block also seems to be increased, especially when the acute phase of the infarction has been complicated by a transient AV block.

Owing to the lack of large randomized studies after acute MI in patients with intraventricular conduction defects and transient high-grade AV block, firm recommendations regarding the use of permanent cardiac pacing in these patients cannot be given at the present time.

Prophylactic Temporary Pacing During Surgical and Invasive Procedures

Theoretically, patients with BFB could be at higher risk for the development of high-grade AV block during surgery or invasive procedures. It is reasonable to believe that hypotension, ischaemia, electrolyte disturbances or pharmacological agents given during these procedures could stress the intraventricular conduction system in vulnerable patients. The insertion of a prophylactic temporary pacemaker lead could limit the haemodynamic consequences of such an event and may be considered in certain patients. An important question is whether patients with an increased risk can be easily identified and whether this risk is high enough to motivate the insertion of a temporary pacemaker lead.

Bellocci *et al.*[105] addressed this question in a study of 98 patients with BFB who underwent general anaesthesia and surgery. Prior to the surgery all patients were examined by an invasive electrophysiological study in which the HV interval was measured. Patients with an increased HV interval had significantly more complications but these were all related to a higher prevalence of underlying heart diseases in this group. In no patient did a high-grade AV block occur during surgery or postoperatively, and the authors did not recommend prophylactic temporary pacing or electrophysiological studies before surgery in patients with BFB. This supports the findings of previous studies, although these did not include an electrophysiological element.[106–110] There are, however, some reports showing that the risk of high-grade AV block in conjunction with noncardiac surgery could be substantial, especially at advanced age and in regions which promote stimulation of vagal activity.[111] In cardiac surgery the incidence of complete heart block in patients with BBB has been less well studied. Emlein et al.[112] showed that left BBB was an independent risk factor for the development of complete heart block which required permanent pacemaker treatment after bypass surgery.

In a study by Gilchrist and Cameron,[113] the use of temporary pacemaker treatment in patients with BBB undergoing coronary angiography was investigated. Only one of 217 patients (0.5%) had an episode of high-grade AV block requiring temporary backup pacing. Patients with a temporary pacing lead had, however, significantly higher incidence of ventricular fibrillation than patients without. A similar result was found by Morris et al.,[114] who studied the incidence of complete heart block in patients with left BBB undergoing pulmonary artery catheterization.

In conclusion, temporary pacing is not recommended during noncardiac surgery or invasive procedures in patients with BBB, but may instead place the patients at risk for malignant ventricular arrhythmias.

Choice of Pacemaker

When the decision to implant a permanent pacemaker is made, the selection of pacemaker is very much dependent on the estimated risk of high-grade AV block progression. If this risk is substantial and a chronic AV block can be expected within a short period, a dual-chamber pacemaker should be chosen as a first-line treatment. If the likelihood of high-grade AV block progression is lower, the additional cost of implanting a dual-chamber pacemaker can be substantial. In those cases a single-chamber VVI pacemaker with a programmed lower rate or hysteresis would be sufficient. If the patient later develops pacemaker dependence, an upgrading to a dual-chamber system can be performed in suitable patients.

If a VVI pacemaker is chosen, an interesting alternative is one with diagnostic functions. This feature represents a safe and accurate diagnostic tool in the management of patients with infrequent episodes of syncope in whom bradycardias are suspected but not proven. Not only can a ventricular standstill be documented, but it can also be ruled out as a cause of symptoms if the patient has syncope without a pacemaker-detected bradycardia.

Several authors have reported on the use of pacemakers with diagnostic capacity from various manufacturers.[58,115–117] Figure 8.5 shows an example of how one of these devices operates. When the bradycardia-detecting function is activated, the pulse generator remains inhibited until the spontaneous rate has fallen below the

Heart rate

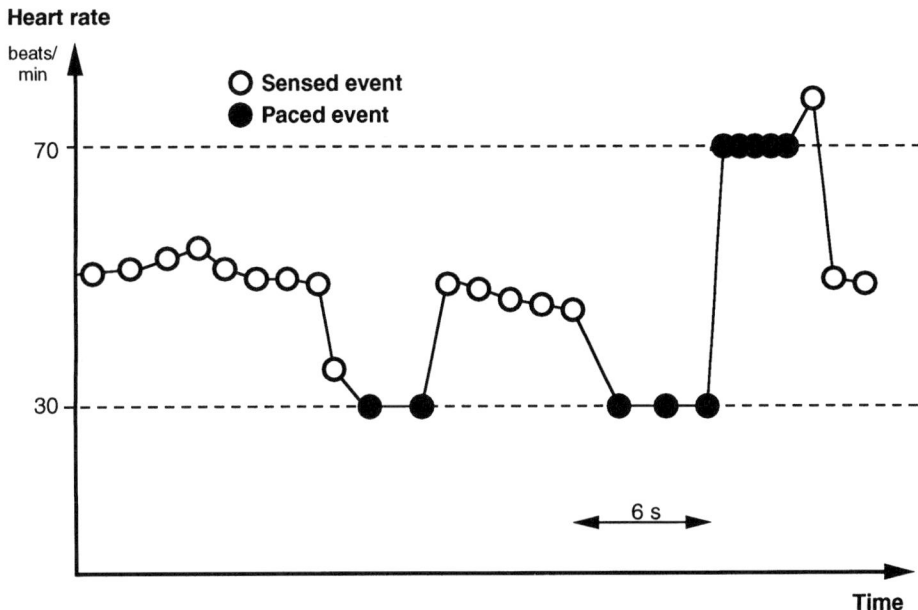

Figure 8.5 Schematic of the function of a bradycardia-detecting pacemaker (Siemens-Elema 738). The example shows a sequence of nine spontaneous beats followed by two paced beats at the bradycardia-detection rate of 30 bpm. The spontaneous activity returns for five beats and then drops below 30 bpm. No spontaneous activity is detected for 6 seconds and the pacemaker delivers three consecutive beats at 30 bpm then starts to operate at the programmed basic rate of 70 bpm. This is termed a bradycardia episode. The pacemaker continues to pace at the basic rate until a spontaneous beat occurs above 70 bpm; this resets the pacemaker, which will remain inhibited until a new episode of bradycardia <30 min occurs. See text for further explanation.

programmed bradycardia-detection rate (in this example programmed to 30 bpm, i.e. an RR interval >2 s). A bradycardia test sequence is then initiated and the pacemaker will deliver three consecutive impulses at the rate of 30 bpm unless spontaneous activity is detected. This is defined as a bradycardia episode and implies that the spontaneous rate has fallen below 30 bpm for more than 6 seconds. After this sequence the pulse generator starts to operate at the basic rate, usually programmed to 70 bpm, until a spontaneous beat is detected. This resets the pacemaker and the bradycardia-detecting function is again activated. An infinite number of bradycardia test sequences can be delivered and the number of paced beats at the bradycardia detection rate as well as the numbers of bradycardia episodes can be disclosed via internal telemetry. Using this device we have found a high concordance of pacemaker-detected bradycardia and documented AV block.[7] In nine patients who had a pacemaker-detected bradycardia, a high-grade AV block was documented after a median time of 11 months (Figure 8.6). This result is similar to previous experiences from the bradycardia-detecting pacemaker.[58,115,116] Bergfeldt et al.[58] also showed that the time between a pacemaker-detected bradycardia and a high-grade AV block could be as long as 100 months, although the casual relationship with such a long interval can be questioned.

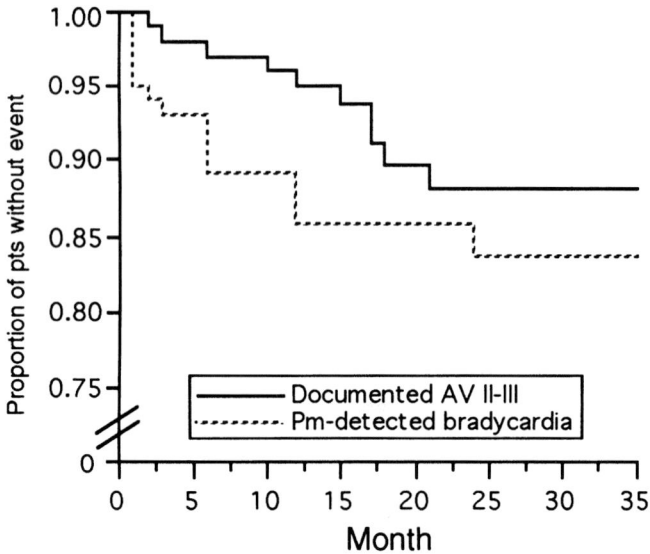

Figure 8.6 Time-relation of pacemaker-detected bradycardia (*n* = 15) and documented high-grade AV block (*n* = 10).

It is, however, important to bear in mind that a bradycardia detected by a VVI pacemaker does not necessarily derive from an intermittent high-grade AV block. A sinus bradycardia could also be the underlying arrhythmia, and a bradycardia detected by a VVI pacemaker rather indicates a need for pacemaker treatment than a high-grade AV block. In order to differentiate between the two types of bradycardia, a dual-chamber diagnostic pacemaker is needed. Such a device has been reported by Lascault et al.,[118] and represents an interesting tool for research.

Conclusions

Patients with BFB have an increased risk of developing high-grade AV block. The progression rate is low in asymptomatic individuals and diagnostic or therapeutic procedures are not indicated in this group.

Patients with syncopal or presyncopal attacks should be investigated thoroughly in order to establish the mechanism behind the syncope and to assess the risk of progression to high-grade AV block. A noninvasive investigation is often inconclusive and an invasive electrophysiological study is then indicated. In order to increase the diagnostic and prognostic value of this investigation, a pharmacological stress test can be used in patients with a normal baseline electrophysiological study. In patients with a history of myocardial infarction, ventricular arrhythmias are common and pro-grammed ventricular stimulation should be part of the protocol.

Patients with BFB and acute myocardial infarction have a poor prognosis, mostly owing to loss of left ventricular function. The risk of high-grade AV block is increased during the acute phase and the patients should be carefully monitored. Prophylactic temporary pacemaker treatment is, however, not indicated, especially not if a thrombolytic agent is given.

The implantation of a permanent pacemaker after a myocardial infarction should be considered in patients with a transient high-grade AV block during the acute phase. In patients without transient AV block a permanent pacemaker is not indicated.

Temporary pacing is not recommended during noncardiac surgery or during invasive procedures in patients with BBB. It may place the patients at risk for malignant ventricular arrhythmias.

When the decision to implant a permanent pacemaker is made, the selection of pacemaker is very much dependent on the estimated risk of high-grade AV block progression. If this risk is substantial and a chronic AV block can be expected within a short period, the patient should be treated with a dual-chamber device. In patients where pacemaker treatment is motivated despite a lower risk of AV block progression, a VVI pacemaker is sufficient, preferably with a diagnostic function.

References

1. Rosenbaum MB, Elizari MV, Lazzari JO. *Los Hemibloqueos*. Parados: Buenos Aires.
2. Anderson RH. Cardiac morphology: the conduction system. In: Julian DG, Camm AJ, Fox KM, Hall RJC, Pool-Wilson PA (eds), *Diseases of the Heart*. London: Baillière Tindall, 1989: 19–23.
3. Fahy GJ, Pinski SL, Miller DP, McCabe N, Pye C, Walsh MJ, Robinson K. Natural history of isolated bundle branch block. *Am J Cardiol* 1996; **77**: 1185–90.
4. Schneider JF, Thomas HE, Kreger BE, McNamara PM, Kannel WB. Newly acquired left bundle branch block: the Framingham Study. *Ann Intern Med* 1979; **90**: 303–10.
5. Schneider JF, Thomas HE, Kreger BE, McNamara PM, Sorlie P, Kannel WB. Newly acquired right bundle branch block: the Framingham Study. *Ann Intern Med* 1980; **92**: 37–44.
6. Rotman M, Triebwasser JH. A clinical and follow-up study of right and left bundle branch block. *Circulation* 1995; **51**: 477–84.
7. Englund A, Bergfeldt L, Rehnqvist N, Astrom H, Rosenqvist M. Diagnostic value of programmed ventricular stimulation in patients with bifascicular block: a prospective study of patients with and without syncope. *JACC* 1995; **26**: 1508–15.
8. Dhingra RC, Palileo E, Strasberg B, Swiryn S, Bauernfeind RA, Wyndham CR, Rosen KM. Significance of the HV interval in 517 patients with chronic bifascicular block. *Circulation* 1981; **64**: 1265–71.
9. McAnulty JH, Rahimtoola SH, Murphy E, DeMotes H, Ritzmann L, Kanarek PE, Kauffman S. Natural history of 'high risk' bundle branch block: final report of a prospective study. *N Eng J Med* 1982; **307**: 137–43.
10. Scheinman MM, Peters RW, Morady F, Sauvé MJ, Malone P, Modin G. Electrophysiologic studies in patients with bundle branch block. *PACE* 1983; **6**: 1157–65.
11. McAnulty JH, Rahimtoola SH. Bundle branch block. *Prog Cardiovasc Dis* 1984; **26**: 333–54.
12. Denes P, Dhingra RC, Wu D, Wyndham CR, Amat-y-Leon F, Rosen KM. Sudden death in patients with chronic bifascicular block. *Arch Intern Med* 1977; **137**: 1005–10.
13. Rabkin SW, Mathewson FA, Tate RB. Natural history of left bundle branch block. *Br Heart J* 1980; **43**: 164–9.
14. Zehender M, Buchner C, Meinertz T, Just H. Prevalence, circumstances, mechanisms, and risk stratification of sudden cardiac death in unipolar single-chamber ventricular pacing. *Circulation* 1992; **85**: 596–605.

15. Dhingra RC, Denes P, Wu D, Chuquimia R, Amat-y-Leon F, Wyndham C, Rosen KM. Syncope in patients with chronic bifascicular block: significance, causative mechanisms, and clinical implications. *Ann Intern Med* 1974; **81**: 302–6.
16. Wiberg TA, Richman HG, Gobel FL. The significance and prognosis of chronic bifascicular block. *Chest* 1977; **71**: 329–34.
17. Scheinman MM, Peters RW, Sauvé MJ, Desai J, Abbott JA, Cogan J, Wohl B, Williams K. Value of the H-Q interval in patients with bundle branch block and the role of prophylactic permanent pacing. *Am J Cardiol* 1982; **50**: 1316–22.
18. Englund A. Electrophysiological studies in patients with bifascicular block (thesis). Stockholm: Karolinska Institute.
19. Gibson TC, Heitzman MR. Diagnostic efficacy of 24-hour electrocardiographic monitoring for syncope. *Am J Cardiol* 1984; **53**: 1013–17.
20. Reiffel JA, Wang P, Bower R, Bigger JT, Livelli F, Ferrick K, Glicklich J, Zimmerman J. Electrophysiologic testing in patients with recurrent syncope: are results predicted by prior ambulatory monitoring? *Am Heart J* 1985; **110**: 1146–53.
21. Lacroix D, Dubuc M, Kus T, Savard P, Shenesa M, Nadeau R. Evaluation of arrhythmic cause of syncope: correlation between Holter monitoring, electrophysiologic testing, and body surface potential mapping. *Am Heart J* 1991; **122**: 1346–54.
22. Kinlay S, Leitch JW, Neil A, Chapman BL, Hardy DB, Fletcher PJ. Cardiac event recorders yield more diagnoses and are more cost-effective than 48-hour Holter monitoring in patients with palpitations: a controlled clinical trial. *Ann Intern Med* 1996; **124**: 16–20.
23. Leitch J, Klein G, Yee R, Lee B, Kallok M, Combs W, Erickson M, Bennett T. Feasibility of an implantable arrhythmia monitor. *PACE* 1992; **15**: 2232–5.
24. Krahn AD, Klein GJ. Norris C, Yee R. The etiology of syncope in patients with negative tilt table testing and electrophysiological testing. *Circulation* 1995; **92**: 1819–24.
25. Byrne JM, Marais HJ, Cheek GA. Exercise-induced complete heart block in a patient with chronic bifascicular block. *J Electrocardiol* 1994; **27**: 339–42.
26. Berkowitz WD, Lau SH, Patton RD, Rosen KM, Damato AN. The use of His bundle recordings in the analysis of unilateral and bilateral bundle branch block. *Am Heart J* 1971; **81**: 340–50.
27. Denes P, Dhingra RC, Wu D, Chuquimia R, Amat-y-Leon F, Wyndham C, Rosen KM. H-V interval in patients with bifascicular block (right bundle branch block and left anterior hemiblock): clinical, electrocardiographic and electrophysiologic correlations. *Am J Cardiol* 1975; **35**: 23–9.
28. Vera Z, Mason DT, Fletcher RD, Awan NA, Massumi RA. Prolonged His-Q interval in chronic bifascicular block: relation to impending complete heart block. *Circulation* 1976; **53**: 47–55.
29. Bloch Thomsen PE. Intracardiac electrography in patients with bifascicular bundle branch block (thesis). *Acta Med Scand* 1981; (suppl 653).
30. Rosen KM, Rahimtoola SH, Chuquimia R, Loeb HS, Gunnar RM. Electrophysiological significance of first-degree atrioventricular block with intraventricular conduction disturbance. *Circulation* 1971; **43**: 491–502.
31. Dhingra RC, Wyndham C, Bauernfeind R, Swiryn S, Deedwania PC, Smith T, Denes P, Rosen KM. Significance of block distal to the His bundle induced by atrial pacing in patients with chronic bifascicular block. *Circulation* 1979; **60**: 1455–64.
32. Petrac D, Radic B, Birtic K, Gjurovic J. Prospective evaluation of infrahisal second-degree AV block induced by atrial pacing in the presence of chronic bundle branch block. *PACE* 1996; **19**: 784–92.
33. Kleinsorge H, Gaida P. Das Verhalten des Serumspiegels nach Intravenöser Injection von Ajmalin. *Klin Wochensch* 1962; **40**: 149–51.
34. Padrini R, Piovan D, Javarnaro A, Cucchini F, Ferrari M. Pharmacokinetics and electrophysiological effects of intravenous ajmaline. *Clin Pharmacokinet* 1993; **25**: 408–14.
35. Chiale PA, Pryzbylski J, Laino RA, Halpern MS, Nau GJ, Sanchez GJ, Lazzari JO, Elizari MV, Rosenbaum M. Usefulness of the ajmaline test in patients with latent bundle branch block. *Am J Cardiol* 1982; **49**: 21–6.

36. Guerot C, Coste A, Valere PE, Tricot R. Ajmaline test in the diagnosis of paroxysmal atrioventricular block (in French). *Arch Mal Coeur Vaiss* 1973; **66**: 1241–53.
37. Guerot C, Valere PE, Laffay N, Lehner JP, Gryman R, Tricot R. Predictive value of the ajmaline test for the diagnosis of distal paroxysmal atrioventricular (in French). *Ann Med Interne Paris* 1981; **132**: 246–51.
38. Puglisi A, Ricci R, Angrisani G. The ajmaline test in identifying patients at high risk of developing complete paroxysmal atrioventricular block (in Italian). *G Ital Cardiol* 1982; **12**: 866–72.
39. Gronda M, Magnani A, Occhetta E, Sauro G, D'Aulerio M, Carfora A, Rossi P. Electrophysiological study of atrio-ventricular block and ventricular conduction defects: prognostic and therapeutical implications. *G Ital Cardiol* 1984; **14**: 768–73.
40. Wunderlich E, Hetze A. Provocation of higher-degree atrioventricular blocks by ajmaline and rapid ventricular pacing in patients with fascicular block. *Cor Vasa* 1984; **26**: 281–8.
41. Kaul U, Kothari SS, Mohan JC, Talwar KK, Bhatia ML. Ajmaline 'stress testing' in chronic bifascicular block. *Ind J Chest Dis Allied Sci* 1986; **28**: 126–34.
42. Kaul U, Dev V, Narula J, Malhotra A, Talwar KK, Bhatai ML. Evaluation of patients with bundle branch block and 'unexplained syncope': a study based on comprehensive electrophysiologic testing and ajmaline test. *PACE* 1988; **11**: 289–96.
43. Saoudi N, Berland J, Hocq R, Cave D, Cribier A, Letac B. Comparison of the effects of ajmaline and procainamide in the diagnosis of paroxysmal atrioventricular block (in French). *Ann Cardiol Angeiol Paris* 1987; **36**: 13–17.
44. Corsini G, Pette R, Cardillo A, Quintiliano G, Di Donna V, Malvezzi A, Mascia F, Correale E. Spontaneous Grade I bundle of His block: clinical, electrocardiographic and electrophysiological studies in 37 patients (in Italian). *G Ital Cardiol* 1989; **19**: 19–27.
45. Poupet JY, Allal J, Vieyres C, Gallimard JF, Coisne D, Barraine R. Development at 5 years of chronic branchial blocks in 164 patients fitted with pacemakers without documented spontaneous atrioventricular block: study of predictive criteria (in French). *Arch Mal Coeur Vaiss* 1989; **82**: 533–40.
46. Gaggioli G, Bottoni N, Brignole M, Menozzi C, Lolli G, Oddone D, Gianfranchi L. Progression to 2nd and 3rd grade atrioventricular block in patients after electrostimulation for bundle-branch block and syncope: a long-term study (in Italian). *G Ital Cardiol* 1994; **24**: 409–16.
47. Scheinman MM, Weiss AN, Shafton E, Benowitz N, Rowland M. Electrophysiological effects of procaine amide in patients with intraventricular conduction delay. *Circulation* 1974; **49**: 522–9.
48. Josephson ME, Caracta AR, Ricciuti MA, Lau SA, Damato AN. Electrophysiological properties of procainamide. *Am J Cardiol* 1974; **33**: 596–603.
49. Tonkin AM, Heddle WF, Tornos P. Intermittent atrioventricular block: procainamide administration as a provocative test. *Aust NZ J Med* 1978; **8**: 594–602.
50. Twidale N, Heddle WF, Tonkin AM. Procainamide administration during electrophysiology study: utility as a provocative test for intermittent atrioventricular block. *PACE* 1988; **11**: 1388–97.
51. Ezi M, Lerman BB, Marchlinski FE, Buxton AE, Josephson ME. Electrophysiologic evaluation of syncope in patients with bifascicular block. *Am Heart J* 1983; **106**: 693–7.
52. Click RL, Gersh BJ, Sugrue DD, Holmes DJ, Wood DL, Osborn MJ, Hammill SC. Role of invasive electrophysiologic testing in patients with symptomatic bundle branch block. *Am J Cardiol* 1987; **59**: 817–23.
53. Birkhead JS, Vaughan Williams EM. Dual effects of disopyramide on atrial and atrioventricular conduction and refractory periods. *Br Heart J* 1977; **39**: 657–60.
54. Desai JM, Scheinman M, Peters RW, O'Young J. Electrophysiological effects of disopyramide in patients with bundle branch block. *Circulation* 1979; **59**: 215–25.
55. Desai JM, Scheinman MM, Hirschfeld D, Gonzalez R, Peters RW. Cardiovascular collapse associated with disopyramide therapy. *Chest* 1981; **79**: 545–51.
56. Timins BI, Gutman JA, Haft JI. Disopyramide-induced heart block. *Chest* 1981; **79**: 477–9.

57. Bergfeldt L, Rosenqvist M, Vallin H, Edhag O. Disopyramide induced second and third degree atrioventricular block in patients with bifascicular block: an acute stress test to predict atrioventricular block progression. *Br Heart J* 1985; **53**: 328–34.
58. Bergfeldt L, Edvardsson N, Rosenqvist M, Vallin H, Edhag O. Atrioventricular block progression in patients with bifascicular block assessed by repeated electrocardiography and a bradycardia-detecting pacemaker. *Am J Cardiol* 1994; **74**: 1129–32.
59. Englund A, Bergfeldt L, Rosenqvist M. Disopyramide stress test: a sensitive and specific tool for predicting impending high-degree atrioventricular block in patients with bifascicular block. *Br Heart J* 1995; **74**: 650–5.
60. Morady F, Higgins J, Peters RW, Schwartz AB, Shen EN, Bhandari A, Scheinman MM, Sauvé MJ. Electrophysiologic testing in bundle branch block and unexplained syncope. *Am J Cardiol* 1984; **54**: 587–91.
61. Twidale N, Heddle WF, Ayres BF, Tonkin AM. Clinical implications of electrophysiology study findings in patients with chronic bifascicular block and syncope. *Aust NZ J Med* 1988; **18**: 841–7.
62. Zipes DP, Akhtar M, Denes P, DeSanctis R, Garson A, Gettes LS, Mason JW, Myerburg RJ, Ruskin JN, Wellens HJJ. Guidelines for clinical intracardiac electrophysiologic studies: a report of the American College of Cardiology/American Heart Association Task Force on Assessment of Diagnostic and Therapeutic Cardiovascular Procedures (Subcommittee to Assess Clinical Intracardiac Electrophysiologic Studies). *JACC* 1989; **14**: 1827–42.
63. Dreifus LS, Griffin JC, Gilette PC, Fisch JC, Mason JW, Parsonnet V. Guidelines for implantation of permanent cardiac pacemakers and antiarrhythmia devices: a report of the American College of Cardiology/American Heart Association Task Force on Assessment of Diagnostic and Therapeutic Cardiovascular Procedures (Committee on Pacemaker Implantation). *JACC* 1991; **18**: 1–13.
64. Canaveris G, Nau GJ. Intraventricular conduction disturbances in flying personnel: development and prognosis of bifascicular blocks. *Aviat Space Environ Med* 1987; **58**: 683–9.
65. Iesaka Y, Nogami A, Aonuma K, Nitta J, Chun YH, Fujiwara H, Hiraoka M. Prognostic significance of sustained monomorphic ventricular tachycardia induced by programmed ventricular stimulation using up to triple extrastimuli in survivors of acute myocardial infarction. *Am J Cardiol* 1990; **65**: 1057–63.
66. Bourke JP, Richards DAB, Ross DL, Wallace EM, McGuire MA, Uther JB. Routine programmed electrical stimulation in survivors of acute myocardial infarction for prediction of spontaneous ventricular tachyarrhythmias during follow-up: results, optimal stimulation protocol and cost-effective screening. *JACC* 1991; **18**: 780–8.
67. Ward DE, Camm AJ. Atrioventricular conduction delays and block. In: *Clinical Electrophysiology of the Heart*. London: Edward Arnold, 1987: 79–93.
68. Sutton R. Syncope. In: Julian DG, Camm AJ, Fox KM, Hall RJC, Poole-Wilson PA (eds), *Diseases of the Heart*. London: Baillière Tindall, 1989: 1431–9.
69. Danforth J, Goldschlager N. Indications for cardiac pacing in the adult. In: Saksena S, Goldschlager N (eds), *Electrical Therapy for Cardiac Arrhythmias*. Philadelphia: WB Saunders, 1990: 91–107.
70. Tolentino AO, Javier RP, Samet P. Indications for cardiac pacing in bradyarrhythmias. In: El-Sherif N, Samet P (eds), *Cardiac Pacing and Electrophysiology*. Philadelphia: WB Saunders, 1991; 652–61.
71. Beck JR, Salem DN, Estes NA, Pauker SG. A computer-based Markov decision analysis of the management of symptomatic bifascicular block: the threshold probability for pacing. *JACC* 1987; **9**: 920–35.
72. Masters AM, Dack S, Jaffe HL. Bundle branch and intraventricular block in acute coronary occlusion. *Am Heart J* 1938; **16**: 285–90.
73. Ginks WR, Sutton R, Oh W, Leatham A. Long-term prognosis after anterior infarction with atrioventricular block. *Br Heart J* 1977; **39**: 186–9.
74. Hindman MC, Wagner GS, Jaro M, Atkins JM, *et al*. The clinical significance of bundle branch block complicating acute myocardial infarction. 1: Clinical characteristics, hospital mortality, and one-year follow-up. *Circulation* 1978; **58**: 679–88.

75. Hauer RN, Lie KI, Liem KL, Durrer D. Long-term prognosis in-patients with bundle branch block complicating acute anteroseptal infarction. *Am J Cardiol* 1982; **49**: 1581–5.
76. Hollander G, Nadiminti V, Lichstein E, Greengart A, Sanders M. Bundle branch block in acute myocardial infarction. *Am Heart J* 1983; **105**: 738–43.
77. Dubois C, Pierard L, Smeets J. Foidart G, Legrand V, Kulbertus H. Short and long term prognostic importance of complete bundle branch block complicating acute myocardial infarction. *Clin Cardiol* 1988; **11**: 292–6.
78. Dubois C, Pierard L, Smeets J, Carier J, Kulbertus H. Long term prognostic significance of atrioventricular block in inferior acute myocardial infarction. *Eur Heart J* 1989; **10**: 816–20.
79. Heras M, Sanz G, Betriu A, Mont L, de Flores T, Navarro-López F. Does left ventricular aneurysm influence survival after acute myocardial infarction? *Eur Heart J* 1990; **11**: 441–6.
80. Ricou F, Nicod P, Gilpin E, Henning H, Ross J. Influence of right bundle branch block on short- and long-term survival after anterior myocardial infarction. *JACC* 1991; **17**: 858–63.
81. Ricou F, Nicod P, Gilpin E, Henning H, Ross J. Influence of right bundle branch block on short- and long-term survival after inferior-wall Q-wave myocardial infarction. *Am J Cardiol* 1991; **67**: 1143–6.
82. Hod H, Goldbourt U, Behar S, and the Study SPRINT Group. Bundle branch block in acute Q wave inferior wall myocardial infarction: a high risk subgroup of inferior myocardial infarction patients. *Eur Heart J* 1995; **16**: 471–7.
83. Godman MJ, Lassers BW, Julian DG. Complete bundle branch block in acute myocardial infarction. *N Engl J Med* 1970; **282**: 237–40.
84. Ross J, Duning A. Right bundle branch block and left axis deviation in acute myocardial infarction. *Br Heart J* 1970; **32**: 847–51.
85. Rizzon P, Biase M, Baissus C. Intraventricular conduction defects in acute myocardial infarction. *Br Heart J* 1972; **36**: 660–8.
86. Scheidt S, Killip T. Bundle branch block complicating acute myocardial infarction. *JAMA* 1972; **222**: 919–24.
87. Atkins JM, Leshin SJ, Blomqvist G, Mullins CB. Ventricular conduction blocks and sudden death in acute myocardial infarction. *N Engl J Med* 1973; **288**: 281–4.
88. Lie KI, Wellens HJJ, Schullenburg RM, Becker AE, Durrer D. Factors influencing prognosis of bundle branch block complicating acute anteroseptal infarction. *Circulation* 1974; **50**: 935–41.
89. Gann D, Balachandran PK, Sherif NE, Samet P. Prognostic significance of chronic versus acute bundle branch block in acute myocardial infarction. *Chest* 1975; **67**: 298–303.
90. Nimetz A, Shubrooks S, Hutter A, DeSanctis R. The significance of bundle branch block during acute myocardial infarction. *Am Heart J* 1975; **90**: 439–44.
91. Hindman MC, Wagner GS, Jaro M, Atkins JM, *et al.* The clinical significance of bundle branch block complicating acute myocardial infarction. 2: Indications for temporary and permanent pacemaker insertion. *Circulation* 1978; **58**: 689–98.
92. Scheinman MM. Treatment of cardiac arrhythmias in patients with acute myocardial infarction. *Am J Surg* 1983; **145**: 707–10.
93. Klein R, Zakauddin V, Mason D. Intraventricular conduction defects in acute myocardial infarction: incidence, prognosis and therapy. *Am Heart J* 1984; **108**: 1007–13.
94. Rosenfeld LE. Bradyarrhythmias, abnormalities of conduction, and indications for pacing in acute myocardial infarction. *Cardiol Clin* 1988; **6**: 49–61.
95. Alpman A, Guldal M, Erol C, Akgun G, Kervancioglu C, Sonel A, Akyol T. The role of arrhythmia and left ventricular dysfunction in patients with acute myocardial infarction and bundle branch block. *Jpn Heart J* 1993; **34**: 145–57.
96. Newby KH, Geiger MJ, Stinnet S, Wildermann N, Pisano E, Natale A. Clinical relevance and outcome of AV block in patients treated with thrombolysis (abstract). *PACE* 1996; **19**: 602.
97. Roth A, Borsuk Y, Keren G, Sheps D, Glick A, Reicher M, Laniado S. Right bundle branch block of unknown age in the setting of acute anterior myocardial infarction: an attempt to define who should be paced prophylactically. *PACE* 1995; **18**: 1496–508.
98. Altamura G, Toscano S, Lo Bianco F, Catalano F, Pistolese M. Emergency cardiac pacing for severe bradycardia. *PACE* 1990; **13**: 2038–43.

99. Opolski G, Kraska T, Ostrzycki A, Zielinski T, Korewicki J. The effect of infarct size on atrioventricular and intraventricular conduction disturbances in acute myocardial infarction. *Int J Cardiol* 1986; **10**: 141–7.

100. Scanlon PJ, Pryor R, Blount SG. Right bundle branch block associated with left superior or inferior intraventricular block: associated with acute myocardial infarction. *Circulation* 1970; **42**: 1135–42.

101. Waugh RA, Wagner GS, Haney TL, Rosati RA, Morris JJ. Immediate and remote prognostic significance of fascicular block during acute myocardial infarction. *Circulation* 1973; **47**: 765–75.

102. Ritter WS, Atkins JM, Blomqvist CG, Mullins CV. Permanent pacing in patients with trifascicular block during acute myocardial infarction. *Am J Cardiol* 1976; **38**: 205–8.

103. Edhag O, Bergfeldt L, Edvardsson N, Holmberg S, Rosenqvist M, Vallin H. Pacemaker dependence in patients with bifascicular block during acute anterior myocardial infarction. *Br Heart J* 1984; **52**: 408–12.

104. Watson RD, Glover DR, Page AJ, Littler WA, Davies P, de Giovanni J, Penntecost BL. The Birmingham trial of permanent pacing in patients with intraventricular conduction disorders after acute myocardial infarction. *Am Heart J* 1984; **108**: 496–501.

105. Bellocci F, Santarelli P, Di Gennaro M, Ansalone G, Fenici R. The risk of cardiac complications in surgical patients with bifascicular block: a clinical and electrophysiologic study in 98 patients. *Chest* 1980; **77**: 343–8.

106. Berg RG, Kottler MN. The significance of bilateral bundle branch block in the preoperative patients. *Chest* 1971; **59**: 62–7.

107. Kunstadt D, Punja M, Cagin N, Fernandez P, Levitt B, Yuceoglu YZ. Bifascicular block: a clinical and electrophysiologic study. *Am Heart J* 1973; **86**: 173–81.

108. Venkataraman K, Madias JE, Hood WJ. Indications for prophylactic preoperative insertion of pacemakers in patients with right bundle branch block and left anterior hemiblock. *Chest* 1975; **68**: 501–6.

109. Rooney JM, Goldiner PL, Muss E. Relationship of RBBB and marked left axis deviation to complete heart block during anaesthesia. *Anaesthesiology* 1976; **44**: 64–6.

110. Pastore JO, Yurchak PM, Janis KM, Murphy JD, Zir LM. The risk of advanced heart block in surgical patients with right bundle branch block and left axis deviation. *Circulation* 1978; **57**: 677–80.

111. Boezaart AP, Clinton CW, Stanley A. Pre-operative prophylactic transvenous cardiac pacing for bifascicular heart block. *S Afr J Surg* 1989; **27**: 103–5.

112. Emlein G, Huang SK, Pires LA, Rofino K, Okike ON, Vander ST. Prolonged brady-arrhythmias after isolated coronary artery bypass graft surgery. *Am Heart J* 1993; **126**: 1084–90.

113. Gilchrist IC, Cameron A. Chronic bundle branch block and use of temporary transvenous pacemakers during coronary arteriography. *Cathet Cardiovasc Diagn* 1988; **15**: 229–32.

114. Morris D, Mulvihill D, Lew WY. Risk of developing complete heart block during bedside pulmonary artery catheterization in patients with left bundle-branch block. *Arch Intern Med* 1987; **147**: 2005–10.

115. Edhag O, Elmqvist H, Vallin H. An implantable pulse generator indicating asystole or extreme bradycardia. *PACE* 1983; **6**: 166–70.

116. Rosenqvist M, Edhag O, Vallin H. Clinical experience with a bradycardia indicating pacemaker. *PACE* 1983; **6**: 515–24.

117. Shaw DB, Kekwick CA, Veale D, Whistance TW. Unexplained syncope: a diagnostic pacemaker? *PACE* 1983; **6**: 720–5.

118. Lascault G, Barnay C, Cazeau S, Frank R, Medvedowsky JL. Preliminary evaluation of a dual chamber pacemaker with bradycardia diagnostic functions. *PACE* 1995; **18**: 1636–43.

9

Pacing in Vasovagal Syncope

D. G. Benditt and K. G. Lurie*

In general, vasovagal syncopal symptoms tend to be solitary events without long-term consequences. From a diagnostic perspective, the nature of the problem can often be readily suspected by an experienced physician based on medical history alone. Nevertheless, selected testing (especially tilt-table testing) may be prudent to confirm this suspicion in certain patients.[1-3] On the other hand, complex diagnostic studies are needed only infrequently.[1,2,5] In terms of prevention, many vasovagal syncopal episodes are clearly related to circumstances which may be avoided (e.g. venipuncture, hot stuffy environments); in other instances, patients quickly learn to recognize potential 'triggers' (e.g. emotional upset, pain) and take protective action in advance so as to either minimize the chance of harm or possibly abort the event entirely. In those patients in whom vasovagal symptoms are recurrent, the episodes are rarely very frequent and recurrences are usually separated by extended asymptomatic periods. In essence, therapeutic interventions (apart from education) are not a consideration in the vast majority of patients experiencing vasovagal syncope.

Notwithstanding the generally 'benign' nature of vasovagal syncope, there is nevertheless a subset of afflicted individuals in whom prevention of recurrences is important enough to require medical intervention. For example, some patients may have already suffered injury or economic loss owing to their susceptibility to recurrent faints. In others, syncope may have occurred without warning, and consequently similar recurrences may be expected to result in unacceptable risk of accident and physical injury. The latter scenario (i.e. absence of usual premonitory symptoms) is particularly prevalent in older patients with vasovagal spells.[6] Similarly, even infrequent recurrences may be unacceptable in certain occupational or avocational settings (e.g. airline pilots, surgeons, heavy machinery operators, commerical vehicle operators, window-washers, sky-divers, scuba divers, etc.). Finally, some 'high profile' circumstances force initiation of attempts at prophylaxis (e.g. prominent public figures, highy paid professional athletes). Consequently, while only a small percentage of affected individuals may be candidates for therapy, there is nonetheless a subset of the vasovagal syncope population in which there is a clear-cut need for effective preventive treatments.

*The authors would like to thank Barry L. S. Detloff for technical assistance, and Wendy Markuson for preparation of the manuscript.

Currently, strategies for prophylactic treatment of vasovagal syncope may be divided into three general categories: (1) pharmacological interventions; (2) non-pharmacological methods (including cardiac pacing); and (3) combined therapies. Pharmacological approaches, although not without controversy, have become relatively widely accepted as first-line treatment when more than education and/or reassurance is needed. The role of cardiac pacing remains less well established. This chapter examines published reports addressing pacing in vasovagal syncope, and attempts to define the current state-of-the-art and identify elements in need of further consideration.

Prevention of Recurrent Vasovagal Syncope: General Concepts

Overview of Treatment Options

In recent years, clinical investigation into the prevention of vasovagal syncope recurrences has largely focused on pharmacological interventions.[2,7–17] This topic, which for the most part lies outside the scope of this chapter, has been the subject of numerous published reports and reviews (see for example references 3 and 4). In brief, a wide range of drugs have been evaluated in this setting. In uncontrolled studies, beta-adrenergic blocking drugs, disopyramide, certain vasoconstrictor agents (e.g. etilephrine, midodrine) and serotonin reuptake blockers have been reported to be helpful in preventing syncope recurrences. On the other hand, with the exception of atenolol, the few controlled studies which have been undertaken have not been so encouraging. Other agents, such as volume expanders (e.g. fludrocortisone, salt tablets), although less well studied, have nonetheless taken on a lesser but useful supportive role in treatment regimens. Belladonna alkaloids (e.g. scopolamine) and purinergic antagonists (e.g. theophylline) have met with even less enthusiasm, although they are apparently helpful in selected cases. Unfortunately, in the absence of large placebo-controlled trials, there remains uncertainty regarding the effectiveness of any of these agents.

Apart from cardiac pacing for selected patients, nonpharmacological treatments for vasovagal syncope prevention include a variety of broadly applicable educational and physical manoeuvres. The latter are among the most important strategies for dealing with vasovagal faints, and include stress and anxiety management, as well as education regarding recognition and avoidance of provoking events and awareness of useful evasive actions (e.g. lying down). In some cases, exposure to a 'controlled' faint using tilt-table technique can be beneficial by facilitating earlier and more accurate recognition of warning symptoms, and by reducing anxiety and apprehension.[17] Another treatment in this category, but one which tends to be less acceptable to patients with vasovagal syncope than is the case in patients with orthostatic hypotension, is use of antigravity clothing. The latter is an uncomfortable inconvenience which is difficult to justify given the unpredictable intermittency of vasovagal events.

The notion of combination therapy reasonably encompasses the use of both oral medications as well as nonpharmacological treatments (especially education and reassurance) in patients with recurrent vasovagal symptoms. However, since educa-tion is probably better considered a basic aspect of all medical treatment, combined treatment is more usefully interpreted at the present time as the addition of cardiac pacing to a drug regimen. In the not too distant future, implantable pacing/drug infusion systems may further enhance the sophistication of combined therapies. Such an innovation may prove particularly beneficial in cases that are difficult to treat, as well as in those patients who are reluctant to take daily oral medication for prevention of rare events, or who are otherwise noncompliant.

Considerations in Treatment Selection

Although the essential clinical features of vasovagal syncope have become widely appreciated since the landmark description by Sir Thomas Lewis in the early 1930s,[18] it was only with the advent of tilt-table testing that substantial numbers of patients could be conveniently evaluated in the clinical laboratory during induced vasovagal episodes. It is on these observations that recently evolving strategies for prevention of vasovagal syncope are predicated.

Tilt-table testing has been used to better understand the pathophysiology associated with vasovagal syncope, and to try to verify the efficacy of proposed pharmacological and pacing therapies. Findings suggest that the electrophysiologi-cal and haemodynamic picture varies among patients, and may even vary markedly from episode to episode within a given individual.[19–22] Thus, in terms of a specific single syncopal event, a few patients may be characterized as exhibiting either a predominantly cardioinhibitory picture (i.e. bradycardia being the principal cause of the faint), or a 'pure' vasodepressor syndrome (i.e. vascular dilation is the crucial factor causing systemic hypotension). The vast majority of patients, however, exhibit a mixed picture in which the relative importance of cardioinhibitory and vasodepressor components may be difficult to ascertain.[20–22] In fact, in the 'mixed' form, the heart rate may seem to be entirely 'normal', yet when placed in the context of a falling systemic pressure it is inappropriately low (i.e. 'relative bradycardia').

A detailed classification[21] of the various vasovagal responses, as observed during tilt-table testing, has been provided by a multicentre European working group (see Table 9.1). In this scheme, individuals with either Type 2A or 2B 'cardioinhibitory' forms of vasovagal faint would seem to be the most appropriate for pacing interven-tion. However, it is crucial that this hypothesis be carefully tested. For example, if it were shown that the electrophysiological/haemodynamic features of induced faints were not reproducible in individual patients, or were not indicative of the course of events during spontaneous episodes in the same patient, or were widely variable from time to time, the utility of tilt-testing for predicting appropriate treatment would be undermined.

The reproducibility of tilt-table testing in terms of inducing syncope has been the subject of a number of studies. In general there has been a relatively high concordance of outcomes within individuals (approximately 80–85%) for two tests carried out

Table 9.1　Vasovagal international study classification for tilt-induced cardioneurogenic (vasovagal) syncope[a]

Type 1: mixed
Heart rate initially increases with head-up tilt and later decreases, but remains above 40 bpm or is less than 40 bpm only briefly (<10 s), and without asystole ⩾3 s. Blood pressure may increase initially but later decreases before heart rate decreases.

Type 2A: cardioinhibitory
Heart rate increases with tilting, then decreases to <40 bpm for >10 s, or has asystole >3 s. Blood pressure may increase initially but decreases before the heart rate decreases.

Type 2B: cardioinhibitory
Heart rate increases initially, then decreases to <40 bpm for >10 s, or has asystole >3 s. Blood pressure decreases to hypotensive levels only at or after the time at which heart rate decreases.

Type 3: pure vasodepressor
Heart rate increases initially and decreases less than 10% from peak value at time of syncope. Blood pressure decreases to account for syncope.

[a] This table does not include the exceptions catalogued by the Vasovagal International Study Investigators.[21]

either on the same day or even many days apart.[23–26] However, the intrapatient reproducibility of electrophysiological and haemodynamic characteristics during induced vasovagal spells has been less well characterized. In this regard, Chen *et al.*[23] reported outcomes of two sequential 80-degree head-up tilt tests (approximately 1 hour apart) in 23 patients (6.5 to 74 years) undergoing evaluation for recurrent syncope of unknown origin. Overall, 15 individuals (65%) developed syncope in either the first or second tilt procedure, while 8 patients remained asymptomatic. The findings in the two tests were concordant with respect to provocation of syncope (i.e. positive in both tests or negative in both tests) in 20 cases (87%). Furthermore, there was a strong correlation between heart rate and haemodynamic findings in both the tests, suggesting that the characteristics of the induced episodes were very similar within a given patient. Similarly, review of the findings presented by Grubb *et al.*,[25] also suggest that repeat tilts 3–7 days apart tend to exhibit a strong intrapatient concordance for heart rate and blood pressure.

On the other hand, Fish *et al.*,[20] came to a somewhat different conclusion during evaluation of a younger group of patients (8 to 19 years). In their study, a series of 90-degree tilts for 15 min each were undertaken in the baseline state followed if necessary by isoproterenol provocation. Findings revealed that syncope or presyncope was reproduced in 14 of 21 cases, with a further 4 patients exhibiting milder symptoms in the second test. However, the pattern of physiological response (i.e. cardioinhibitory, vasodepressor, mixed) varied. Thus, despite their 67% reproducibility rate (with respect to syncopal symptoms), these investigators were less convinced of the utility of head-up tilt as a useful method for assessing therapeutic interventions. Similar concerns have been raised by de Mey and Enterling.[27] Additional studies providing even more careful evaluation of moment-to-moment heart rate and blood pressure changes would be helpful in clarifying the potential utility of tilt-table testing for predicting the optimal treatment avenue, and later assessing efficacy.

Evaluating Treatment Efficacy: Clinical End-points

The evaluation of candidate therapies for vasovagal syncope is not straightforward. First, it is probably unrealistic to expect any treatment to eliminate all events entirely. Indeed, other than in conditions which have a high probability of a fatal outcome (e.g. the resuscitated out-of-hospital arrest victim who is a candidate for implantable cardioverter–defibrillator therapy), such a treatment requirement would almost certainly expose patients to excessively high risk of adverse treatment effects (e.g. drug toxicity). Therefore 'syncope recurrence' alone is an inadequate end-point in this setting. Techniques comparable to those proposed for evaluation of drug treatment in supraventricular tachycardias should be considered.[28–30] Thus, the number of episodes, the duration of symptom-free intervals, the presence or absence of a premonitory phase and the occurrence of physical injury or accident, should be reported. Second, the effectiveness of a treatment based solely on the results of follow-up tilt-table testing relies on an as yet unproven relationship. In this regard, despite the fact that the conversion of a 'positive' tilt to a 'negative' tilt has been thought to indicate an effective treatment, the accuracy of such testing for predicting long-term treatment benefit (or inadequacy) is unknown. Finally, placebo-controlled trials of relatively long duration are essential given the sporadic nature of syncopal episodes and the potentially powerful placebo effect of any proposed treatment. In essence, all currently available clinical studies of treatment efficacy suffer from important end-point assessment limitations, and consequently interpretation of their results must be undertaken with caution.

Current Status of Pacing for Vasovagal Syncope

Overview

Stimulating the heart to prevent syncope is not a new concept, but in fact was initially contemplated more than a century ago. In 1887, MacWilliam wrote that 'in certain forms of cardiac arrest there appears to be a possibility of restoring by artificial means the rhythmic beat, and tiding over a sudden and temporary danger'.[31] In an even more prescient speculation, he went on to state that 'such is especially the case in those instances where cardiac failure assumes the form of an inhibition of the heart beat by impulses reaching the organ along the vagus nerves'. Of course, it was not possible to test this concept until approximately 80 years later. Even then, despite more than three decades of experience with implantable pacemakers, substantial controversy remains regarding appropriate pacing modes for – and overall efficacy of – pacemaker therapy in those forms of syncope to which MacWilliam was alluding (i.e. neurally mediated syncope including carotid sinus syndrome and vasovagal syncope). Nevertheless, current American Heart Association/American College of Cardiology guidelines,[32] as well as those of the British Pacing and Electrophysiology Working Group,[33] provide a Class II indication for pacing as a treatment for vasovagal syncope.

In carotid sinus syndrome, cardiac pacing is a standard element in the treatment plan when there is evidence of an important cardioinhibitory component, whether or not a substantial concomitant vasodepressor element is present.[34–41] Such is not the case, however, for vasovagal syncope where treatment is heavily (and for the most part appropriately) focused on education and reassurance, with pharmacological agents (see earlier) being the principal 'backup' if needed. Several factors account for the marked difference in therapeutic approach to these two forms of neurally mediated syncope.

First, although fatal or near-fatal outcomes are rare in either case, syncope-related physical injury is a greater concern in the usually older patients with carotid sinus syndrome and a lesser issue in most (generally somewhat younger) vasovagal syncope patients.

Second, since vasovagal syncope is typically accompanied by an identifiable set of warning symptoms which patients can be taught to recognize (theoretically thereby permitting their undertaking evasive action) it tends to be accorded a more benign prognosis than is the case for the typically abrupt (without substantial warning) loss of consciousness associated with carotid sinus syndrome. The less severe the presumed prognosis, the greater the barrier against proceeding with a procedure which has such important economic, psychological and lifestyle consequences.

Third, there is a widespread clinical impression that the cardioinhibitory component is more consistent and important in carotid sinus syndrome than in vasovagal syncope where a clinically significant concomitant vasodepressor response is almost universally present. The latter, of course, would not be expected to be altered by conventional pacing techniques.

Fourth, a substantial percentage of vasovagal fainters are relatively young, otherwise healthy, and more concerned about body image than are most older individuals. As a result, vasovagal fainters may be less inclined to accept a recommendation for pacemaker implantation.

Finally, in contrast to carotid sinus syndrome,[34–41] there have been relatively few published reports examining the effects of pacing in vasovagal syncope (see later). Further, most of the studies that do exist incorporate only a small number of patients followed for a brief period of time. Additionally, the treatment 'end-points' used in these reports have varied, leading to some considerable confusion among clinicians as to the meaningfulness of the results.

Clinical Investigations of Cardiac Pacing in Vasovagal Syncope

Although a wide array of potentially beneficial pharmacological measures for treatment of patients with recurrent vasovagal spells are available, there remains an important subset of individuals in whom symptom control continues to be a problem. As a rule, these patients are currently best identified by failure of pharmacological means to prevent spontaneous symptom recurrences (see section on 'end-points' earlier). However, drug-related side-effects and compliance issues may detract from the effectiveness of pure pharmacological strategies and lead towards earlier consideration of cardiac pacing in some cases. Findings which additionally support such a consideration include evidence of overt or relative bradycardia at the time of symptoms. On the other hand, pacing therapy does not yet seem to be warranted as a first step for treatment of solitary faints (see earlier caveat regarding occupational/ avocational status), even in the face of lengthy asystolic pauses. In fact, the duration of documented asystole does not appear to impact the clinical picture of prognosis associated with these types of faint.[42-44]

Only within the last few years has the potential utility of cardiac pacing for treatment of patients with recurrent vasovagal syncope become the subject of clinical study. In an initial consideration of this problem, Fitzpatrick *et al.*,[45] reported findings in two patients who originally received single-chamber ventricular pacemakers in an attempt to prevent syncope of unknown origin. However, symptoms subsequently recurred in both cases. Tilt-table testing not only confirmed susceptibility to neurally mediated hypotension/bradycardia (i.e. vasovagal mechanism) in these individuals, but also suggested that symptomatic hypotension was actually aggravated by ventricular pacing (the 'pacemaker effect'). Subsequently, the pacing systems in both patients were converted to dual-chamber modes (DDI mode, with a basic rate of 50 bpm and a hysteresis feature in which bradycardia (< 50 bpm) triggered the device to pace at a higher rate (80 bpm). Following this change, one of the two patients became asymptomatic while the other continued to experience symptoms.

Somewhat later, in a prospective evaluation of the effects of temporary dual-chamber pacing in vasovagal syncope, Fitzpatrick *et al.*,[46] reported haemodynamic and symptom status in seven patients with recurrent syncope who underwent tilt-table testing, and in whom vasovagal reactions were inducible on two successive days. The pacing protocol in this study utilized a hysteresis feature in which the base rate was 50 bpm with the subsequent intervention pacing rate being 90 bpm. Among all patients, pacing significantly improved cardiac index (baseline 1.0 ± 0.2 L/min/ m^2 *vs* paced 1.6 ± 0.3 L/min/m^2) and mean arterial blood pressure (baseline 30 ± 11 mmHg *vs* paced 48 ± 12 mmHg) during induced vasovagal reactions. Further, pacing reduced the rate at which blood pressure tended to decrease and prolonged head-up tilt tolerance (i.e. potentially offering a longer period in which patients have the opportunity to take evasive action). In five cases syncope was prevented despite evident onset of a vasovagal reaction as attested to by both haemodynamic recordings, and the evolution of sufficient bradycardia to initiate pacing. Two other patients exhibited no apparent symptomatic benefit. Quantitatively, following onset of the vasovagal reaction the duration of upright posture tolerated was longer during pacing than in the baseline state (unpaced 0.9 ± 1.2 min *vs* paced 3.2 ± 1.6 min; $p < 0.01$). These findings provided considerable encouragement to the notion that pacing may be a potentially useful therapy. However, this study addressed neither the reproducibility of benefit nor whether benefit could be sustained in the long term.

In a similar study using temporary pacing, Samoil *et al.*,[47] provided further support for the utility of cardiac pacing for prevention of vasovagal syncope. They reported findings in six patients (average age 31 ± 12 years) in whom hypotension and bradycardia were reproducibly inducible during tilt-table study. Patients were evaluated in the baseline unpaced state, during single-chamber ventricular pacing, and again during dual-chamber cardiac pacing. The pacing algorithm employed rate-hysteresis; i.e. after sufficiently severe bradycardia (< 60 bpm) had been detected, the intervention pacing rate was set to 20 bpm above resting rate. Findings indicated that with respect to end-points such as time to onset of symptoms or total tolerated upright tilt time, ventricular pacing proved to be essentially ineffective. On the other hand, dual-chamber pacing significantly improved upright tilt tolerance (dual-chamber pacing 25 ± 6 min *vs* unpaced 12 ± 6 min; $p < 0.001$). In addition, dual-chamber pacing prevented syncope during tilt-table testing in three patients (50%).

In a somewhat larger study, Sra *et al.*,[48] examined the impact of temporary conventional cardiac pacing techniques for prevention of tilt-induced hypotension and bradycardia in 22 syncope patients in whom an initial tilt-test was associated with bradycardia of presumably sufficient magnitude (heart rate nadir <60 bpm) to trigger a pacing system. The pacing intervention was undertaken at a rate approximately 20% higher than the supine resting heart rate, and was initiated while the patient was supine, and was continued throughout the tilt. Twenty patients were evaluated during atrioventricular sequential mode pacing, while two others with atrial fibrillation were tested in a single-chamber ventricular pacing mode. Findings revealed that despite pacing, mean arterial pressure fell significantly during upright tilt (97 ± 19 mmHg to 57 ± 19 mmHg). However, the magnitude of tilt-induced hypotension was less during pacing than during tilt-testing undertaken in the baseline untreated state (blood pressure decline: paced 41 ± 19 *vs* unpaced 59 ± 16). Furthermore, symptoms were much improved. One patient remained asymptomatic and one other complained of dizziness but was not hypotensive during pacing. Fifteen patients had only presyncopal symptoms while five developed syncope. In contrast, all had been syncopal in the baseline state. These results, despite the investigators' scepticism, are quite encouraging in regard to the potential utility of cardiac pacing in vasovagal syncope. In essence, using a relatively simple pacing algorithm, pacing proved to be remarkably effective in converting syncope to less severe manifestations of vasovagal reactions (i.e. presyncope) in a considerable percentage of patients in this study.

The most important available evidence supporting the potential utility of pacing in vasovagal syncope is found in the report by Petersen *et al.*[49] This study reviewed an experience with implantable pulse generators programmed to the DDI mode in 37 patients in whom vasovagal syncope appeared to exhibit a predominantly cardio-inhibitory character as assessed during tilt-testing. The devices were programmed to detect heart rates in the 40–50 bpm range, and respond with pacing rates of 80–90 bpm. Patients were followed for 39 ± 19 months. Symptomatic improvement was noted in 84% of cases, with complete resolution of symptoms in 35%. The overall frequency of syncopal episodes (annual syncope burden) was reported to be reduced from 125.8 to 12.6 episodes per year. Clinical features predicting the usefulness of pacing included: younger patient age (58 *vs* 70 years), lower supine systolic blood pressure (135 *vs* 163 mmHg) and absence of prodromal symptoms.

Automatic Detection of Vasovagal Syncope in Implantable Pacemakers

The studies summarized above generally support the notion that cardiac pacing may benefit selected patients with recurrent (predominantly cardioinhibitory) vasovagal syncope. However, reliable automatic detection of imminent vasovagal events is a necessity in order to bring the promise of pacing into reality.

At present, pacing systems used in vasovagal syncope patients rely solely on recognition of marked bradycardia in order to trigger an intervention. As a result, such systems are only likely to be of benefit in a given patient if distinct heart rate slowing is a definitive marker signalling onset of symptomatic hypotension. Unfortunately, this is not always the case. Indeed, 'pathological' bradycardia often occurs only after substantial hypotension has already become manifest in many vasovagal patients. For example, in a study from our laboratory, Chen *et al.*,[50] pointed out that the evolution of hypotension often began many seconds before onset of asystole in patients being evaluated on the tilt-table (Figure 9.1). Somewhat later, Sra *et al.*[48] reported essentially the same finding. In 17 of 22 patients (77%) in the latter study, onset of hypotension was noted on average 42 ± 29 seconds before development of significant bradycardia. In the remaining 23%, the findings were coincident. Consequently, pacing interventions based on heart rate changes alone may not be optimally timed to achieve the best result in the majority of cases. Alternative or supplementary sensors appear to be essential (see later).

Despite the evident limitation associated with relying solely on heart rate changes as the diagnostic tool, it is certainly the most practicable first step. In this context, preliminary reports assessing the utility of a rate drop response (RDR) diagnostic algorithm along with a relatively rapid pacing intervention have been encouraging.[51–54] The current RDR algorithm utilizes a programmable 'Window' (defined by a 'Top' heart rate, a 'Bottom' heart rate, and 'Width' in 'beats') to identify heart rate changes suggestive of an evolving vasovagal event (Figure 9.2). When the 'Window' criteria are met and confirmed by a programmable number of 'Confirmation' beats at a rate lower than the 'Bottom' rate, a pacing 'Intervention' is initiated. The pacing intervention rate is typically selected to be relatively rapid, and of a sufficient duration to support the circulation until the acute episode has presumably subsided. Thereafter, the rate slowly decrements back to the atrial-tracking or sensor-indicated rate depending on which is the faster at the time.

Programming of the RDR algorithm appears to be reasonably easy. In a recently reported multicentre study, programming and effectiveness of the algorithm were assessed in 28 patients (14 to 81 years) with recurrent cardioinhibitory vasovagal syncope.[54] Prior to pacing, patients averaged 1.1 syncopal episodes per month; physical injury occurred in 13 (46%) and automobile accidents in 2 (7%). Following pacemaker therapy (mean follow-up 6.6 months), the mean syncope burden was 0.3/month ($p < 0.05$ *vs* pre-pacemaker). At last follow-up, 75% or more of the patients were programmed to a Window height (Top rate minus Bottom rate) $\leqslant 20$ bpm, two or three Confirmation beats, an Intervention rate $\geqslant 100$ bpm and an Intervention duration of 1 or 2 min. Only Top and Bottom rates showed widespread selection variability, suggesting that these are the most patient-specific of the programmable parameters.

Pacing Mode and Algorithm

Assuming pacing therapy is to be instituted, a dual-chamber pacing mode is essential. Furthermore, atrial pacing (AAI or AAIR) alone is contraindicated owing to the

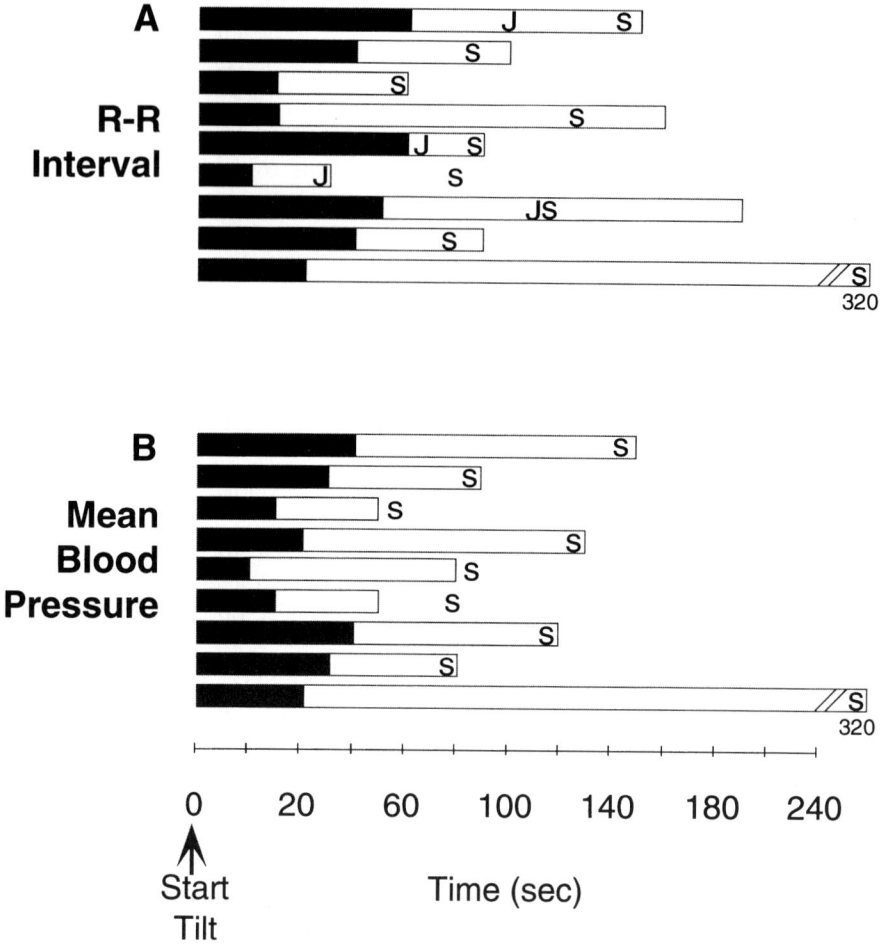

Figure 9.1 Graphs summarizing the temporal relation of changes in cardiac rhythm (A) and changes in systemic mean blood pressure (B) with development of syncope (S) in each tilt-positive isoproterenol patient ($n = 9$). The filled bars in the upper panel represent the time (seconds) from start of upright tilt to onset of measurable RR interval prolongation or blood pressure decline. The open bars represent the time from onset of PR prolongation to maximal observed RR interval. In four patients the heart rhythm changed from sinus to AV junctional (J) rhythm before or during syncope. Onset of syncope was not closely associated with maximal RR interval prolongation. In the lower panel, the filled bars represent the time from assumption of upright tilt to first measurable sustained decrease of systemic pressure. The open bars represent the time taken until nadir of blood pressure decrease was observed. Note the generally close association of the onset of syncopal symptoms with nadir of the blood pressure. (Reproduced from reference 50 with permission)

potential for transient AV block during vasovagal events (a concern also well known in carotid sinus syndrome). In addition, pure atrial-tracking modes (e.g. VDD or VDDR) are generally undesirable since the atrial rate is almost always inappropriately slow for the magnitude of hypotension, and in the presence of atrial bradycardia the onset of ventricular pacing (possibly with intact retrograde conduction) may aggravate hypotension. The findings of Petersen et al.[55] with VDD pacing support this view.

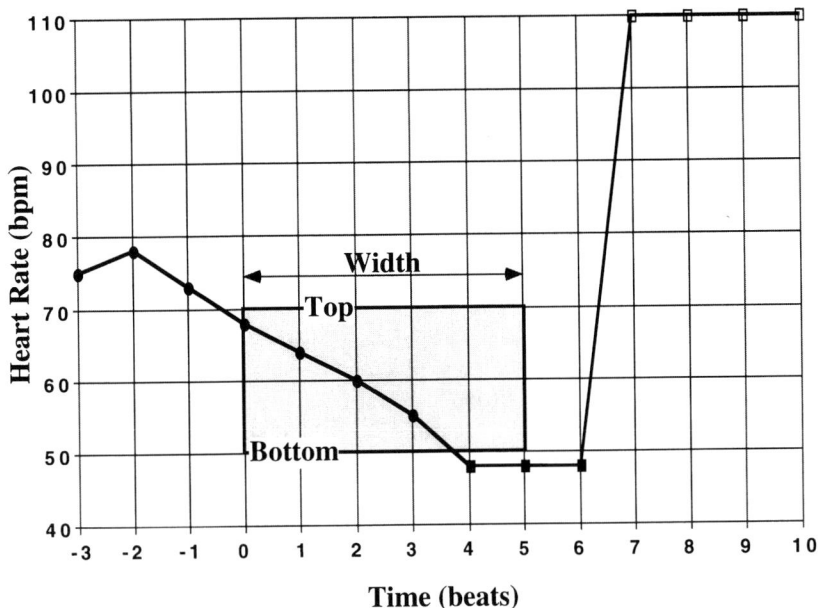

Figure 9.2 Schematic illustrating the programmable Window used in the rate-drop response algorithm. The Top and Bottom rates as well as the Width (number of beats) are programmable. In order to trigger a pacing intervention, the native heart rate must fall through the Window (Top to Bottom) in a time frame less than the programmed Window duration. In addition, a preselected number of beats (confirmation beats) must occur at a rate less than the Bottom rate. In this example, the Window is indicated by the box. During a vasovagal episode, the heart rate falls through the Window and a predetermined number of Confirmation beats (in this case 3) are detected before pacing Intervention (in this instance at 110 bpm) is initiated. The duration of the pacing intervention is programmable, with the usual setting being 2 or 3 min.

During paired tilt-table tests in patients with an implanted dual-chamber pacemaker, there was no difference in either the number of patients who developed syncope (unpaced 7/11 *vs* paced 9/11), or the time to syncope (paced 23 ± 11 min *vs* unpaced 21 ± 13 min). Prodrome may have been somewhat extended by pacing. Therefore, a modified DDI or DDI(R) pacing mode appears to be the best option to turn to after detection of an event. At other times, the patient should be permitted to remain in a more physiological DDD or DDD(R) pacing mode.

Pacing Algorithms

The optimum pacing algorithm for prevention of vasovagal syncope has not yet been developed. At present, a form of rate hysteresis appears to offer benefit (see the RDR discussion earlier). Essentially, after the vasovagal syncope detection algorithm is triggered (i.e. detects a vasovagal event), the pulse generator responds by pacing at a rate rapid enough to be appropriate to the degree of hypotension present. Based on available clinical experience, the intervention rate needs to be ⩾100 bpm (more likely 110–120 bpm). Periodically, the device will need to terminate pacing and assess native heart rate. If the latter has returned to normal, the pacing sequence will terminate. If not, a further period of pacing support will be offered. Unfortunately, it is not yet possible to monitor and respond to an even more crucial parameter, systemic pressure.

Future Developments

Detection Algorithms

As noted above, current detection of vasovagal syncope relies on heart rate slowing, a marker which for reasons discussed earlier may not be sufficiently sensitive in many cases. Additionally, specificity is a concern. Abrupt heart rate slowing may accompany several important nonvasovagal conditions, such as intrinsic sick sinus syndrome, sleep, or acute myocardial infarction. In such circumstances, inappropriate initiation of a high-rate pacing intervention may be undesirable. Consequently, it is imperative that future pacing systems collect additional information and correlate this information with the heart rate findings. For example, theoretical considerations suggest that markers of systemic pressure, oxygen saturation, myocardial fibre shortening, respiratory and heart rate variability and PR or QT interval changes could prove helpful in this context. The goal is to provide more sensitive and specific recognition of vasovagal syndromes at an earlier stage in the progression of events. Furthermore, application of one or more of these alternative sensors would allow extension of pacing therapy to those patients who never develop severe bradycardia during their spells (although 'relative' bradycardia may indeed be present).

Pacing Interventions

At present, pacing interventions are restricted to the time period after onset of an abrupt bradycardia. By this time, however, considerable vasodilatation has already occurred, and pacing may not be able to compensate sufficiently. Potentially, intervention at an earlier stage (i.e. before hypotension has become too severe) could prove more effective in stabilizing the circulation. The report by Sra et al.,[48] in which pacing was initiated in the supine posture prior to tilt, is somewhat encouraging in this regard. On the other hand, Sutton and coworkers had less success when pacing was manually triggered in the upright patient at what appeared to be an early stage of the vasovagal event (R. Sutton, personal communication). Further study of this concept is needed.

Combined Interventions

The combination of drug and device therapy is likely to be a necessary strategy in the most difficult-to-control patients with recurrent vasovagal spells, and may also prove useful in other forms of neurally mediated syncope such as cough syncope and postmicturition syncope.[3,4] At present, the administration of oral mediations in conjunction with an implantable pulse generator is the most reasonable direction to pursue. However, for reasons outlined earlier, many patients with vasovagal syncope may be reluctant to accept conventional daily pharmacological treatment regimens, especially when serious symptomatic vasovagal events have been infrequent. Consequently, the concept of combining pacing and drug infusion capability into a single automatic treatment device may have merit. Agents such as midodrine, ephedrine, or perhaps even disopyramide, could be candidates for parenteral delivery. However, before such an approach becomes feasible, considerable progress must be made in both the development of diagnostic algorithms and our understanding of drug dosing and routes of delivery.

Conclusion

Controversy continues to surround the current role and potential future impact of cardiac pacing in management of patients with recurrent vasovagal syncope. At the present time several lines of clinical investigation point towards potential effectiveness in selected patients. However, maximum benefit from this therapeutic avenue will not be attained until we achieve greater understanding of the spectrum of manifestations of vasovagal syncope and devise techniques to recognize its onset at an early stage. In this regard, implantable pacing systems with sophisticated sensors and extended memories may facilitate obtaining the necessary 'natural history' information. Perhaps these insights, along with a broader base of clinical experience, will lead to more optimal pacing algorithms and/or allow combining pacing systems with allied disciplines such as neural recording and drug infusion in order to provide even more effective treatment options.

References

1. Benditt DG, Ferguson DW, Grubb BP, *et al*. Tilt-table testing for assessing syncope: an American College of Cardiology expert consensus document. *JACC* 1996; **28**: 263–75.
2. Raviele A, Gasparini G, Di Pede F, *et al*. Usefulness of head-up tilt test in evaluating patients with syncope of unknown origin and negative electrophysiologic study. *Am J Cardiol* 1990; **65**: 1322–7.
3. Benditt DG, Sakaguchi S, Schultz JJ, Remole S, Adler S, Lurie KG. Syncope: diagnostic considerations and the role of tilt-table testing. *Cardiol Rev* 1993; **1**: 146–56.
4. Kosinski DJ, Grubb BP. Neurally mediated syncope with an update on indications and usefulness of head-up tilt table testing and pharmacologic therapy. *Curr Opin Cardiol* 1994; **9**: 53–64.
5. Kapoor W. Evaluation and outcome of patients with syncope. *Medicine* 1990; **69**: 160–75.
6. Fitzpatrick A, Theodorakis G, Vardas P, Kenny RA, Travill CM, Ingram A, *et al*. The incidence of malignant vasovagal syndrome in patients with recurrent syncope. *Eur Heart J* 1991; **12**: 389–94.
7. Milstein S, Buetikofer J, Dunnigan A, Benditt DG, Gornick C, Reyes WJ. Usefulness of disopyramide for prevention of upright tilt-induced hypotension–bradycardia. *Am J Cardiol* 1990; **65**: 1339–44.

8. Fitzpatrick AP, Ahmed R, Williams S, Sutton R. A randomised trial of medical therapy in 'malignant vasovagal syndrome' or 'neurally-mediated bradycardia hypotension syndrome'. *Eur J Cardiac Pacing Electrophysiol* 1991; **2**: 99–102.

9. Nelson S, Stanley M, Love C, *et al.* Autonomic and hemodynamic effects of oral theophylline in patients with vasodepressor syncope. *Arch Int Med* 1991; **90**: 2425–9.

10. Brignole M, Menozzi C, Gianfranchi L, Lolli G, Bottoni N, Oddone D. A controlled trial of acute and long-term medical therapy in tilt-induced neurally-mediated syncope. *Am J Cardiol* 1992; **70**: 339–42.

11. Sra JS, Murthy VS, Jazayeri MR, Shen Y-H, Troup P, Avitall B, Akhtar M. Use of intravenous esmolol to predict efficacy of oral adrenergic blocker therapy in patients with neurocardiogenic syncope. *JACC* 1993; **19**: 402–8.

12. Morillo C, Leitch JW, Yee R, Klein GJ. A placebo-controlled trial of intravenous and oral disopyramide for prevention of neurally mediated syncope induced by head-up tilt. *JACC* 1993; **22**: 1843–8.

13. Grubb BP, Wolfe D, Samoil D, Temesy-Armos P, Hahn H, Elliott L. Usefulness of fluoxetine hydrochloride for prevention of resistant upright tilt induced syncope. *PACE* 1993; **16**: 458–64.

14. Kosinski DJ, Grubb BP, Temesy-Armos PN. The use of serotonin re-uptake inhibitors in the treatment of neurally mediated cardiovascular disorders. *J Serotonin Res* 1994; **1**: 85–90.

15. Mahanonda N, Bhuripanyo K, Kangkagate C, *et al.* Randomized double-blind placebo-controlled trial of oral atenolol in patients with unexplained syncope and positive upright tilt table results. *Am Heart J* 1995; **130**: 1250–3.

16. Moya A, Permanyer-Miralda G, Sagrista-Sauleda J, *et al.* Limitations of head-up tilt test for evaluating the efficacy of therapeutic interventions in patients with vasovagal syncope: results of a controlled study of etilefrine versus placebo. *JACC* 1995; **25**: 65–9.

17. Jankovic J, Hiner BC, Brown DC, Rubin M. Neurogenic orthostatic hypotension: a double-blind placebo-controlled study with midodrine. *Am J Med* 1993; **95**: 38–48.

18. Lewis T. Vasovagal syncope and the carotid sinus mechanism; with comments on Gower's and Nothnagel's syndrome. *Br Med J* 1932; **1**: 873–8.

19. Almquist A, Goldenberg IF, Milstein S, *et al.* Provocation of bradycardia and hypotension by isoproterenol and upright posture in patients with unexplained syncope. *N Engl J Med* 1989; **320**: 346–51.

20. Fish FA, Strasburger JF, Benson DW. Reproducibility of a symptomatic response to upright tilt in young patients with unexplained syncope. *Am J Cardiol* 1992; **70**: 605–9.

21. Sutton R, Petersen M, Brignole M, *et al.* Proposed classification for tilt induced vasovagal syncope. *Eur J Cardiac Pacing Electrophysiol* 1992; **2**: 180–3.

22. Benditt DG, Goldstein MA, Adler S, Sakaguchi S, Lurie KG. Neurally mediated syncopal syndromes: pathophysiology and clinical evaluation. In: Mandel WJ (ed.), *Cardiac Arrhythmias*, 3rd edn. Philadelphia: JB Lippincott Co, 1995: 879–906.

23. Chen XC, Chen MY, Remole S, *et al.* Reproducibility of head up tilt table testing for eliciting susceptibility to neurally-mediated syncope in patients without structural heart disease. *Am J Cardiol* 1992; **69**: 755–60.

24. Sheldon R, Splawinski J, Killam S. Reproducibility of upright tilt-table tests in patients with syncope. *Am J Cardiol* 1992; **69**: 1300–5.

25. Grubb BP, Wolfe D, Temesy-Armos P, Hahn H, Elliott L. Reproducibility of head upright tilt table test results in patients with syncope. *PACE* 1992; **15**: 1477–81.

26. Brooks R, Ruskin JN, Powell AC, Newell J, Garan H, McGovern BA. Prospective elevaluation of day-to-day reproducibility of tilt-table testing in unexplained syncope. *Am J Cardiol* 1993; **71**: 1289–92.

27. de Mey C, Enterling D. Variant responses impair the usefulness of passive upright tilt in drug research. *Meth Find Exptl Clin Pharmacol* 1988; **10**: 57–64.

28. Pritchett EL, Smith MS, McCarthy EA, Lee K. The spontaneous occurrence of paroxysmal supraventricular tachycardia. *Circulation* 1984; **70**: 1–6.

29. Greer GS, Wilkinson WE, McCarthy EA, Pritchett EL. Random and nonrandom behaviour of symptomatic paroxysmal atrial fibrillation. *Am J Cardiol* 1989; **64**: 339–42.

30. Clair WK, Wilkinson WE, McCarthy EA, Page RL, Pritchett ELC. Spontaneous occurrence of symptomatic paroxysmal atrial fibrillation and paroxysmal supraventricular tachycardia in untreated patients. *Circulation* 1993; **87**: 1114–22.
31. MacWilliam JA. Electric stimulation of the mammalian heart. *J Int M Congr* 1887; **3**: 253–5.
32. Dreifus LS, Fisch C, Griffin JC, Gillette PC, Mason JW, Parsonnet V. Guidelines for implantation of cardiac pacemaker and antiarrhythmic devices: American Heart Association/American College of Cardiology Task Force report. *JACC* 1991; **18**: 1–13.
33. British Pacing and Electrophysiology Group Working Party. Recommendations for pacemaker prescription for symptomatic bradycardia. *Br Heart J* 1991; **66**: 185–91.
34. Sugrue DD, Gersh BJ, Holmes DR, Wood DL, Osborn MJ, Hammill SC. Symptomatic 'isolated' carotid sinus hypersensitivity: natural history and results of treatment with anticholinergic drugs or pacemaker. *JACC* 1986; **7**: 158–62.
35. Morley CA, Perrins EJ, Grant P, Chan SL, McBrien DJ, Sutton R. Carotid sinus syncope treated by pacing: analysis of persistent symptoms and role of atrioventricular sequential pacing. *Br Heart J* 1982; **47**: 411–18.
36. Morley CA, Perrins EJ, Chan SL, Sutton R. Long-term comparison of DVI and VVI pacing in carotid sinus syndrome. In: Steinbach K (ed.), *Cardiac Pacing: Proceedings of the Seventh World Symposium on Cardiac Pacing.* Darmstad: Steinkopff Verlag, 1983; 929–35.
37. Madigan NP, Flaker GC, Curtis JJ, Reid J, Mueller KJ, Murphy TJ. Carotid sinus hypersensitivity: beneficial effects of dual-chamber pacing. *Am J Cardiol* 1984; **53**: 1034–40.
38. Brignole M, Sartore B, Barra M, Menozzi C, Lolli G. Is DDD superior to VVI pacing in mixed carotid sinus syndrome? An acute and medium-term study. *PACE* 1988; **11**: 1902–10.
39. Brignole M, Sartore B, Barra M, Menozzi C, Lolli G. Ventricular and dual chamber pacing for treatment of carotid sinus syndrome. *PACE* 1989; **12**: 582–90.
40. Deschamps D, Richard A, Citron B, Chaperon A, Binon JP, Ponsonaille J. Hypersensibilite sino-carotidienne: evolution a moyen et a long terme des patients traites par stimulation ventriculaire. *Arch Mal Coeur* 1990; **83**: 63–7.
41. Brignole M, Menozzi C, Lolli G, Oddone D, Gianfranchi L, Bertulla A. Validation of a method for choice of pacing mode in carotid sinus syndrome with or without sinus bradycardia. *PACE* 1991; **14**: 196–203.
42. Brignole M, Menozzi C, Gianfranchi L, *et al.* The clinical and prognostic significance of the asystolic response during the head-up tilt test. *Eur J Cardiac Pacing Electrophysiol* 1992; **2**: 109–13.
43. Folino AF, Buja GF, Martini B, *et al.* Prolonged cardiac arrest and complete AV block during up-right tilt test in young patients with syncope of unknown origin – prognostic and therapeutic implications. *Eur Heart J* 1992; **13**: 1416–21.
44. Dhala A, Natale A, Sra J, *et al.* Relevance of asystole during head up tilt testing. *Am J Cardiol* 1995; **75**: 251–4.
45. Fitzpatrick AP, Travill CM, Cardas PE, Hubbard WN, Wood A, Ingram A, Sutton R. Recurrent symptoms after ventricular pacing in unexplained syncope. *PACE* 1990; **13**: 619–24.
46. Fitzpatrick A, Theodorakis G, Ahmed R, Williams T, Sutton R. Dual chamber pacing aborts vasovagal syncope induced by head-up 60 degree tilt. *PACE* 1991; **14**: 13–19.
47. Samoil D, Grubb BP, Brewster P, Moore J, Temesy-Armos P. Comparison of single and dual chamber pacing techniques in prevention of upright tilt induced vasovagal syncope. *Eur J Cardiac Pacing Electrophysiol* 1993; **1**: 36–41.
48. Sra J, Jazayeri MR, Avitall B, Dhala A, Deshpande S, Blanck Z, Akhtar M. Comparison of cardiac pacing with drug therapy in the treatment of neurocardiogenic (vasovagal) syncope with bradycardia or asystole. *N Engl J Med* 1993; **328**: 1085–90.
49. Petersen MEV, Chamberlain-Webber R, Fitzpatrick AP, Ingram A, Williams T, Sutton R. Permanent pacing for cardio-inhibitory malignant vasovagal syndrome. *Br Heart J* 1994; **71**: 274–81.
50. Chen M-Y, Goldenberg IF, Milstein S. Buetikofer J, Almquist A, Lesser J, Benditt DG. Cardiac electrophysiologic and hemodynamic correlates of neurally-mediated syncope. *Am J Cardiol* 1989; **63**: 66–72.

51. Ahmed R, Guneri S, Ingram A, *et al*. Double blind comparison of DDI, DDI with rate hysteresis, VVI and VVI with rate hysteresis in control of symptoms in carotid sinus syndrome (abstract). *Br Heart J* 1991; **66**: 63.
52. Zhu W-X, Rizo-Patron C, Berrier HB, *et al*. Value of dual chamber pacemakers with rate drop response/search hysteresis in the management of vasovagal syncope and carotid sinus hypersensitivity (abstract). *PACE* 1995; **18**: 907.
53. Petersen M, Hess M, Markowitz T, *et al*. Acute human investigation of an algorithm to treat vasovagal syncope using a computer based simulator (abstract). *PACE* 1995; **18**: 825.
54. Benditt DG, Sutton R, Fetter J, *et al*. Cardiac pacing in vasovagal syncope: multicenter assessment of a rate-drop response algorithm (abstract). *PACE* 1996; **19**: 592.
55. Petersen MEV, Price D, Williams T, *et al*. Short AV interval DDD pacing does not prevent tilt induced vasovagal syncope in patients with cardioinhibitory vasovagal syndrome. *PACE* 1994; **17**: 882–91.

10

Pacing in the Long-QT Syndrome

W. Zareba and A. J. Moss

Pathophysiology of the Congenital Long-QT Syndrome

The hereditary long-QT syndrome (LQTS) is a genetic cardiac disorder manifested by an abnormally prolonged duration of ventricular repolarization (QT interval prolongation) and a propensity to arrhythmogenic syncope and fatal ventricular arrhythmias.[1,2] As a result of the collaborative efforts of several investigators associated with the International LQTS Registry, significant progress has been made in the understanding of the mechanisms underlying this disease.[3-6] Recent advances in molecular biology have allowed researchers to determine that LQTS disorder is linked to abnormalities in at least four different chromosomal loci on chromosomes: 3, 4, 7 and 11[4,6-8] (Table 10.1). There are numerous LQTS families which are not linked to the above chromosomal loci, providing further evidence for genetic heterogeneity of this disease.

The specific gene mutations have been recently identified on chromosome 3 involving the SCN5A sodium channel gene,[5] and on chromosome 7 involving the HERG potassium channel gene.[6] The SCN5A mutation has been shown to be associated with impaired inactivation of sodium membrane channels. The HERG mutation was demonstrated to be associated with abnormal kinetics of putative potassium channels. A similar mechanism is believed to be responsible for LQTS linked to a chromosome 11 abnormality.[7] The different genetic abnormalities are represented by distinct ECG patterns of repolarization morphology, described by different T-wave shape and duration of repolarization parameters.[9] These recent developments provided a direct link between genetic cellular abnormalities and cardiac electrophysiology, opening a new area of research focusing on new forms of

Table 10.1 Genetic background of LQTS

LQTS types	Chromosomal loci	Ionic current abnormalities
LQT1	Chr. 11	KVLQT1 potassium current gene (I_{Ks})
LQT2	Chr. 7	HERG potassium current gene (I_{Kr})
LQT3	Chr. 3	SCN5A Sodium current gene (I_{Na})
LQT4	Chr. 4	?

therapy directed to correcting the ionic defects of genetic disorders.[10–13] Providing the above introductory background seems to be relevant for the complex issue of the role of pacemaker therapy in patients with LQTS, the disease which is no longer considered to be a uniform pathophysiological entity.

Cardiac Events in Long-QT Syndrome

Risk of Cardiac Events in Patients with LQTS

The long-QT syndrome is a serious arrhythmic disorder with over 80% of probands experiencing cardiac events: syncope, aborted cardiac arrest or cardiac death.[1–3] The mortality rate in untreated LQTS probands is as high as 70%, with the highest risk of death in children, adolescents and young adults.[14] The occurrence of cardiac events in LQTS probands is independently associated with longer QTc duration and a history of cardiac events in the past.[3,14] These independent predictors of cardiac events may serve to identify LQTS patients at particularly high risk for arrhythmic events. The family members of LQTS probands are also at increased risk of cardiac events, with female first-degree relatives being at the highest risk.[15] Figure 10.1 shows the prevalence of cardiac events in the 1996 population of patients enrolled in the International LQTS Registry.

The high risk of cardiac events in LQTS patients can be substantially decreased with beta-blocker therapy, but this therapeutic measure is not sufficient to protect all LQTS patients. Approximately 6–10% of this group taking beta-blockers suffer life-threatening cardiac events.[2] Left cervicothoracic sympathectomy (LCTS) is an additional helpful intervention in high-risk LQTS patients – i.e. in those with a history of aborted cardiac arrest, or with arrhythmias resistant to beta-blocker therapy.[16,17] However, a number of LQTS patients treated with beta-blockers and LCTS require more aggressive therapy with implantation of permanent pacemakers or sometimes implantation of cardioverter–defibrillators.

Torsade de Pointes: a Tachyarrhythmia of the LQTS

Torsade de pointes (TdP) polymorphic ventricular tachycardia is the leading life-threatening arrhythmia in patients with LQTS.[18] This ventricular arrhythmia, characterized by twisting QRS morphology, has been recorded in patients with both idiopathic and acquired QT prolongation. The mechanism of TdP is most likely to be related to increased dispersion of refractoriness and development of early after-depolarizations (EADs). Slow heart rate in association with prolongation of QT interval create favourable conditions for TdP to occur.[19–21] The presence of sudden RR cycle length changes (usually long–short–long series) is an additional factor precipitating TdP.[19,22,23] Patients with LQTS frequently present with bradycardia that is known to enhance both dispersion of refractoriness and EADs. An example of pause-dependent TdP in a LQTS patient is shown in Figure 10.2.

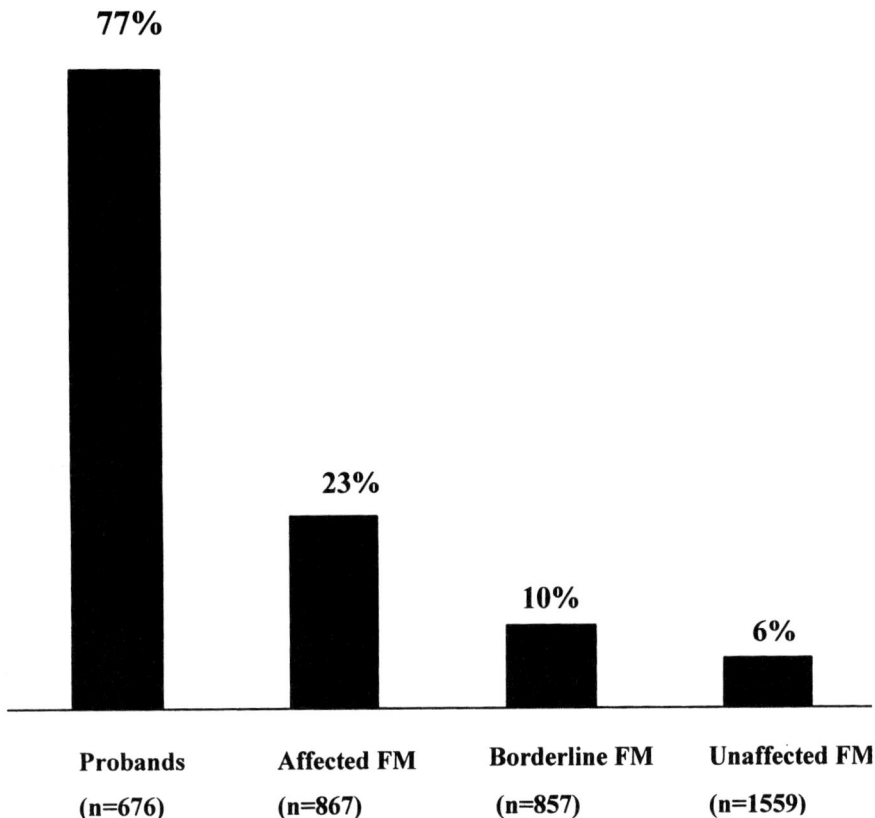

Figure 10.1 Prevalence of pre-enrolment cardiac events in LQTS probands and their family members (FM) enrolled in the International LQTS Registry. The family members are categorized based on age- and gender-specific cut-offs of the QTc duration.

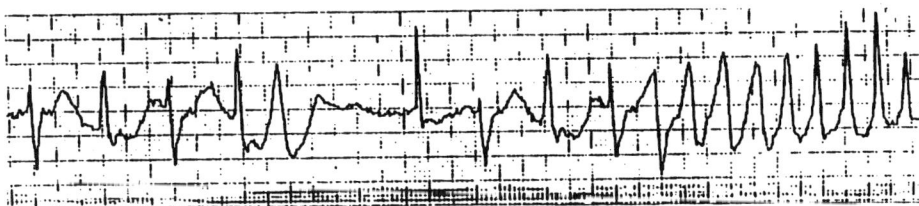

Figure 10.2 ECG of an LQTS patient with a pause-dependent episode of torsade de pointes.

Bradycardia in Long-QT Syndrome

Incidence and Clinical Significance of Bradyarrhythmias in LQTS

Bradycardia below 60 bpm, recorded on the enrolment ECG, was observed in 31% of 328 LQTS probands and in 16% of 688 affected family members from the International

LQTS Registry.[3] In a study of 637 family members, bradycardia was found to be independently associated with an increase in risk of cardiac events.[15] The LQTS family members with heart rate below 25th percentile in this population had a higher incidence of cardiac events than patients with normal (between 25th and 90th percentiles) range of heart rate. The age-dependent cut-off values for identifying bradycardia (heart rate below 25th percentile) were as follows: for age below 2 years, <110 bpm; for age from 2 to below 5 years, <95 bpm; for age 5 to below 10 years, <75 bpm; and for age 10 and above, <60 bpm. These values were somewhat higher than conventionally accepted criteria for definition of bradycardia for the age groups.[24] Nevertheless, in the LQTS patient population the above heart rate values were able to identify bradycardic individuals at increased risk for cardiac events.

Bradyarrhythmias were found on routine ECG in 20% of 287 LQTS children enrolled in the multicentre study conducted by the Pediatric Electrophysiology Society.[14] Of the 156 patients who had a Holter monitoring, 19% had a minimum heart rate that was below the normal for age. One-hundred and three patients had an exercise test and 36% of them presented with a maximum heart rate lower than normal for age. In this study, LQTS patients with bradycardia had a significantly higher incidence of cardiac events than patients without bradycardia (17% vs 7%, respectively; $p < 0.05$).

Pathomechanism of Bradyarrhythmias

The above studies in large LQTS patient populations provide evidence that brady-cardia is a quite common ECG abnormality that may predispose to life-threatening ventricular arrhythmias. Although bradycardia is frequently observed in LQTS patients, its pathomechanism is still not fully understood. Two clinical presentations of bradycardia are reported in LQTS patients: atrioventricular (AV) conduction block and sinus bradycardia (or bradyarrhythmia).

Atrioventricular 2:1 block in LQTS

In 1993, Garson and coworkers reported a 5% incidence of AV conduction block among 287 LQTS children. Patients, usually infants, with AV 2:1 block present a particularly high-risk subset of the LQTS population.[14,25] In a review of the literature in 1995, Trippel and coworkers reported that LQTS infants with 2:1 AV block had a 50% mortality rate at 6 months and 67% at 2 years. As shown in Figure 10.3, in LQTS

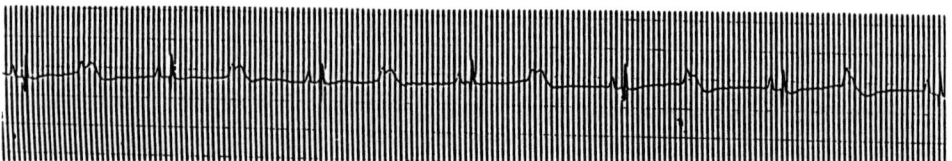

Figure 10.3   ECG of an LQTS patient with 2:1 atrioventricular block (QT = 0.60 s; PP = 0.54 s).

patients with an extremely long QT interval that exceeds the sinus node cycle length, a 2:1 AV block may occur when every second sinus beat is blocked due to prolonged ventricular refractoriness. Increase in heart rate with QT interval shortening usually leads to 1:1 AV conduction in these patients. This rate-dependency implies that the site of AV block in LQTS infants is below the His-bundle, at the level of the myocytes, which show a prolonged effective refractory period.[26–28] Further support for the theory of the functional AV block in LQTS patients is provided by electrophysiological studies which demonstrated normal His–Purkinje (HV) conduction time.[27,29] According to the literature, there is no evidence to claim that specific histological abnormalities of the AV conduction system are responsible for AV 2:1 conduction block in LQTS infants.[14,25,30]

Sinus bradycardia

Resting sinus bradycardia is a common finding in patients with the long-QT syndrome.[1,31,32] Approximately 20–25% of patients with LQTS present with sinus bradycardia, which is believed to result from a sinus node dysfunction.[33] In the study of 14 young LQTS patients (aged 3 to 16 years), Kugler observed one or more features of sinus node dysfunction in 13 of them. The corrected sinus node recovery time (CSNRT) was found to be prolonged in 8 of 14 patients and the sinoatrial conduction time (SACT) was long in 6 of 9 in whom it was calculable. The maximum heart rate during exercise testing was abnormally low in 6 of 12 tested children and an abnormally low heart rate on Holter monitoring was found in 4 of the 12 patients. The possible explanations for sinus node dysfunction in LQTS patients include a deficiency of right-sided sympathetic activity[31,32] and histological abnormalities of the sinus node.[30,34] Considering recent genetic LQTS findings, a more likely explanation would be that sinus node function in some LQTS patients demonstrating bradycardia may result from abnormal ionic current kinetics in pacemaker cells of the sinus node.

Both beta-blocker therapy and left cervicothoracic sympathectomy may lead to excessive bradycardia, increasing the risk of like-threatening arrhythmias. In a recent study of 320 LQTS patients treated with beta-blockers, the heart rate decreased on average from 73 bpm before beta-blocker therapy to 63 bpm on beta-blocker therapy ($p < 0.001$).[35] In over one-third of these patients a heart rate below 60 bpm was observed.

Rationale for Cardiac Pacing in LQTS

Benefit of Cardiac Pacing in Patients with Torsade de Pointes

Torsade de pointes, a polymorphic ventricular tachycardia, is a characteristic arrhythmia complicating QT prolongation. There is a substantial literature documenting torsade de pointes in both idiopathic LQTS and secondary (usually iatrogenic) QT prolongation.[22,36–38] Two major mechanisms are believed to be responsible for torsade de pointes: re-entry due to dispersion of refractory periods, and triggered activity

Table 10.2   Role of cardiac pacing in preventing torsade de pointes (TdP)

Pathogenic TdP factors	Effects of cardiac pacing
Slow heart rate	Selecting optimal pacing rate decreases risk of bradycardia-dependent TdP
Prolonged QT interval	Pacing-increased heart rate shortens QT interval
Sudden rate change	Pacing stabilizes the rhythm, decreasing the likelihood of short–long–short cycle-length patterns
Presence of EADs	Pacing suppresses EADs, decreasing the likelihood of arrhythmias
Dispersion of refractoriness	Pacing decreases the magnitude of dispersion, lowering the chances of re-entrant arrhythmias

initiated by early after-depolarizations (EADs). The electrophysiological conditions contributing to the torsade de pointes ventricular tachycardia also include: slow heart rate, prolonged QT interval, sudden change in heart rate.[22,38,39]

Pacemaker therapy seems to be the appropriate treatment to alleviate the above arrhythmogenic conditions (Table 10.2). Thirty years ago, Han et al.,[40] showed that pacing may decrease dispersion of refractoriness. Permanent pacing may also decrease increased automacity which is also believed to contribute to torsade de pointes.[36,41] The beneficial role of cardiac pacing in patients with torsade de pointes ventricular tachycardia has been proved by a common therapeutic approach consisting of temporary overdrive pacing applied in an acute arrhythmic setting.[42,43] Permanent cardiac pacing is an accepted treatment in bradycardia-dependent torsade de pointes and is also becoming an important part of the therapy in LQTS patients.

QT Interval and Cardiac Pacing

Rate-dependency of the QT interval has been a recognized electrophysiological phenomenon since the beginning of electrocardiography.[44] Recordings of monophasic action potentials (MAPs) showed a close association between the duration of the action potential and heart rate,[45,46] with a reported average 23 ms increase in the action potential duration per 100 ms cycle length increase. Recently Hirao et al.[47] studied the rate-dependency of MAP duration and dispersion in 11 LQTS and 10 control subjects in baseline conditions and after infusion of epinephrine. As shown in Figure 10.4, both the dispersion and duration of MAPs showed significant decreases with incremental pacing. The degree of MAP shortening, however, was much higher in LQTS than in control subjects. Epinephrine prolonged MAPs and increased the dispersion of MAPs significantly at all paced heart rates in the LQTS patients, but did not produce these changes in the control group. This observation emphasizes:

(a) the benefit of cardiac pacing that decreases bradycardia-dependent phenomena, i.e. prolonged duration and increased dispersion of repolarization;
(b) the need for a pacemaker therapy combined with antiadrenergic measures (beta-blockade and left cervicothoracic sympathectomy).

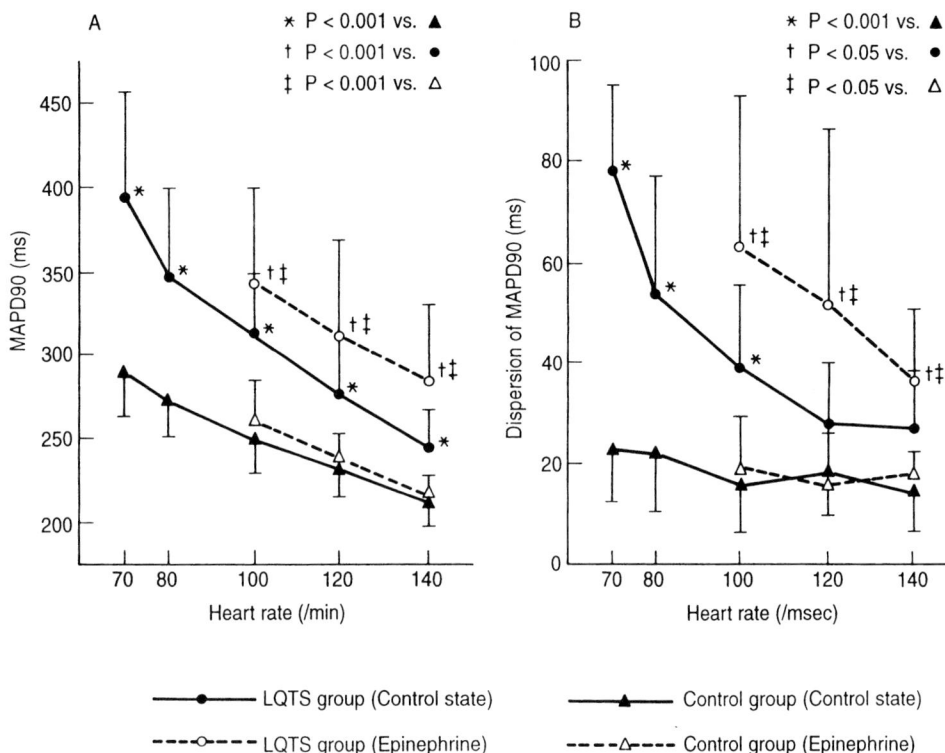

Figure 10.4 Changes in MAPD90 and dispersion of MAPD90 in relation to paced heart rate and effect of epinephrine infusion on MAPD90 and dispersion of MAPD90 in 11 patients with LQTS and 10 control subjects. MAPD90 = monophasic action potential duration at 90% repolarization. (Reproduced from reference 47 with permission)

Indications for Pacing in Patients with LQTS

In 1987, Eldar *et al.*[48] described their experience with permanent cardiac pacing in 8 female LQTS patients with ages 16–57 years. All these patients had recurrent syncope and 4 of them had at least one episode of aborted cardiac arrest despite beta-blocker therapy or left cervicothoracic sympathectomy. Six patients had documented episodes of torsade de pointes ventricular tachycardia. A few years later, Eldar *et al.*[49] added their observations on an additional 13 LQTS patients, making the total 21 patients. Again, history of syncopal episodes or aborted cardiac arrest was the most common indication (20 patients; 95%); 11 patients (52%) had a family history of syncope or aborted cardiac arrest; 5 patients (25%) had episodes of atrioventricular block.

The efficacy of permanent pacing in the management of high-risk patients with LQTS was investigated by Moss *et al.*,[50] in a group of 30 patients enrolled in the International LQTS Registry. Specific indications for pacemaker implantation included: recurrent syncope or aborted cardiac arrest refractory to antiadrenergic therapy in 14 patients (47%); symptomatic bradycardia with beta-blockers in 3

Table 10.3 Indications for permanent pacing in LQTS patients to prevent pause- or bradycardia-dependent arrhythmias

1. Recurrent cardiac events (episodes of serious ventricular arrhythmias, syncope or cardiac arrest), especially if refractory to antiadrenergic therapy
2. History of aborted sudden death
3. Prolonged QT with 2:1 atrioventricular conduction block
4. Prolonged QT with spontaneous or treatment-dependent (beta-blockers, LCTS) bradycardia (defined according to patient age)
5. Noncompliant LQTS patients likely to interrupt beta-blocker therapy
6. Intolerance to beta-blocker treatment

patients (10%); recurrent syncope or aborted cardiac arrest without antiadrenergic therapy in 11 patients (36%); and in 2 patients (7%) sinus bradycardia without antiadrenergic therapy.

Based on the above experience from the two largest reports of LQTS patients treated with permanent pacing,[49,50] a number of indications for pacemaker implantation in LQTS patients should be considered (Table 10.3). All these indications have a common goal, i.e. to prevent pause- or bradycardia-dependent phenomena triggering cardiac events in LQTS patients.

LQTS patients with recurrent cardiac events despite antiadrenergic therapy (beta-blockers, LCTS) is the first priority group of candidates for pacemaker implantation. The likelihood of repeated events in patients with a history of recurrent episodes of syncope is extremely high (3–6 times higher than in LQTS patients without a history of cardiac events[50]), and a combined therapy consisting of antiadrenergic treatment, pacemaker implantation, or even better implantation of a cardioverter–defibrillator with pacemaker capabilities, is the primary choice for these patients. A documented history of cardiac arrest aborted by resuscitation should definitely be considered as an indication for a combined therapy including permanent pacing. Young children, especially newborns with LQTS, are at extremely high risk of cardiac death.[14] They frequently present with 2:1 functional AV block precipitating the episodes of torsade de pointes. The reported 2-year mortality of LQTS newborns with functional AV block is as high as 67%.[25] Despite some technical difficulties, a combination therapy with pacemaker implantation in such LQTS infants is the treatment of choice in order to help them survive the most dangerous period of their life. Nevertheless, the episodes of 2:1 AV block may also occur in adult LQTS patients (as reported by Eldar *et al.*,[49] in 3 out of 15 adults), increasing the risk of cardiac events. As described earlier in this chapter, sinus bradycardia is frequently observed in LQTS patients and may be exaggerated by antiadrenergic therapy. Since bradycardia may contribute to excessive QT prolongation and increased dispersion of refractoriness, and may precipitate EADs, cardiac pacing is a highly recommended measure to alleviate these unfavourable conditions. It is worth emphasizing that bradycardia should be defined for the age of the patient instead of using an arbitrary cut-off below 60 bpm.

Some LQTS families present with an especially malignant course of the disease characterized by a history of sudden death or aborted cardiac death in several members of the family. Symptomatic patients coming from such high-risk families should undergo pacemaker implantation as a part of the combined therapy. Finally, since LQTS is a disease affecting young people – frequently children and adolescents – the issue of patient compliance should always be considered. There is enough evidence from clinical practice to prove that interruption of beta-blocker therapy may be fatal in LQTS patients. Implanting pacemakers in noncompliant patients does not solve the problem, but at least it decreases the likelihood of fatal consequences associated with sudden drug withdrawal. While Table 10.3 points out the most frequent reasons for pacemaker implantation in LQTS patients, clinical decisions have to be made on an individual patient basis after accounting for several possible factors and conditions influencing the course of the disease.

Efficacy of Cardiac Pacing in LQTS Patients

In a series of 30 high-risk LQTS patients described by Moss et al.,[50] permanent cardiac pacing was associated with a significant reduction in recurrent cardiac events (Figure 10.5).

Nevertheless, 9 of these patients experienced cardiac events after pacemaker implantation despite beta-blocker therapy in 8 of them. A similar observation was reported by Eldar et al.,[49] who evaluated a long-term follow-up of 21 LQTS patients with implanted pacemakers. Twenty patients had syncopal or cardiac arrest episodes before pacemaker implantations, and 5 of them experienced cardiac events during a

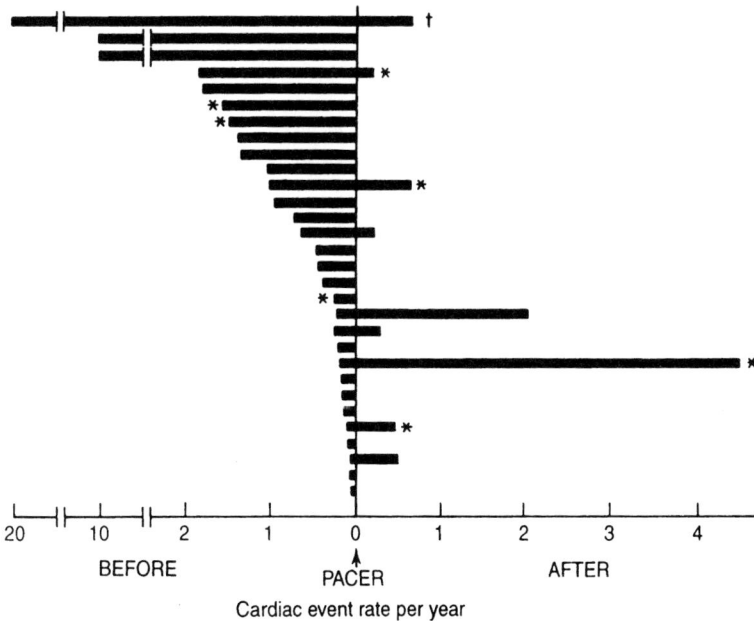

Figure 10.5 Cardiac event rates before (syncope or aborted cardiac arrest) and after (syncope, aborted cardiac arrest or death) permanent pacemaker in LQTS patients. †Cardiac death; *left cervicothoracic sympathectomy. (Reproduced from reference 50 with permission)

mean 55-month follow-up. Two patients had cardiac events despite beta-blocker therapy combined with permanent cardiac pacing, and 3 other patients experienced cardiac events associated with lapses in the combined therapy (beta-blocker withdrawn or lead fracture).

These observations, made in independent series of LQTS patients, indicate that in a high-risk subset of LQTS patients, permanent cardiac pacing is a very helpful therapeutic measure, although it does not provide complete protection against cardiac events. In patients with cardiac events despite beta-blocker treatment combined with permanent cardiac pacing, additional therapeutic modalities including LCTS and an implanted cardioverter–defibrillator should be considered.

Pacing Rate and Mode in LQTS Patients

Pacing Rate

Permanent cardiac pacing in LQTS patients should not be considered just as a 'backup' for a very slow heart rate or heart block. In addition to providing such protection, cardiac pacing in LQTS aims to diminish conditions (Table 10.2) that could precipitate arrhythmic events. To achieve these goals, the pacing rate in LQTS patients should be optimized to provide a maximal benefit of pacing therapy.

Eldar et al.,[48] based on their first series of eight LQTS patients treated with permanent pacing, proposed setting the pacing rate at the level when a clear-cut shortening of QT interval occurs. In their adult LQTS patients (ages 16–57 years), pacing rates between 70 and 85 bpm caused a significant QT interval shortening from 534 ± 51 ms to 426 ± 19 ms ($p < 0.001$). The QTc interval shortened too, but not significantly (526 ± 36 ms to 483 ± 43 ms). However, the rate-dependency of the QT interval has a gene-specific pattern,[51,52] with LQTS patients linked to sodium-channel abnormalities (LQT3) showing greater extent of shortening in comparison with patients linked to potassium-channel abnormalities (LQT1 or LQT2). These recent observations suggest that a benefit of cardiac pacing in these three genotypes might be quite different, but further long-term studies are required to address this point.

In a retrospective analysis of 19 LQTS patients, Moss et al.[50] found that pacing rates were lower in 6 patients with cardiac events after pacemaker implantation in comparison with 13 patients without cardiac events during follow-up (69 ± 8 vs 75 ± 11 bpm, respectively; $p = 0.18$). This difference, although nonsignificant, may further suggest a beneficial role of higher pacing rates.

Further support for a need for elevated pacing rates is provided by an analysis of cardiac events in relation to the heart rate in LQTS patients.[15] As shown in Figure 10.6, there is a curvilinear association between the odds ratio for cardiac events and heart rate.

A bimodal relationship between the risk of cardiac events and heart rate was observed in LQTS family members: both elevated and low heart rates were associated with an increased risk of cardiac events. A logistic regression model, with continuous values of RR and RR^2 included, yielded a statistically significant curvilinear association between cardiac events and heart rate. Since clinical interpretation of quadratic

**Odds Ratio for
Cardiac Events**

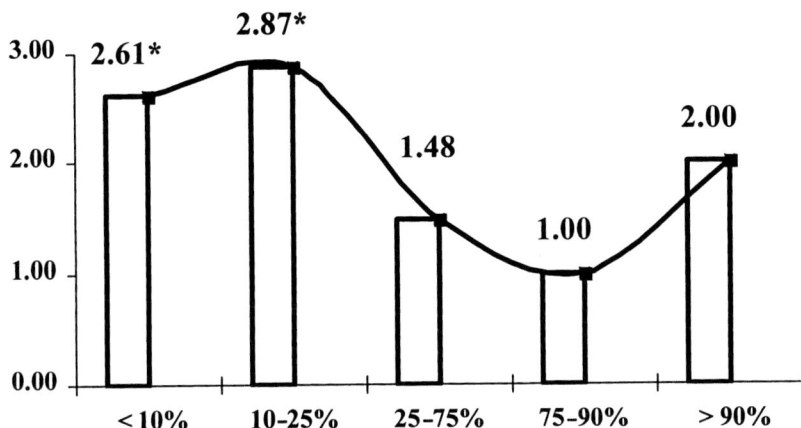

Figure 10.6   Odds ratio for cardiac events in relation to the percentile of heart rate in LQTS patients in a multivariate logistic regression model adjusting for QTc, gender, and relationship to the proband. The curvilinear association between cardiac events and heart rate was proved in the modal with RR^2. Percentiles of the heart rate in the population studied are determined according to the age group shown in Table 10.4.

Table 10.4   Age-adjusted heart rates associated with the low risk for cardiac events in LQTS patients, and recommended age-adjusted pacing rates

Age group	Number of patients studied	Heart rates (25–90th percentiles) (bpm)	Recommended pacing rates (bpm)
0–2 years	73	111–150	120–140
2–5 years	49	97–120	105–115
5–10 years	100	73–107	80–100
>10 years	962	60–86	70–80

terms in risk stratification models is impractical, simpler age-adjusted criteria to define relative tachycardia and bradycardia were proposed. The heart rates associated with lower risk of cardiac events were defined between 25th and 90th percentiles for the LQTS population values (Table 10.4). These data suggest the setting of age-adjusted pacing rates in LQTS patients above standard back-up pacing rates.

Pacing Mode

There are not enough published data to determine the long-term efficacy of specific pacing modes in LQTS patients. Atrial (AAI), ventricular (VVI) and dual-chamber (DDD) pacing modes have been described as effective in these patients. Failures of pacing therapy have also been reported in all three pacing modes without a particular preponderance of any one of them. The extent of QT shortening in response to AAI, VVI and DDD pacing seems also to be similar.[48,49] Nevertheless, dual-chamber pacing should be considered as the pacing mode of choice, especially in patients with QTc > 0.55 seconds who may develop a functional 2:1 AV block. In newborns and infants with LQTS and functional AV conduction block, permanent pacing and beta-blocker therapy should be implemented as soon as the diagnosis is made. If for technical reasons DDD pacemaker implantation is not feasible, a VVI pacemaker with a high pacing rate (usually > 120 bpm) is the treatment of choice.

Complications of Pacemaker Therapy in LQTS Patients

As in any other group of patients with permanent pacing, a number of problems may emerge. Lead fracture is an uncommon complication, but can be associated with recurrence of cardiac events. Therefore, whenever an LQTS patient on permanent cardiac pacing experiences a syncopal episode, a careful inspection of lead continuity and connections is needed. Another reported problem is T-wave oversensing, which can be managed by pacemaker reprogramming. In some LQTS patients with implanted AAI pacemakers, AV conduction block may occur leading to bradycardia and RR-interval instability, which may trigger episodes of torsade de pointes. This problem can be alleviated by implanting a DDD or VVI pacemaker.

Combined Therapy in LQTS: Pacing, Beta-blockers, LCTS, ICD

LQTS patients with a history of cardiac events have an at least threefold higher chance of developing subsequent cardiac events than patients without such a history.[3] Patients belonging to families with a history of sudden death at a young age and those with marked QT prolongation also have high odds ratios for cardiac events. In such high-risk LQTS patients, a combined therapy is strongly recommended and in some cases even mandatory. The combined therapy usually consists of full beta-blockade (usually achieved by administration of 3 mg/kg of propranolol per day) and pacemaker implantation. In some patients, beta-blockers may precipitate bradycardia but permanent cardiac pacing is not reserved only for beta-blocker-related brady-cardic LQTS patients. High-risk LQTS patients with normal range of the heart rate on beta-blockers should also be qualified to dual therapy. Additional therapeutic measures, used in patients with episodes refractory to dual therapy, include left cervicothoracic sympathectomy (LCTS) and implantation of a defibrillator. Both these methods are beneficial, but neither provides full protection against cardiac events. More hope is being seen in gene-specific therapeutic approaches.

Gene Specific Approach to LQTS Patients

Recent findings in the molecular biology of the LQTS have opened new directions in the therapy of these patients. The phenotypical differences between patients linked to different chromosomal loci include: distinct repolarization morphology,[9] distinct

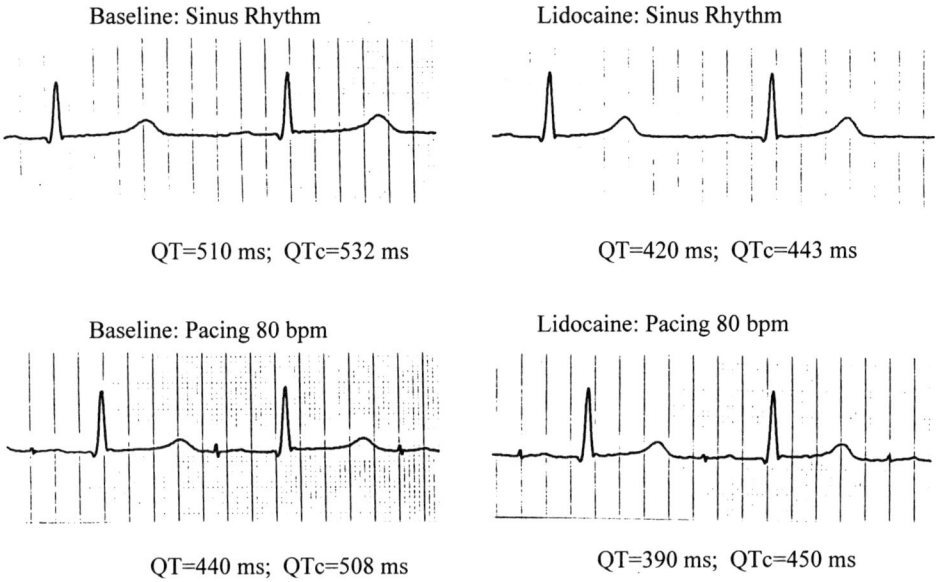

Baseline: Sinus Rhythm

QT=510 ms; QTc=532 ms

Lidocaine: Sinus Rhythm

QT=420 ms; QTc=443 ms

Baseline: Pacing 80 bpm

QT=440 ms; QTc=508 ms

Lidocaine: Pacing 80 bpm

QT=390 ms; QTc=450 ms

Figure 10.7 QT and QTc intervals in patients with LQT3 (SCN5A sodium-channel gene mutation) in baseline conditions and during cardiac pacing at 80 bpm, before and after lidocaine infusion (paper speed 50 mm/s). Note a greater degree of QTc shortening due to lidocaine administration in comparison with cardiac pacing itself (443 ms and 508 ms, respectively).

dispersion of repolarization[53] and different heart-rate adaptation of the QT interval.[52,54] The distinct heart-rate dependency of the QT interval may suggest that not all LQTS patients will benefit from permanent cardiac pacing to the same degree. The specific ionic current abnormalities are believed to be primarily responsible for these phenotypic expressions. In patients with LQTS linked to abnormalities on chromosomes 11 (LQT1) and 7 (LQT2), premature closing of potassium outward currents extends repolarization. In patients with abnormalities on chromosome 3 (LQT3), an impaired inactivation of inward sodium currents contributes to QT-interval prolongation. These ionic current abnormalities are likely to be corrected with drugs targeting specific ionic dysfunctions. For example, sodium-channel blockers (e.g. lidocaine) may close a prolonged inward sodium ion leakage with subsequent shortening of the action potential (and QT interval). Figure 10.7 shows ECGs of an LQT3 patient before and after lidocaine infusion during sinus rhythm and paced rhythm at 80 bpm.

Major QT and QTc shortening is attributed to sodium-channel blockade rather than to pacing itself. This example illustrates that pacemaker therapy is still a palliative therapeutic measure, whereas the main efforts should be focused on developing specific ionic-related treatments.

Summary

Clinical experience of the last decade has proved that permanent cardiac pacing is an accepted method of treatment in selected LQTS patients. Beneficial effects of cardiac pacing are related to reduction in bradycardia-dependent phenomena, including pause-dependent torsade de pointes, increased dispersion of refractoriness, and development of early after-depolarizations. Beta-blocker therapy, a standard therapeutic approach in LQTS patients, may in some of them exaggerate bradycardia-dependent phenomena. Permanent cardiac pacing should be considered in high-risk LQTS, especially those with: recurrent cardiac events, history of aborted cardiac arrest, AV conduction blocks and those with fatal LQTS family history (see Table 10.3 for details). Pacing rates should be age-adjusted and set above standard backup pacing rates. A dual-chamber pacemaker is the mode of choice, preventing AV blocks and providing flexible programming relevant for T-wave oversensing problems.

Finally, permanent pacing in LQTS patients should be combined with other therapeutic measures: primarily with beta-blockade, and in selected cases with left cervicothoracic sympathectomy and an implanted cardioverter–defibrillator. New gene-specific therapy is being developed and tested, and the role of cardiac pacing in combination with treatment correcting ionic abnormalities remains to be examined.

References

1. Moss AJ, Schwartz PJ, Crampton RS, Locati E, Carleen E. The long QT syndrome: a prospective international study. *Circulation* 1985; **71**: 17–21.
2. Schwartz PJ, Locati EH. The idiopathic long QT syndrome: pathogenetic mechanisms and therapy. *Eur Heart J* 1985; **6** (suppl D): 103–14.
3. Moss AJ, Schwartz PJ, Crampton RS, *et al*. The long QT syndrome: prospective longitudinal study of 328 families. *Circulation* 1991; **84**: 1136–44.
4. Keating M, Atkinson D, Dunn C, Timothy K, Vincent GM, Leppert M. Linkage of cardiac arrhythmia, the long QT Syndrome, and the Harvey ras-1 gene. *Science* 1991; **252**: 704–6.
5. Wang Q, Shen J, Splawski I, Atkinson D, Li Z, Robinson JL, Moss AJ, Towbin JA, Keating MT. SCN5A mutations cause an inherited cardiac arrhythmia, long QT syndrome. *Cell* 1995; **80**: 805–11.
6. Curran ME, Splawski I, Timothy K, Vincent GM, Green E, Keating MT. A molecular basis for cardiac arrhythmia: HERG mutations cause long QT syndrome. *Cell* 1995; **80**: 795–803.
7. Wang Q, Curran ME, Splawski I, *et al*. Positional cloning of a novel potassium channel gene: KVLQT1 mutations cause cardiac arrhythmias. *Nat Gen* 1996; **12**: 17–23.
8. Schott JJ, Charpentier F, Peltier S, *et al*. Mapping of gene for long QT syndrome to chromosome 4q25-27. *Am J Hum Genet* 1995; **57**: 1114–22.
9. Moss AJ, Zareba W, Benhorin J, *et al*. Electrocardiographic T-wave patterns in genetically distinct forms of the hereditary long QT syndrome. *Circulation* 1995; **92**: 2929–34.
10. Bennett PB, Yzawa K, Meklte N, Gearge AL. Molecular mechanism for an inherited cardiac arrhythmia. *Nature* (Lond.) 1995; **375**: 583–5.
11. An RH, Bangalore R, Rosero SZ, Kass RS. Lidocaine block of LQT-3 mutant human Na$^+$ channels. *Circ Res* 1996; **79**: 103–8.
12. Schwartz PJ, Priori SG, Locati EH, *et al*. Long QT syndrome patients with mutations of the SCN5A and HERG genes have differential responses to Na$^+$ channel blockade and to increases in heart rate: implications for gene-specific therapy. *Circulation* 1995; **92**: 3381–6.
13. Compton SJ, Lux RL, Ramsey MR, Strelich KR, Sanguinetti MC, Green LS, Keating MT, Mason JW. Genetically defined therapy of inherited long-QT syndrome: correction of abnormal repolarization by potassium. *Circulation* 1996; **94**: 1018–22.
14. Garson A, Dick M, Fournier A, Gillette PC, Hamilton R, Kugler JD, Van Hare GF, Vetter V, Vick GW. The long QT syndrome in children: an international study of 287 patients. *Circulation* 1993; **87**: 1866–72.

15. Zareba W, Moss AJ, le Cessie S, Locati E, Robinson JL, Hall WJ, Andrews ML. Risk of cardiac events in long QT syndrome family members. *JACC* 1995; **26**: 1685–91.
16. Moss AJ, McDonald J. Unilateral cervicothoracic sympathetic ganglionectomy for the treatment of long QT interval syndrome. *N Engl J Med* 1970; **285**: 903–4.
17. Schwartz PJ, Locati EH, Moss AJ, Crampton RS, Trazzi R, Ruberti U. Left cardiac sympathetic denervation in the therapy of congenital long QT syndrome: a worldwide report. *Circulation* **84**: 503–11.
18. Moss AJ, Schwartz PJ. Delayed repolarization (QT and Q-U prolongation) and malignant ventricular arrhythmias. *Mod Concepts Cardiovasc Dis* 1982; **51**: 85–90.
19. Brachman J, Scherlag BJ, Rosenshtraukh LV, Lazzara R. Bradycardia-dependent triggered activity: relevance to drug-induced multiform ventricular tachycardia. *Circulation* 1983; **68**: 846–56.
20. Roden DM, Woosley RL, Primm RK. Incidence and clinical features of the quinidine-associated long QT syndrome: implications for patient care. *Am Heart J* 1986; **111**: 1088–94.
21. El-Sherif N, Zeiler RH, Craelius W, Gough WB, Henkin R. QTU prolongation and polymorphic ventricular tachyarrhythmias due to bradycardia-dependent early after-depolarizations. *Circ Res* 1988; **62**: 286–305.
22. Locati EH, Maison-Blanche P, Dejode P, Cauchemez B, Coumel P. Spontaneous sequences of onset of torsade de pointes in patients with acquired prolonged repolarization: quantitative analysis of Holter recordings. *JACC* 1995; **25**: 1564–75.
23. Kay GN, Plumb VJ, Arciniegas JG, Henthorn RW, Waldo AL. Torsade de pointes: the long–short initiating sequence and other clinical features. *Am J Cardiol* 1983; **52**: 806–17.
24. Garson A. *The Electrocardiogram of Infants and Children: A Systematic Approach*. Philadelphia: Lea & Febiger, 1983: 396.
25. Trippel DL, Parsons MK, Gillette PC. Infants with long-QT syndrome and 2:1 atrioventricular block. *Am Heart J* 1995; **130**: 1130–4.
26. Scott AW, Dick M. Two:one atrioventricular block in infants with congenital long QT syndrome. *Am J Cardiol* 1987; **60**: 1409–10.
27. Van Hare GF, Franz MR, Roge C, Scheinman MM. Persistent functional atrioventricular block in two patients with prolonged QT intervals: elucidation of the mechanism of block. *PACE* 1990; **13**: 608–18.
28. Rosenbaum MB, Acunzo RS. Pseudo 2:1 AV block and T wave alternans in the long QT syndrome. *JACC* 1991; **18**: 1362–6.
29. Saoudi N, Bozio A, Kirkorian G, Attalah G, Normand J, Touboul P. Prolonged QT, atrioventricular block, and sudden death in the newborn: an electrophysiologic evaluation. *Eur Heart J* 1991; **12**: 838–41.
30. Bharati S, Dreifus L, Buchelers G, Molthan M, Covitz W, Isenberg HS, Lev M. The conduction system in patients with a prolonged QT interval. *JACC* 1985; **6**: 1110–19.
31. Schwartz PJ. Idiopathic long QT syndrome: progress and questions. *Am Heart J* 1985; **109**: 399–411.
32. Vincent GM. The heart rate of Romano–Ward syndrome patients. *Am Heart J* 1986; **112**: 61–4.
33. Kugler JD. Sinus nodal dysfunction in young patients with long QT syndrome. *Am Heart J* 1991; **121**: 1132–6.
34. James TN, Froggatt P, Atkinson WJ, Lurie PR, McNamara DG, Miller WM, Schloss GT, Carrol JF, North RL. Observations on the pathophysiology of the long QT syndrome with special reference to the neuropathology of the heart. *Circulation* 1978; **57**: 1221–31.
35. Zareba W, Moss AJ, Benhorin J, *et al.* The influence of beta-blockers on QT interval in patients with long QT syndrome (abstract). *JACC* 1996; **27**: 121A.
36. Dessertenne F. La tachycardie ventriculaire a deux foyers opposes variables. *Arch Mal Coeur* 1966; **59**: 263–72.
37. Tzivoni D, Keren A, Stern S, Gotlieb S. Disopyramide-induced torsade de pointes. *Arch Intern Med* 1981; **141**: 946–7.
38. Viskin S, Alla SR, Barron HV, *et al.* Mode of onset of torsade de pointes in congenital long QT syndrome. *JACC* 1996; **28**: 1262–8.

39. Vos MA, Verduyn SC, Gorgels APM, Lipcsei GC, Wellens HJJ. Reproducible induction of early afterdepolarizations and torsade de pointes arrhythmias by D-sotalol and pacing in dogs with chronic atrioventricular block. *Circulation* 1985; **91**: 864–72.

40. Han J, Millet D, Chizzonitti B, Moe GK. Temporal dispersion of recovery of excitability in atrium and ventricle as a function of heart rate. *Am Heart J* 1966; **71**: 481–7.

41. Vassalle M. Electrogenic suppression of automaticity in sheep and dog Purkinje fibers. *Circ Res* 1970; **27**: 361–77.

42. Kahn MN, Logan KR, McComb JM, Adgey JAA. Management of recurrent ventricular tachyarrhythmias associated with QT prolongation. *Am J Cardiol* 1981; **47**: 1301–8.

43. Keren A, Tzivoni D, Gavish D, Levi J, Gottlieb S. Etiology, warning, signs and therapy of torsade de pointes: a study of 10 patients. *Circulation* 1981; **64**: 1167–74.

44. Bazett HC. An analysis of the time relations of electrocardiograms. *Heart* 1920; **7**: 353–67.

45. Franz MR. Long term recording of monophasic action potential from human endocardium. *Am J Cardiol* 1983; **51**: 1629–35.

46. Franz MR, Swerdlow CD, Liem LB, Schaefer J. Cycle length dependence of human action potential duration *in vivo*: effects of single extrastimuli, sudden sustained rate acceleration and deceleration, and different steady-state frequencies. *J Clin Invest* 1988; **82**: 972–9.

47. Hirao H, Shimizu W, Kurita T, Suyama K, Aihara N, Kamakura S, Shimomura K. Frequency-dependent electrophysiologic properties of ventricular repolarization in patients with congenital long QT syndrome. *JACC* 1996; **28**: 1269–77.

48. Eldar M, Griffin JC, Abbott JA, Benditt D, Bhandari A, Herre JM, Benson DW, Scheinman MM. Permanent cardiac pacing in patients with the long QT syndrome. *JACC* 1987; **10**: 600–7.

49. Eldar M, Griffin JC, VanHare GF, Witherell C, Bhandari A, Benditt D, Scheinman M. Combined use of beta-adrenergic blocking agents and long-term cardiac pacing for patients with the long QT syndrome. *JACC* 1992; **20**: 830–7.

50. Moss AJ, Liu JE, Gottlieb S, Locati EH, Schwartz PJ, Robinson JL. Efficacy of permanent pacing in the management of high-risk patients with long QT syndrome. *Circulation* 1991; **84**: 1524–9.

51. Priori SG, Napolitano C, Cantu F, Brown AM, Schwartz PJ. Differential response to Na$^+$ channel blockade, β-adrenergic stimulation, and rapid pacing in a cellular model mimicking the SCN5A and HERG defects present in the long QT syndrome. *Circ Res* 1996; **78**: 1009–15.

52. Locati EH, Stramba-Badiale M, Priors SG, Napolitano C, Towbin JA, Keating MT, Vinolas X, Schwartz PJ. Gene-specific differences in the dynamic relation of QT interval and heart rate in the congenital long QT syndrome (abstract). *JACC* 1996; **27**: 126A.

53. Zareba W, Narins CR, Moss AJ, *et al.* Dispersion of repolarization and the genotype of long QT syndrome (abstract). *JACC* 1996; **27**: 20A.

54. Priori SG, Zareba W, Napolitano C, Locati E, Robinson JL, Diehl L, Schwartz PJ, Moss AJ. The implantable cardioverter defibrillator (ICD) in the long QT syndrome: data from the International Registry (abstract). *PACE* 1996; **19**: 566.

SECTION II

Issues

11

Should Every Patient with High-Grade AV Block have a DDD Device?

K. A. Ellenbogen, D. M. Gilligan, M. A. Wood and C. A. Morillo

In this chapter we will argue that most patients undergoing pacemaker implantation for high-grade AV block should have a dual chamber pacemaker implanted to restore AV synchrony. Exceptions to this general statement include patients with a life expectancy less than 6 months to 1 year, patients with chronic illness that markedly limits their quality of life and level of activity, patients with atrial standstill and patients with chronic or persistent atrial fibrillation. This viewpoint is similar to those published in the last 5 years by the American Heart Association/American College of Cardiology and the British Pacing and Electrophysiology Group.[1,2] We will compare data on the haemodynamics, vascular changes, exercise performance, neurohumoral markers, quality of life, costs, morbidity and mortality associated with dual-chamber pacing and with ventricular pacing in patients with heart block (Table 11.1).

From the outset, it is important to emphasize that we believe that the restoration of AV synchrony in patients with high-grade AV block leads to improved haemo-dynamics, which results in improved exercise performance, and ultimately leads to a more optimal neurohumoral milieu, more optimal vascular responses to changes in cardiac output and an improved quality of life. Future studies will determine if these haemodynamic and neurohumoral changes result in improved survival.

Haemodynamics

The haemodynamic benefit of AV synchrony has been well described in the physiology literature.[3–6] McWilliam is credited with one of the earliest published descriptions of AV synchrony.[7] He documented that a marked fall of blood pressure occurred during periods of AV dyssynchrony during an experiment with a cat's heart using vagal stimulation to alter contraction of the auricles and ventricles. He

Table 11.1   AV sequential and VVI(R) pacemakers compared

Definite advantages of AV sequential pacemakers over VVI(R) pacemakers
Improved haemodynamics at rest:
  higher systolic and mean arterial pressure
  higher stroke volume and cardiac output
  lower right atrial, pulmonary artery and left ventricular end-diastolic pressures
Improved quality of life
Improved exercise tolerance compared with patients with VVI pacemakers
Lower incidence of pacemaker syndrome

Probable advantages of AV sequential pacemakers
Improved survival in patients with congestive heart failure

Possible advantages of AV sequential pacemakers
Improved survival in patients without congestive heart failure
Lower incidence of atrial fibrillation
Lower incidence of stroke
Lower incidence of admission to the hospital for congestive heart failure
Improved exercise tolerance compared with patients with VVI(R) pacemakers

---

concluded that 'in order that such excitation should be as effective as possible, it is probably best to send the stimulating shocks through the whole heart, so that the auricles may come directly under their influence as well as the ventricles.'

A considerable body of subsequent work has examined the effects of AV synchrony on blood pressure, intracardiac filling pressures and cardiac output. A brief review of the haemodynamic consequences of AV synchrony is valuable in helping to understand changes in the autonomic system with pacing.

The atrium serves as a booster pump to contribute 10–50% of resting cardiac output.[3,6] Improved cardiac output with AV synchrony has been demonstrated in a wide variety of patient populations, including patients with NYHA Class IV heart failure as well as those with hypertrophic cardiomyopathy and aortic stenosis.[8–10] The atrial contribution to cardiac output has been noted over a wide range of paced heart rates, in the supine and upright positions and in the presence of inotropic stimulation. The variable contribution of the atrial 'kick' to cardiac output depends on heart rate, AV delay, myocardial function (both diastolic and systolic), presence of valvular heart disease and left atrial size.[11–13]

Restoration of AV synchrony has been shown by many investigators to result consistently in lower left ventricular end-diastolic pressures, lower left ventricular end-diastolic volumes, lower mean and phasic right atrial pressures, lower mean and phasic pulmonary artery pressures and higher mean arterial pressures (Figure 11.1). These haemodynamic changes have been noted in patients with and without clinical congestive heart failure, and are independent of left atrial size. Optimal timing of left atrial and left ventricular contraction is the goal of DDD pacing. Optimization of the AV interval may be especially important in patients with severe left ventricular systolic or diastolic function. Several groups have shown that stroke volume may be augmented by 25–46% by changes in the programmed AV delay from the least to most optimal values.[13,14]

The 'pacemaker syndrome' is the clinical consequence of haemodynamic changes that occur in patients who do not have restoration of AV synchrony in response to

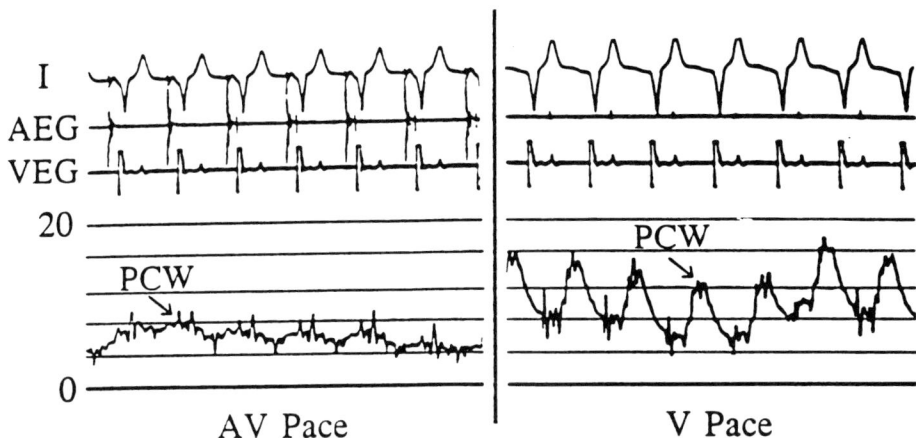

Figure 11.1 Surface electrocardiographic lead I, atrial electrogram (AEG), ventricular electrogram (VEG) and pulmonary capillary wedge pressure (PCW) recordings from a single patient during AV pacing (AV Pace) and ventricular pacing (V Pace) at 80 bpm with an AV interval of 150 ms. The cannon A wave is noted (arrow) on the PCW tracing. (Reproduced from reference 65 with permission)

single- or dual-chamber pacing.[14] The symptoms associated with pacemaker syndrome vary from mild to severe, and in many patients are not even realized until AV synchrony is restored.[14–16] A list of possible symptoms associated with pacemaker syndrome is shown in Table 11.2.

The relationship between haemodynamic changes that occur during VVI pacing and the resultant clinical symptoms may at times be difficult to discern. For example, the increased mean and phasic right and left atrial pressure with AV dyssynchrony

Table 11.2 Clinical symptoms of 'pacemaker syndrome'

Mild
Pulsations or pain in neck
Pulsations or pain in jaw
Pulsations in abdomen
Lump in throat or neck
Chest fullness or chest pain
Cough
Headache
Fatigue, malaise, tiredness, weakness
Choking sensation
Palpitations

Moderate
Shortness of breath on exertion
Dizziness
Vertigo
Orthopnoea
Paroxysmal nocturnal dyspnoea

Severe
Presyncope
Syncope
Shortness of breath at rest

may result in headaches, fullness in the head or neck, pulsations in the neck or abdomen, cough and jaw pain. In more severe cases cannon A waves are visible on haemodynamic tracings and correlate with symptoms of neck discomfort in many patients. More severe symptoms of pacemaker syndrome include dizziness, confusion, presyncope, syncope or decreased exercise tolerance. These more severe symptoms correlate with decreased cardiac output and blood pressure in patients without restoration of AV synchrony. Since many elderly patients complain of a variety of nonspecific symptoms, VVI pacemaker patients complaining of tiredness or weakness may have these complaints ignored or attributed to other medical problems. As a result, the 'true' incidence of pacemaker syndrome is probably under-estimated.[14–17]

Failure to restore AV synchrony may result in an increased incidence and degree of mitral and tricuspid regurgitation. Furman *et al.*[18] reported a 69% incidence of tricuspid valve regurgitation in patients with VVI(R) pacemakers at the end of 6 months. Reynolds *et al.*[19] used left ventricular angiography to compare the effects of AV sequential pacing with ventricular pacing. Thirty percent of patients with VVI pacemakers had a slight or mild worsening of mitral regurgitation during ventricular pacing. Naito *et al.*[20] demonstrated angiographic evidence of retrograde blood flow in the pulmonary venous system in dogs during ventricular but not AV sequential pacing.

Ishikawa *et al.*[21] studied the acute effects of AV sequential pacing on left atrial dimensions. Immediately following implantation of DDD pacemakers in 22 patients with AV block, the left atrial size decreased and reached a plateau by 1 min. The decrease in left atrial dimensions was maintained for up to a week. Stambler *et al.*[22] compared the effects of AV sequential and ventricular pacing on P-wave duration and left atrial size in patients participating in a randomized comparison of VVI(R) to DDD(R) pacing (the PASE trial). A significant increase in left atrial size and P-wave duration was noted in patients programmed to the VVI(R) mode compared with patients programmed to the DDD(R) mode. These results are similar to those reported in patients with sick sinus syndrome from the Danish trial of physiological pacing.[23] Another recent report of patients with VVI(R) pacemakers showed left atrial appendage dysfunction to be particularly common in patients with ventriculoatrial conduction.[24]

Exercise Capacity

A 'superior' pacing mode should demonstrate an improvement in exercise capacity in addition to improved haemodynamics measured at rest or exercise. Multiple studies have compared the effects of different pacing modes on exercise capacity. Exercise capacity has been measured in both the supine and upright positions, and is best gauged by metabolic stress testing. Objective measurements of exercise capacity generally consist of maximal oxygen consumption during exercise, preferably at the anaerobic threshold. This measurement is believed to represent a reliable and reproducible method for determination of exercise capacity. In addition to cardiac output, factors that influence exercise capacity include inspired oxygen concentration, muscle mechanics, alveolar gas exchange, oxygen-carrying capacity of blood, local tissue factors and systemic regional blood flow.

There is a considerable body of work showing acute improvements in exercise capacity for DDD compared with VVI pacing. Perrins et al.[25] showed that VDD pacing was associated with a 27% increase in exercise capacity compared with VVI pacing. Sutton et al.[26] also demonstrated a 34% improvement in bicycle ergometry exercise tolerance with VDD pacing at an average of 33 months. Kristensson et al.[27] demonstrated a 14% improvement in exercise tolerance in 44 patients who were randomly assigned to VVI or VDD pacing for 3 weeks.

Comparisons of exercise capacity of patients randomized to either DDD(R) or VVI(R) pacing have not been clear-cut. Several small trials of patients with pacemakers programmed either to the DDD or VVI(R) mode have been inconclusive. Linde-Edelstam et al.[28] compared submaximal exercise capacity in VVI(R) and DDD modes in 17 patients: patients programmed to the DDD pacing mode did not show any difference in exercise time compared with patients programmed to the VVI(R) pacing mode. Fannapazir et al.,[29] Menozzi et al.,[30] Oldroyd et al.[31] and Jutzy et al.[32] were all unable to show any benefit of DDD pacing (with appropriate chronotropic response) over VVI(R) pacing with respect to exercise capacity.

Vascular Reflexes

The vascular responses to ventricular pacing have important consequences. Alicandri et al.[33] from the Cleveland Clinic studied three patients with severe pacemaker syndrome. These patients suffered from hypotension and presyncope during ventricular pacing. Measurements of arterial pressure, cardiac output, right atrial pressure and total peripheral vascular resistance were compared with a control group. The three patients with hypotension during ventricular pacing manifested a 20% decrease in peripheral resistance, while the control patients did not develop hypotension during ventricular pacing and had an increase or no change in peripheral vascular resistance. Erlebacher et al.[34] made similar observations in patients following bypass surgery. They examined the pulmonary capillary wedge tracing for the presence or absence of cannon A waves during ventricular pacing in 20 patients following uncomplicated bypass surgery or aortic valve replacement. The patients with cannon A waves were more likely to have ventriculoatrial conduction compared with patients without cannon A waves. The change in mean systemic blood pressure during ventricular pacing was predicted by the presence of cannon A waves which was associated with inhibition of the normal reflex increases in systemic vascular resistance. The induction of hypotension during ventricular pacing was associated with cannon A waves, suggesting that atrial inhibitory reflexes may play a role in pacemaker syndrome.

Ellenbogen et al.[35] have also studied changes in vascular tone during different pacing modes. They used the technique of forearm venous plethysmography to measure forearm blood flow and changes in forearm vascular resistance during atrial, ventricular and simultaneous ventricular and atrial pacing with a VA interval of 100–150 ms. Forearm blood flow provides an accurate measure of changes in regional blood flow, reflecting changes in regional vasomotor tone. During ventricular pacing, especially with simulated VA conduction (i.e. VA pacing) forearm vascular resistance increased. These changes in regional vascular resistance were striking, occurring within 30 seconds of the onset of ventricular pacing while patients were studied in the supine relaxed state. Intra-arterial phentolamine blocked regional vasoconstriction confirming that changes in vascular tone are mediated by sympathetic vasoconstriction. These changes in vascular tone can also be demonstrated with peroneal microneurography. Arterial baroreceptors primarily modulate these changes in vascular tone through the sympathetic nervous system. Recently, the technique of peroneal microneurography has been used to provide additional instantaneous information about the changes in measured sympathetic nerve activity during single-chamber ventricular pacing and dual-chamber pacing. We recorded arterial pressure, respiration and muscle sympathetic nerve activity during ventricular pacing and AV synchronous pacing in 13 patients, while pacing at 60 and 100 bpm.[36] Acute atrioventricular synchronous pacing resulted in higher arterial pressure and lower sympathetic nerve activity than during ventricular pacing. This indicates that the cardiac pacing mode may influence sympathetic outflow through the arterial baroreflexes.

Based on these observations, we hypothesize that ventricular pacing, but not AV sequential pacing, results in a decrease in stroke volume, cardiac output and arterial pressure, subsequently resulting in activation of the sympathetic nervous system to maintain constriction of blood vessels and preservation of vascular tone (Figure 11.2). This is opposed by the elevation in filling pressures and atrial distension during ventricular pacing that leads to inhibition of vasoconstriction and vasodilatation. In some patients, these two opposing reflexes result in an inadequate vasoconstrictor response and an overall decrease in vascular tone, which finally leads to symptoms suggestive of pacemaker syndrome and hypotension from vasodilatation. These reflexes may be further exaggerated or altered by changes in position, as well as by cardiac drugs and changes in volume status.

Humoral Changes

A variety of humoral changes occur with pacing. We and others have demonstrated that plasma norepinephrine and epinephrine levels are elevated acutely during shifts from normal sinus rhythm to VVI pacing at different rates.[37] Plasma catecholamine levels may correlate poorly with changes in cardiac sympathetic tone during non-steady-state conditions, such as during acute changes in pacing mode. Others have shown that coronary sinus norepinephrine levels and cardiac norepineprine spillover are higher with VVI pacing than during VAT pacing.[38,39] Cardiac norepinephrine spillover is likely to closely reflect cardiac sympathetic tone. VVI pacing caused more marked increases in arterial concentrations of catecholamines than AV synchronous pacing. These findings are consistent with the studies cited above showing that ventricular pacing is associated with greater activation of the sympathetic nervous system than is DDD pacing.

ANP (atrial natriuretic peptide) is a 28-amino-acid polypeptide located in atrial granules. This polypeptide has multiple complex physiological effects, but has been

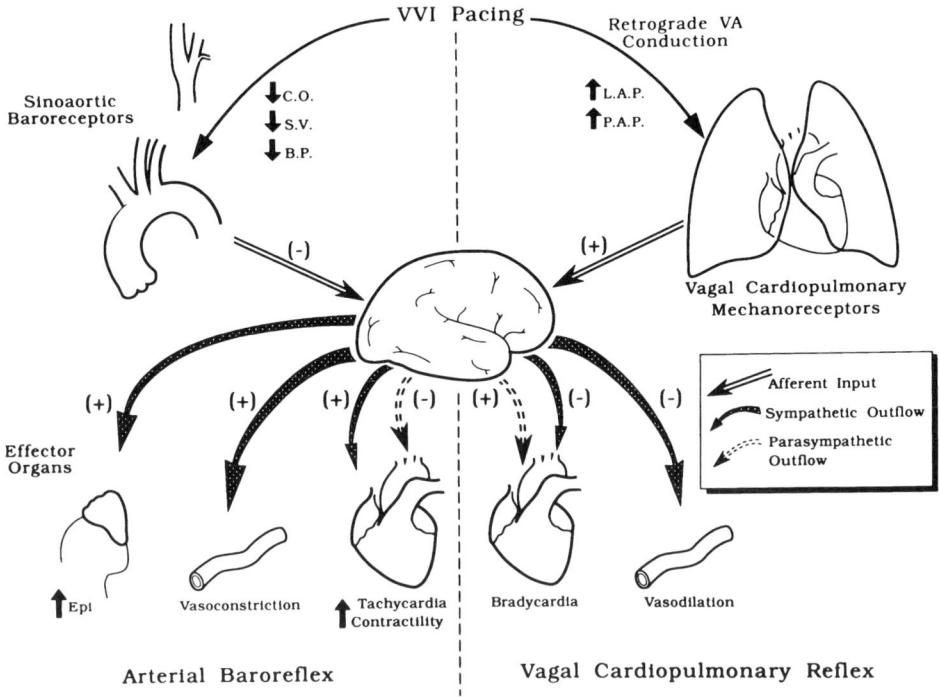

Figure 11.2 Diagrammatic representation of multiple reflex pathways involved in pacemaker syndrome. See text for discussion. The arterial baroreflexes detect a decrease in stroke volume when atrioventricular (AV) dyssynchrony occurs, leading to sympathetic activation and vasoconstriction. AV dyssynchrony leads to atrial wall distension and activation of inhibitory reflex pathways leading to vagally mediated vasodilation (and sympathetic withdrawal) as well as release of humoral substances, including atrial natriuretic peptide (ANP), which may potentiate these inhibitory reflexes. LAP = left atrial pressure; PAP = pulmonary artery pressure; CO = cardiac output; SV = stroke volume; BP = blood pressure; EPI = epinephrine. (Reproduced from reference 14 with permission)

implicated by some to be related to pacemaker syndrome.[40] ANP levels increase acutely and chronically to a greater degree during VVI pacing than with AV pacing.[41–43] Investigators recently reported an increased mean calf capillary filtration coefficient (measured with a modified plethysmographic technique) during ventricular pacing compared with DDD pacing.[44] Increased ANP levels may lead to an enhanced flux of fluid from the intravascular to the extravascular compartment. Elevated ANP levels during VVI pacing have also been noted with exercise and during pacing mode crossover studies associated with AV dyssynchrony.[45] Whether ANP plays an important causative role in any symptoms that patients experience associated with VVI pacing is unknown.

Quality of Life

Permanent pacing prevents syncope or torsade de pointes initiated by bradycardia in some patients, but the goals of pacing should be broader. DDD pacing has its greatest impact on patients in their routine activities of daily life, in particular by improving their quality of life and decreasing symptoms during these activities. More importantly, VVI or VVI(R) pacing has a negative impact on many patients' quality of life. The precise incidence of 'suboptimal' function in patients with ventricular pacing has only recently become recognized.

The 'true' incidence of pacemaker syndrome is realized when one avoids 'strict' definitions of the situation. We believe that pacemaker syndrome includes any and all symptoms related to the loss of AV synchrony.[14,17] These symptoms may be manifested by an impaired quality of life, decreased exercise tolerance or complaints related to AV dyssynchrony.

In one study, investigators from the Mayo Clinic reported that 20% of 50 patients with DDD pacemakers had a mean decrease in systolic blood pressure of 24 ± 11 mmHg during VVI pacing compared with DVI pacing or sinus rhythm.[46] Ten patients experienced dizziness in the standing position during VVI pacing. Heldman and colleagues tried to assess the 'true incidence of pacemaker syndrome' based on symptom questionnaires in 40 unselected DDD pacemaker patients who underwent pacemaker programming to either DDD or DDI compared with VVI for 1 week in each mode. Patients completed a series of questionnaires relating to the presence of symptoms and the severity of those symptoms during each pacing mode. Twelve of 16 symptoms were worse during VVI compared with DDD pacing. The most significant symptoms were shortness of breath, dizziness, fatigue, pulsations in the neck or abdomen, cough and apprehension. Eighty-three per cent of patients paced in the VVI mode had symptoms, and 65% of patients experienced at least moderate or severe symptoms. Only 17% of patients experienced no new or worsened symptoms during VVI pacing. Forty-two per cent of patients were unable to tolerate VVI pacing for even 1 week.

Several crossover trials have compared quality of life between DDD and VVI or VVI(R) pacing. The majority of these studies have demonstrated a convincing improvement in quality of life in patients paced in an AV synchronous mode compared with patients paced either in the VVI or VVI(R) mode[47–49] A criticism of some of these studies is that the quality-of-life instruments used have not been thoroughly scientifically validated. A quality-of-life instrument should be reliable, valid and sensitive. Ideally, these studies should incorporate a quality-of-life instrument appropriate for pacemaker patients, and separate patients with sick sinus syndrome from those with complete heart block. Another concern is that investigators or patients may not be carefully blinded to their therapy, resulting in biased assessments of pacing modes. Sulke *et al.*[15,50] have performed two studies that further explore the relatively high incidence of pacemaker syndrome. They reported on the subjective and objective assessment of a group of 22 patients with heart block programmed to DDD, DDI(R) and VVI(R) pacing modes. Patients were programmed to each pacing mode for a 4-week period of out-of-hospital activity. Subjective assessment of pacing was performed with visual analogue scales to assess patient-perceived general well-being and exercise tolerance. A second questionnaire was used to assess patients' perceived physical limitations and a third questionnaire was used to assess the incidence and frequency of symptoms of pacemaker syndrome. Objective assessments consisted of graded exercise treadmill testing measuring total exercise time, mental stress testing, suitcase lifting, staircase ascent and descent, as well as measurement of pulmonary artery systolic pressure and stroke volume by echocardiographic techniques. Seventy-three per cent of patients found the VVI(R) mode to be the least acceptable pacing mode (Figure 11.3). General well-being, functional status, perceived exercise capacity and specific symptom scores were lower with VVI(R) pacing than with any other pacing mode. Five of the 22 patients programmed to the VVI(R) mode demanded early crossover to DDD pacing because of symptoms of dyspnoea, dizziness, tiredness and palpitations. In another study, these investigators reported on 16 patients with VVI pacemakers who had generally felt well for at least 3 years prior to the time of their pulse generator change for battery depletion.[50]

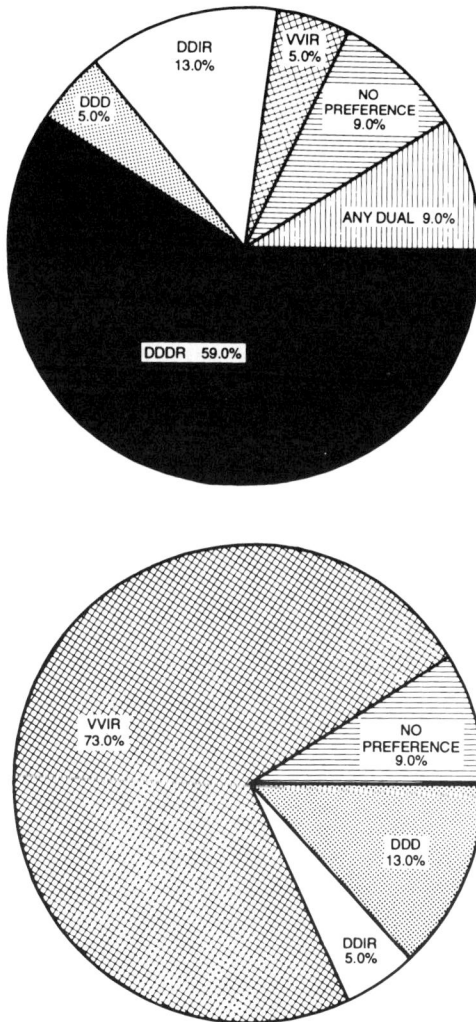

Figure 11.3 Preferred (*top*) and least acceptable pacing modes based on symptom questionnaire. (Reproduced from reference 15 with permission)

Table 11.3   Clinical predictors of 'pacemaker syndrome'

Definite
None

Probable
Retrograde VA conduction
Cannon A waves
Increase in stroke volume with DDD pacing
Decrease in stroke volume during VVI pacing
Relatively higher atrial contribution to ventricular filling or stroke volume
Change in blood pressure with ventricular pacing

Not predictive
Presence of congestive heart failure
Left ventricular function
Aetiology of conduction system disease; sick sinus syndrome *vs* AV block
Left atrial size
Left ventricular size
Ejection fraction
Age
Baseline stroke volume
Baseline pulmonary capillary pressure

All these patients were upgraded to DDD pacemakers at the time of battery replacement by atrial lead implantation. The authors used the same methodology to characterize the changes in subjective and objective responses during pacing mode changes. Seventy-five per cent of patients preferred the DDD mode and 68% found the VVI mode to be the least acceptable. Only 12% expressed no pacing mode preference. Perceived general well-being, symptom scores, and exercise treadmill times were all improved with DDD pacing. The authors concluded that a 'subclinical' pacemaker syndrome is present in up to 75% of patients with VVI pacemakers who do not have 'overt' or severe symptoms of pacemaker syndrome.

Ideally, clinical, electrocardiographic or echocardiographic variables that predict the development of intolerance to VVI pacing could be discerned. Multiple studies have failed to consistently confirm any individual clinical or laboratory variable that reliably predicts the development of pacemaker syndrome. Variables that have been clearly shown *not* to predict the development of pacemaker syndrome include the presence of congestive heart failure, the indication for pacing (sick sinus syndrome *vs* AV block), ejection fraction, left atrial size, left ventricular function and left ventricular size (Table 11.3). Several investigators have suggested that the presence of VA conduction or the percentage change in cardiac output or stroke volume with VVI versus DDD pacing are two variables that appear to be somewhat predictive of a higher incidence of developing pacemaker syndrome.[51,52]

Practice Patterns

A recent publication evaluated patterns of pacemaker selection in elderly Medicare pacemaker recipients in the United States. This analysis was based on a 20% random national sample of all Medicare beneficiaries older than 65 years who underwent pacemaker implantation.[53] In 1990, 37% of patients undergoing pacemaker implantation had a dual-chamber pacemaker implanted. Patients were more likely to get a DDD pacemaker if they were men, younger, had AV block and had a diagnosis of congestive heart failure. A survey of cardiac pacing practices in 1993 extended these findings. The authors noted an increase in DDD pacemaker implantation, from 32% to 68%, in patients undergoing a primary pacemaker implant procedure receiving DDD pacemakers.[54] An increase in dual-chamber pacing has been noted in other countries as well.

Mortality and Morbidity

Changes in mortality or the incidence of stroke, atrial fibrillation or hospitalization for congestive heart failure with different pacing modes are increasingly required to justify clinical practices in an ever-increasing cost-conscious environment. There are no conclusive data regarding these issues comparing VVI with DDD pacing. Retrospective nonrandomized trials have reported a worse prognosis in patients undergoing VVI pacing compared with patients receiving atrial synchronous pacing. Alpert et al.[55] in a study of 132 patients with pre-existing congestive heart failure noted an improved survival in the patients who received dual-chamber pacemakers. Linde-Edelstram et al.[56] performed a case–control study of 74 patients who received DDD pacemakers and 74 patients with VVI pacemakers during a mean follow-up of 5.4 years. The overall survival rate was not different between the two patient groups, and was similar to the survival of a matched group of individuals from the general population. An increased mortality was seen in a subgroup of their patients with congestive heart failure who underwent VVI pacing. These two studies suggest that patients with congestive heart failure who have a VVI pacemaker implanted have an increased mortality, but the studies have been criticized because of the nonrandom patient selection, possibly leading to exclusion of the sickest patients from receiving DDD pacemakers. Many other nonrandomized studies assessing patient survival and other 'hard' objective end-points (e.g. heart failure, atrial fibrillation, stroke) suffer from similar limitations, as well as small sample size, inadequate duration of follow-up and inclusion of mostly patients with sick sinus syndrome.

The Danish trial was a prospective, randomized comparison of atrial versus ventricular based pacing but included only patients with sick sinus syndrome.[23] In the trial, patients receiving VVI(R) pacemakers had a higher incidence of systemic thromboembolism (stroke and peripheral arterial emboli). A recent report of platelet activation in patients paced with VVI(R) suggests that increased platelet activation is related to loss of AV synchrony and not atrial fibrillation.[57] The PASE trial which randomized 403 elderly patients to VVI(R) or DDD(R) pacing showed no significant improvement of DDD(R) over VVI(R) when subgroups of patients with sick sinus syndrome and complete heart block were analysed separately. A composite secondary end-point consisting of mortality, stroke, atrial fibrillation and exacerbation of congestive heart failure showed a trend towards an improvement with DDD(R) pacing ($p = 0.05$). A striking finding in this study was that 30% of patients programmed to VVI(R) were crossed over to DDD(R) pacing, thus limiting the power of the study.

The UK-PASE trial will provide additional information about mortality and other 'hard' end-points in patients receiving DDD(R) or VVI(R) pacemakers.[58] This trial will enrol patients over age 70 with complete or high-grade AV block and randomize them to dual-chamber or ventricular pacing. The primary end-point is mortality, the secondary end-points are the development of atrial fibrillation, stroke, congestive heart failure and pacemaker syndrome. Quality of life, exercise tolerance and costs of pacing and follow-up will also be addressed.

Another randomized trial comparing DDD(R) with VVI(R) pacing is the Canadian Trial of Physiological Pacing (CTOPP). This multicentre trial is examining the risk of the combined outcome of cardiovascular death or stroke in patients receiving a dual-chamber or single-chamber pacemaker for sick sinus syndrome or complete AV block. The rate of occurrence of atrial fibrillation, systemic embolism and admission to a hospital with congestive heart failure is a secondary end-point. Additional quality-of-life and economic evaluations are being performed.

Cost Considerations

Until the results of prospective randomized studies like UK-PASE and CTOPP are available, issues of cost-effectiveness of DDD pacing will be based on analyses of nonrandomized published studies.[58] One issue often raised is that DDD pacemakers are inherently more expensive in part because of a relatively high incidence of atrial lead dislodgement or atrial lead malfunction. These arguments are largely based on early studies shortly after the introduction of atrial leads. Improvements in lead technology have made atrial lead dislodgement and atrial lead failure relatively uncommon. One recent study from a tertiary referral centre with experienced operators failed to show a difference in the overall complication rate for DDD pacing compared with VVI pacing.[59] There was no difference in electrode displacement rates or need for reoperation for dual- compared with single-chamber replacement rates.

A cost analysis based on the recommendations of the British Pacing and Electrophysiology Group guidelines was performed by two groups and showed that implementation of this group's pacing recommendations would lead to an estimated 75–94% increase in pacemaker budgets. Additional costs would probably be incurred by increased costs of follow-up.[60,61] A recent cost–benefit analysis comparing DDD pacing with VVI pacing was performed based on a literature review and found a different result.[62] A computer model was set up based on the calculated incidence and prevalence of stroke, atrial fibrillation, permanent disability, heart failure and mortality in patients with AV block. The costs of procedures, hospitalization and medication were based on UK prices in 1991. The authors calculated that for patients with AV block, the difference in cumulative cost between VVI and DDD pulse generators was seven times the purchase price of a VVI pulse generator. In other words, at the end of 10 years the increased cost of VVI pacing in terms of increased risk of stroke, death, heart failure, atrial fibrillation, pacemaker syndrome and disability was equal to seven times the purchase price of the single-chamber pulse generator. By the third year after implantation, the cumulative costs of DDD pacing were lower than for VVI pacing. Limitations of this type of analysis include the reliability of data used for calculating the incidence of different outcomes and the accuracy of cost data based on retrospective information. Another limitation of this analysis is that it does not consider the option of implanting VDD single-lead pacemakers in patients with complete heart block, with the resultant decreased cost and complexity of such a system. It is hoped that the results of large prospective trials will provide more information about the costs of VVI and DDD pacing.

Ethics

Recently several investigators have questioned the ethics of performing clinical trials comparing VVI(R) with dual-chamber pacing. Fogoros has argued that data generated by a clinical trial must have a reasonable probability of resolving a dispute or disturbing the clinical 'equipoise'.[63] Fogoros argues that if the issue of DDD versus VVI pacing does not approach a state of clinical equipoise, then why propose and perform a clinical trial that compares patients paced in each pacing mode? He raises the issue that financial factors may be driving enrolment and randomization in clinical trials where 'equipoise' is not present. Ovsyshcher argues that randomization of patients to receive DDD(R) or VVI(R) pacemakers as part of a large multicentre trial may be substituted with outcomes of research trials.[64] She argues that given the differences in clinical care from one implanter or institution to another, tracking of outcomes among a large group of patients of various ages and risk profiles allows one to inexpensively and rapidly compare these two modes of pacing. The databases would have to have detailed information on patient characteristics, outcomes and costs. The concerns about the ethics of implanting VVI(R) pacemakers in patients has raised considerable debate among implanters.

Summary

DDD pacing provides restoration of AV synchrony and superior haemodynamic, exercise and subjective function compared with VVI pacing. The majority of patients will choose AV synchronous pacing over VVI or VVI(R) pacing when programmed to each of these different pacing modes. VVI(R) pacing should be reserved for the infirm, or inactive, or patients with limited life expectancy or chronic atrial dysrhythmias. Clinical and echocardiographic or electrocardiographic predictors of pacemaker syndrome remain unproven, but there is some suggestion that intact retrograde ventriculoatrial conduction predisposes patients to the development of pacemaker syndrome. With an incidence of pacemaker syndrome approaching 80% in some studies, and few reliable clinical predictors of its development, we argue that almost all patients should have DDD pacemakers implanted.

References

1. Dreifus LS, Fisch C, Griffin JC, _et al_. Guidelines for implantation of cardiac pacemakers and antiarrhythmia devices. _JACC_ 1991; **8**: 1–13.
2. Clarke M, Sutton R, Ward D, Camm JA, Rickards A, _et al_. Recommendations for pacemaker prescription for symptomatic bradycardia. _Br Heart J_ 1991; **6**: 185–91.
3. Baig MW, Perrins EJ. The hemodynamics of cardiac pacing: clinical and physiological aspects. _Prog Cardiovasc Dis_ 1991; **33**: 283–98.
4. Buckingham Ta, Janosik DL, Pearson AC. Pacemaker hemodynamics: clinical implications. _Prog Cardiovasc Dis_ 1992; **34**: 347–66.
5. Faerestrand S. Nonivasive hemodynamic evaluation of pacing. In: Barold SS, Mugica J (eds), _New Perspectives in Cardiac Pacing: 3_. Mount Kisco, NY: Futura, 1993: 113–67.
6. Janosik DL, Labovitz AJ. Basic physiology of cardiac pacing. In: Ellenbogen KA, Kay GN, Wilkoff BL (eds), _Clincial Cardiac Pacing_. Philadelphia, PA: WB Saunders, 1995: 367–98.
7. McWilliam JA. Electrical stimulation of the heart in man. _Br Med J_ 1889; **1**: 348–50.
8. Mukharji J, Rehr RB, Hastillo A, _et al_. Comparison of atrial contribution to cardiac hemodynamics in patients with normal and severely compromised cardiac function. _Clin Cardiol_ 1990; **13**: 639–43.
9. Gross JN, Keltz TN, Cooper JA, _et al_. Profound 'pacemaker syndrome' in hypertrophic cardiomyopathy. _Am J Cardiol_ 1992; **70**: 1507–11.
10. Patel AK, Yap VU, Thomsen JH. Adverse affects of right ventricular pacing in a patient with aortic stenosis: hemodynamic documentation and management. _Chest_ 1977; **72**: 103–5.
11. Karlof I. Haemodynamic effect of atrial triggered versus fixed rate pacing at rest and during exercise in complete heart block. _Acta Med Scan_ 1975; **197**: 195.
12. Pearson AC, Janosik DL, Redd RM, _et al_. Hemodynamic benefit of atrioventricular synchrony: prediction from baseline doppler echocardiographic variables. _JACC_ 1989; **13**: 1613.
13. Lascault G, Bigonzi F, Frank R, _et al_. Noninvasive study of dual chamber pacing by pulsed Doppler: prediction of the haemodynamic response by echocardiographic measurements. _Eur Heart J_ 1989; **10**: 525.
14. Ellenbogen KA, Stambler BS. Pacemaker syndrome. In: Ellenbogen KA, Kay GN, Wilkoff BL (eds), _Clinical Cardiac Pacing_. Philadelphia, PA: WB Saunders, 1995: 419–31.
15. Sulke N, Chambers J, Dritsas A, Sowton, E. A randomized double-blind crossover comparison of four rate-responsive pacing modes. _JACC_ 1991; **17**: 696.
16. Ausubel K, Furman S. The pacemaker syndrome. _Ann Intern Med_ 1985; **103**: 420–9.
17. Ellenbogen KA, Wood MA, Stambler B. Pacemaker syndrome: clinical, hemodynamic and neurohumoral features. In: Barold SS, Mugica J (eds), _New Perspectives in Cardiac Pacing: 3_. Mount Kisco, NY: Futura, 1993: 85–112.
18. Furman S, Cooper JA. Atrial fibrillation during AV-sequential pacing. _PACE_ 1982; **5**: 133.
19. Reynolds DW, Olson EG, Burow RD, _et al_. Hemodynamic evaluation of atrioventricular and ventriculoatrial pacing (abstract). _PACE_ 1984; **7**: 476.
20. Naito M, Driefus LS, Mardelli TJ, _et al_. Echocardiographic features of atrioventricular and ventriculoatrial conduction. _Am J Cardiol_ 1980; **46**: 625.
21. Ishikawa T, Kimura K, Yoshimura H, _et al_. Acute changes in left atrial and left ventricular diameters after physiological pacing. _PACE_ 1996; **19**: 143–9.
22. Stambler BS, Lamas GA, Hoffman SW, _et al_. Is atrial refractoriness shorter in VVI than DDD paced patients? (abstract). _PACE_ 1995; **18**: 883.
23. Andersen HR, Thuesen L, Bagger JP, _et al_. Prospective randomised trial of atrial versus ventricular pacing in sick-sinus syndrome. _Lancet_ 1994; **344**: 1523–8.
24. Asanuma T, Tanabe K, Yoshitomi H, _et al_. Left atrial appendage function in patients with single-chamber ventricular pacing. _Am J Cardiol_ 1995; **76**: 840–2.
25. Perrins EJ, Morley CA, Chan SL, _et al_. Randomised controlled trial of physiological and ventricular pacing. _Br Heart J_ 1983; **50**: 112.
26. Sutton R, Perrins EJ, Morley C, _et al_. Sustained improvement in exercise tolerance following physiological cardiac pacing. _Eur Heart J_ 1983; **4**: 781.

27. Kristensson B-E, Arnman K, Smedgard P, *et al*. Physiological versus single-rate ventricular pacing: a double-blind cross-over study. *PACE* 1985; **8**: 73.
28. Linde-Edelstam C, Hjemdahl P, Phehrsson SK,*et al*. Is DDD pacing superior to VVIR? A study on cardiac sympathetic nerve activity and myocardial oxygen consumption at rest and during exercise. *PACE* 1992; **15**: 425.
29. Fananapazir L, Bennett DH, Monks P. Atrial synchronised ventricular pacing: contribution of the chronotropic response to improved exercise performance. *PACE* 1983; **6**: 601.
30. Menozzi C, Brignole M, Moracchini PV, *et al*. Intrapatient comparison between chronic VVIR and DDD pacing in patients affected by high-degree AV block without heart failure. *PACE* 1990; **13**: 1816.
31. Oldroyd KG, Rae AP, Carter R, *et al*. Double-blind cross-over comparison of dual-chamber pacing (DDD) and ventricular rate-adaptive (VVIR) pacing on neroendocrine variables, exercise performance, and symptoms in complete heart block. *Br Heart J* 1991; **65**: 188.
32. Jutzy RV, Florio J, Isaeff DM, *et al*. Comparative evaluation of rate modulated dual chamber and VVIR pacing. *PACE* 1990; **13**(II): 1838.
33. Alicandri C, Fouad F, Farazi RC, *et al*. Three cases of hypotension and syncope with ventricular pacing: possible role of atrial reflexes. *Am J Cardiol* 1978; **42**: 137.
34. Erlebacher JA, Danner RL, Stelzer PE. Hypotension with ventricular pacing: an atrial vasodepressor reflex in human beings. *JACC* 1984; **4**: 550.
35. Ellenbogen KA, Thames MD, Mohanty PK. New insights into pacemaker syndrome gained from hemodynamic, humoral and vascular responses during ventriculo-atrial pacing. *Am J Cardiol* 1990; **65**: 53–9.
36. Taylor JA, Morillo CA, Eckberg DL, Ellenbogen KA. Higher sympathetic nerve activity during ventricular (VVI) pacing than dual chamber (DDD) pacing: a potential mechanism for improved survival with DDD pacing. *JACC* (in press).
37. Hull RW, Snow F, Herre J, *et al*. The plasma catecholamine responses to ventricular pacing: implications for rate-responsive pacing. *PACE* 1990; **13**: 1408.
38. Linde-Edelstam C, Nordlander R, Pehrsson SK, *et al*. A double-blind study of submaximal exercise tolerance and variation in paced rate in atrial synchronous compared to activity sensor modulated ventricular pacing. *PACE* 1992; **15**: 905.
39. Pehrrson SK, Hjemdahl P, Nordlander R, *et al*. A comparison of sympathoadrenal adrenal activity and cardiac performance at rest and during exercise in patients with ventricular demand or atrial synchronous pacing. *Br Heart J* 1988; **60**: 212.
40 Clemo HF, Baumgarten CM, Stambler BS, *et al*. Atrial natriuretic factor: implications for cardiac pacing and electrophysiology. *PACE* 1994; **17**: 70–91.
41. Theodorakis GN, Kremastinos DTH, Markianos M, *et al*. Total sympathetic activity and atrial natriuretic factor levels in VVI and DDD pacing with different atrioventricular delays during daily activity and exercise. *Eur Heart J* 1992; **112**: 1477.
42. Theodorakis G, Kremastinos D, Markianos M, *et al*. C-AMP and ANP levels in VVI and DDD pacing with different AV delays during daily activity and exercise. *PACE* 1990; **13**: 1773.
43. Blanc JJ, Mansourati J, Ritter P, *et al*. Atrial natriuretic factor release during exercise in patients successively paced in DDD and rate matched ventricular pacing. *PACE* 1992; **15**: 397.
44. Mahy IR, Lewis DM, Shore AC, *et al*. Disturbance of peripheral microvascular fluid permeability by the onset of atrioventricular asynchrony in patients with programmable pacemakers. *Heart* 1996; **75**: 509–12.
45. Travill CM, Sutton R. Pacemaker syndrome: an iatrogenic condition. *Br Heart J* 1992; **68**: 163–6.
46. Heldman D, Mulvihill D, Nguyen H, *et al*. True incidence of pacemaker syndrome. *PACE* 1990; **13**: 1742.
47. Lau CP, Tai Y-T, Lee PWH, *et al*. Quality-of-life in DDDR pacing: atrioventricular synchrony or rate adaptation? *PACE* 1994; **17**(II): 1838–43.
48. Lukl J, Doupal V, Heinc P. Quality-of-life during DDD and dual sensor VVIR pacing. *PACE* 1994; **17**(II): 1844–8.

49. Linde C. How to evaluate quality-of-life in pacemaker patients: problems and pitfalls. *PACE* 1996; **19**: 391–7.
50. Sulke N, Dritsas A, Bostock J, *et al.* 'Subclinical' pacemaker syndrome: a randomized study of symptom-free patients with ventricular demand (VVI) pacemakers upgraded to dual-chamber devices. *Br Heart J* 1992; **67**: 57.
51. Stewart WJ, Dicola VC, Hawthorne JW, *et al.* Doppler ultrasound measurement of cardiac output in patients with physiologic parameters. *Am J Cardiol* 1984; **54**: 308.
52. Rediker DE, Eagle KA, Homma S, *et al.* Clinical and hemodynamic comparison of VVI versus DDD pacing in patients with DDD pacemakers. *Am J Cardiol* 1988; **61**: 323.
53. Lamas GA, Pashos CL, Normand SLT, *et al.* Permanent pacemaker selection and subsequent survival in elderly medicare pacemaker recipients. *Circulation* 1995; **91**: 1063–9.
54. Bernstein AD, Parsonnet V. Survey of cardiac pacing and defibrillation in the United States in 1993. *Am J Cardiol* 1996; **78**: 187.
55. Alpert MA, Curtis JJ, Sanfelippo JF, *et al.* Comparative survival after permanent ventricular and dual chamber pacing for patients with chronic high degree atrioventricular block with and without preexisting congestive heart failure. *JACC* 1986; **7**: 925.
56. Linde-Edelstram C, Gullberg B, Nordlander R, *et al.* Longevity in patients with high degree atrioventricular block paced in the atrial synchronous or the fixed-rate ventricular-inhibited mode. *PACE* 1992; **15**: 304.
57. Tse HF, Lau CP, Lee K, *et al.* Rate adaptive ventricular (VVIR) pacing is associated with increased platelet activation in patients with bradyarrhythmia (abstract). *Circulation* 1995; **91**: I-533.
58. Connolly SJ, Kerr C, Gent M, Yusuf S. Dual-chamber versus ventricular pacing: critical appraisal of current data. *Circulation* 1996; **94**: 578–83.
59. Aggarwal R, Connelly DT, Ray SG, *et al.* Early complications of permanent pacemaker implantation: no difference between dual and single chamber systems. *Br Heart J* 1995; **73**: 571–5.
60. Ray SG, Griffith MJ, Jamieson S, Bexton RS, Gold RG. Impact of the recommendations of the British Pacing and Electrophysiology Group's recommendations for pacing. *Br Med J* 1992; **305**: 861–5.
61. DeBelder MA, Linker NJ, Jones S, *et al.* Cost implications of the British Pacing and Electrophysiology Group on pacemaker prescription and on the immediate costs of pacing in the Northern Region. *Br Heart J* 1992; **68**: 531–4.
62. Sutton R, Bourgeois I. Cost benefit analysis of single and dual chamber pacing for sick sinus syndrome and atrioventricular block: an economic sensitivity analysis of the literature. *Eur Heart J* 1996; **17**: 574–82.
63. Fogoros RE. Letter to the editor. *PACE* 1996; **19**: 384–6.
64. Ovsyshcher IE. Matching optimal pacemaker to patient: do we need a large scale clinical trial of pacemaker mode selection? *PACE* 1995; **18**: 1845–52.
65. Reynolds DW. Hemodynamics of cardiac pacing. In: Ellenbogen KA (ed.), *Cardiac Pacing*. Cambridge, MA: Blackwell Scientific, 1992: 120–61.

12

Is There an Optimal AV Delay?

D. Katritsis and A. J. Camm

The 'AV delay' is the programmable time period from the occurrence of an atrial event, either intrinsic (PV) or paced (AV), to a paced ventricular event. The optimal AV delay is probably that interval which provides the delay required for left atrial systole to make its maximum contribution to stroke volume, either at rest or during exercise, maintains AV synchrony up to the highest heart rate achieved, and allows a normal ventricular activation by avoiding unnecessary ventricular pacing.

Following the seminal study of Karlof[1] on the beneficial effects of AV synchrony and the confirmation by Kruse et al.[2] of the long-term maintenance of this benefit, the haemodynamic importance of coordinated atrioventricular contraction has become well established.[3–5] An appropriately timed atrial systole improves left ventricular performance and reduces mean atrial pressure by coordinating atrioventricular valve closure,[6] facilitating venous return[7,8] and increasing preload.[7] Improperly timed paced atrial contractions may cause mitral regurgitation and result in impaired diastolic filling and even a decrease in cardiac output compared with ventricular pacing alone.[9–11] The time of mitral valve closure is inversely related to the AV interval during physiological pacing. Excessively long AV delay intervals may cause early mitral valve closure, thus limiting the diastolic filling period[12–13] as well as diastolic mitral regurgitation.[14,15,51] Very short AV delay intervals (<75 ms) may not allow sufficient time for atrial emptying before the onset of ventricular contraction.[12]

Physiological Considerations

The optimal AV delay, in which atrial contraction occurs in late ventricular diastole and contributes most to left ventricular filling,[16] is influenced by factors such as heart rate,[17,18] left ventricular function,[19,20] atrial size[21] and the interindividual differences in electrical and electromechanical intervals of both the atria and ventricles.[9,22] These intervals are dependent on multiple factors, including interatrial conduction time, electromechanical delay within the right and the left atrium, and the interventricular conduction time.[9,22] Following atrial stimulation, conduction from the right atrial appendage to the left atrium occurs during the programmed AV delay which begins with the atrial pacing artefact. This places left atrial depolarization late in the AV interval, relatively close to the ventricular pacing stimulus. During atrial sensing, the impulse originating in the sinus node is conducted to the left atrium, when it is sensed by the electrode in the right appendage. The programmed AV delay in this case starts with the sensed event in the right atrial appendage. The relatively short time required to complete conduction to the left atrium after sensing in the right atrium places left atrial depolarization earlier within the programmed AV delay, and further from the ventricular pacing stimulus. To avoid, therefore, a change in timing of left atrial contraction with a consequent decrease in stroke volume, the pro-grammed AV delay must be less during atrial triggering than in dual-chamber sequential pacing.[19,22,23] A difference of 30–50 ms may be necessary to optimize cardiac output,[22,24,25] although a number of factors – including electrode position, lead and circuit technology, amplitude and rate of stimulation, P-wave configura-tion, electrolytes, drugs and myocardial disease – may affect the delay between the onset of the native P wave and atrial sensing during atrial tracking. This difference in the optimal AV delay between a paced atrial cycle and a sensed atrial cycle emphasizes the importance of the so-called AV delay hysteresis with altering pacing modes (differential AV delay).[22,24]

The Effect of Exercise

The PR interval shortens progressively on exercise as the heart rate increases.[26–28,43] This decrease is caused by an improvement in nodal conduction induced by sympathetic stimulation and a decrease in vagal tone. In healthy subjects, Daubert *et al.*[28] have demonstrated an almost linear shortening of the atrioventricular interval, measured by intracardiac recordings, with an increase in heart rate during exercise. This adaptation was characterized by a relatively low amplitude and an average AV interval decrease of 27 ± 11 ms for an average heart rate increase of 79 ± 22 bpm. Notably, however, the AV variation was significantly different in individual subjects: the variation was very low for some patients and much faster for others (Figure 12.1). Although the younger patients showed particularly low variation, no significant correlation was found between the AV interval variation curve and the age of the patient or the baseline value of the PR interval. During the recovery phase, AV interval evolution was less uniform. Most patients in this study showed a very rapid decrease within 1 minute following cessation of physical exercise, and the phenom-enon then slowed down and returned to the base value within approximately 15 min. Only one patient displayed a nonlinear relationship between AV interval and heart rate during recovery. The adaptation of the PR interval with increasing heart rate has been shown by several studies: it appears that up to a heart rate of approximately 140 bpm there is an average shortening of the PR interval by 4–5 ms for increments of 10 bpm; the PR interval, however, seldom falls below 100 ms.[26–28] Barbieri *et al.*,[43] in a study of 20 patients with normal exercise tests in the context of exertional chest pain, found that the curve of the PR interval as a function of heart rate appears to be linear within a range of approximately 95–130 bpm; but considering a wider range of 50–155 bpm, the curve is sigmoidal with asymptotes at the low and high rates. Data on the

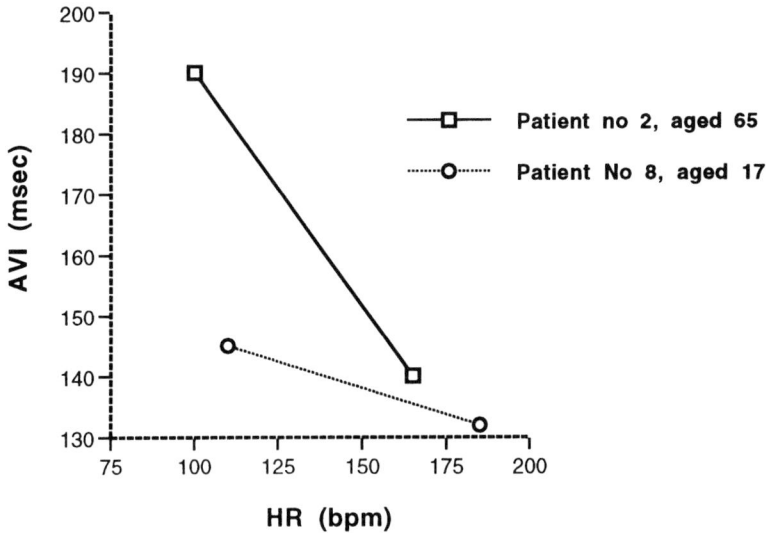

Figure 12.1 Relationship between AV interval and heart rate during exercise in two different patients. There is considerable difference between the slopes of the two curves. (Adapted from data presented by Daubert *et al.*[28])

pattern of PR shortening in special clinical settings, such as increasing age, underlying heart disease and the administration of cardiac medication, are virtually absent.

Most of the modern dual-chamber pacemakers include a programmable algorithm to shorten the AV delay as heart rate increases. However, it is still a matter of controversy whether modulation of the AV delay improves haemodynamic performance during exercise (Table 12.1). In general, the clinical importance of using different AV delays for different heart rates still remains controversial although most of the available studies,[9,23,25,30–32,37–39,44,80] but not all,[33–35,40] are in favour of AV adaptation. Several explanations can be offered for these inconsistent results concerning the benefit or otherwise of a rate-adaptive AV delay during atrioventricular sequential pacing. First, most studies on the effect of different AV intervals on exercise tolerance compared fixed AV delays. When an automatically rate-adaptive AV delay was employed, functional improvement was invariably detected (Figure 12.2). Second, most of the time these AV delays were selected arbitrarily and, as discussed later, no universally accepted method for the selection of the optimal AV delay in individual patients and in particular clinical settings exists. Third, the indices considered for assessment of the offered benefit were not comparable. Frielingsdorf *et al.*[40] have shown that an individually programmed AV delay, although capable of improving left ventricular ejection fraction at rest, failed to achieve any improvement of physical work capacity in patients with complete heart block. Fourth, the exercise capacity was submaximal in some studies and maximal in others. Sheppard *et al.*,[32] in patients with complete heart block and normal left ventricular function, have clearly shown that it is at peak exercise when the benefit of rate-adaptive AV delay becomes prominent. On the other hand, in a group of 631 patients including cases of heart

Table 12.1   Effects of rate-adapted AV delay during exercise

Study	No. of patients	AV delay modification	Results
Leman et al. (1985)[30]	10	100, 150 ms	Improved RNV-derived LV EF
Ryden et al. (1988)[35]	15	50, 100, 200, 250 ms	No change in O_2 consumption and exercise capacity
Haskell et al. (1989)[34]	7	66, 168 ms	No change in O_2 consumption
Mehta et al. (1989)[36]	13	75–80, 100–110, 140–150, 200 ms	Improved Doppler cardiac output and exercise capacity
Ritter et al. (1989)[25]	10	150, 200 ms and rate-adaptive	Improved thermodilution-derived cardiac output
Lau et al. (1990)[33]	7	75, 150 ms	No change in Doppler cardiac output
Ritter et al. (1991)[39]	23	156 ms and rate-adpative	Improved O_2 consumption
Sheppard et al. (1993)[32]	14	156 and rate-adaptive	Improved Doppler cardiac output, exercise capacity
Frielingsdorf et al. (1994)[40]	12	Fixed AV delays selected according to RNV-derived LV EF	No change in maximum workload

AV = atrioventricular; EF = ejection fraction; RNV = radionuclide ventriculography; LV = left ventricular.

failure and patients on antiarrhythmic medication, Luceri et al.[27] found that the PR interval shortening was predominantly observed in the earlier stages of exercise (Figure 12.3). Furthermore, the relative contribution of atrial systole to ventricular filling is more important at rest than during exercise when the relative contribution of atrial systole diminishes concomitantly with a rise in mitral blood flow velocity.

Thus, the available data are controversial; but since they are often derived with varying methodologies and from different patient cohorts, straight comparisons may not be applicable. The majority of the existing evidence shows a haemodynamic

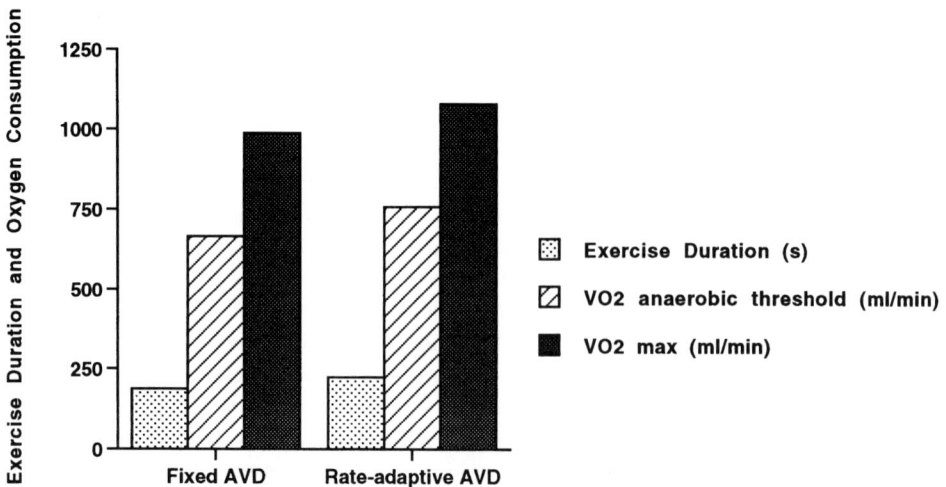

Figure 12.2   Rate-adaptive AV delay (156–63 ms) versus fixed AV delay (156 ms) on exercise capacity and oxygen consumption in 23 patients with complete heart block treated with DDD pacing. (Adapted from Ritter et al.[39])

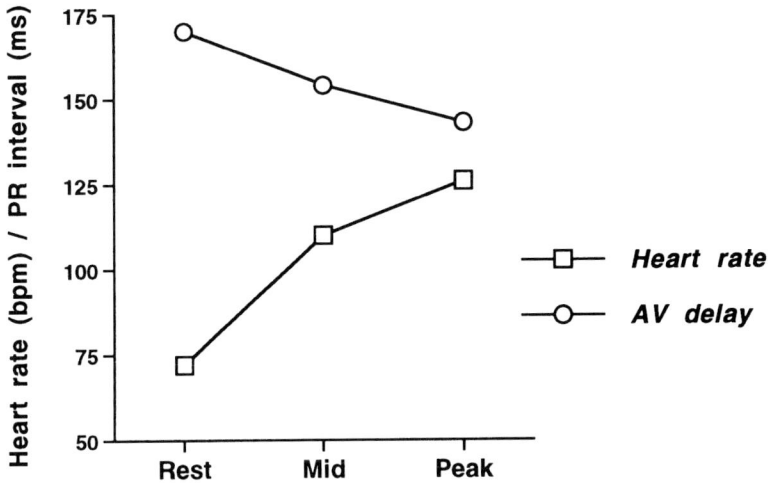

Figure 12.3 PR intervals at rest and at mid and peak exercise in 631 patients with and without heart disease. (Adapted from Luceri *et al.*[27])

improvement with rate-adaptive AV delays, at least in patients with normal left ventricular function.[42] In clinical practice, the haemodynamic benefit from a rate-dependent AV interval may also occur not only because of the optimized AV interval, but also due to the fact that a rate-dependent AV interval may allow a higher ventricular rate by decreasing the total atrial refractory period which is essential at high rates. This is particularly relevant in patients requiring long postventricular atrial refractory periods to avoid pacemaker-mediated tachycardia due to retrograde conduction.

Optimal AV Delay and Pacing Mode

DDD pacing allowing normal ventricular activation

Electrical stimulation of the right ventricle from locations such as the ventricular apex results in asynchronous ventricular contraction which depresses ventricular function;[52-54] histological abnormalities have been demonstrated in the myocardium of puppies and young patients with congenital heart block treated with VVI pacing.[55] In patients with sick sinus syndrome, a reasonable way to avoid unnecessary ventricular stimulation while retaining the benefits of ventricular pacing backup is the use of DDD units programmed to maximum AV delay.[56] An AV delay longer than 200 ms should maximize the likelihood of normal ventricular activation following atrial pacing. Two potential problems should be considered with a long AV delay. First, prolonged AV delays impose a restriction on the upper rate limit provided by DDD units and reprogramming is needed if progression of AV disease results in continuous dual-chamber pacing. A solution to this problem has been achieved by the ELA Chorus™ pacemaker, in which a prolonged AV interval is programmable to allow atrial pacing without ventricular pacing. Once, however, AV conduction has been lost for a single beat and ventricular pacing has intervened, a second shorter and nonphysiological AV delay is instituted with continuous AV pacing until AV conduction has returned and the cycle begins again. Second, with any pacemaker which tracks atrial activity, pacemaker-mediated tachycardia or the so-called AV desynchronization arrhythmia (i.e. unsensed retrograde P waves followed by ineffectual atrial stimulation during atrial refractoriness[57] may occur when retrograde conduction is present. Their occurrence is facilitated by long AV delays or short postventricular atrial refractory periods. In this setting, the presence of a rate-adaptive AV delay appears to offer theoretical advantages. It should be noted, however, that even an adaptive AV delay in the presence of a relatively long total atrial refractory period may be associated with lockout of upper rate behaviour; i.e. the development of sudden 2:1 AV block at high atrial rate exceeding the maximum tracking rate.[58]

DDD(R) pacing

The prevalence of specific atrial chronotropic incompetence is estimated from 25% to 64% in elderly patients,[59] and when dual-chamber pacing is required in this setting the DDD(R) mode is appropriate. In DDD(R) units with ventricular-based lower rate timing, an adaptive AV delay reduces the discrepancy between the atrial pacing rate and the sensor-driven upper rate and thus compensates for a disadvantage of the ventricular-based as compared with the atrial-based lower rate timing.[60] In sick sinus syndrome with intact nodal conduction or intermittent AV block, programming of a long AV delay is recommended. However, this combination may result in T-wave pacing due to undersensing of conducted QRS complexes in pacemakers with a rate-adaptive AV delay.[61] Therefore, in patients prone to ventricular fibrillation due to myocardial disease, programming of short AV delays may be required.[61]

Interestingly, a lack of physiological adaptation of the AV interval to heart rate has been reported in patients chronically paced in the AAI(R) mode.[62]

Optimal AV Delay and Cardiac Disease

Atrial Disease

Approximately 12% of patients with AV block and 35 of patients with atrial disease are estimated to have delayed interatrial conduction times of up to 170 ms.[29] In this situation, atrial stystole is relatively delayed and prolonged AV delays often exceeding 250 ms may be necessary in order to achieve AV synchronization. This, however, inevitably reduces the upper rate limit of the pacemaker and does nothing to avoid interatrial delay which may promote arrhythmias. Recently, the use of two atrial leads, one stimulating the right atrium and the other the left atrium via the coronary sinus, has been proposed. The clinical indications and potential long-term benefit from the use of such 'triple-chamber pacemakers' is under investigation.[63]

Ventricular Disease

In patients with normal left ventricular function, the optimal atrioventricular delay at rest lies between 150 and 200 ms.[10–12,16,19,34] Several studies have suggested a relationship between left ventricular function and optimal AV interval: small changes in the programmed AV delay can have a significant effect on cardiac function at rest.[9,16,22,34,42] In certain patients with first-degree AV block and normal left ventricular function, the so-called 'pacemaker syndrome without pacemaker' or 'pseudopacemaker syndrome' may occur, particularly in the setting of fast pathway ablation for the treatment of AV nodal re-entrant tachycardia.[81] This condition is now an indication for dual-chamber pacing with a short AV delay.[82]

In patients with abnormal ventricular diastolic function, a longer AV delay may be beneficial[45] and significant haemodynamic differences between ventricular and AV sequential pacing in patients with impaired ventricular diastolic function have been reported.[46] In patients with diastolic dysfunction in the context of hypertrophic cardiomyopathy, some studies,[76,77] although not all,[78] have also demonstrated worsened diastolic parameters with a short AV delay. In patients with congestive heart failure and ventricles operating at the extremes of the flattened Frank–Starling curve, rate adaptation appears to be more important than AV delay adaptation, since the stroke volume is not being affected significantly by the atrial contribution.[47] In situations of acute stress such as myocardial infarction[3,4] and postoperative states,[5] where the heart rate is expected to be faster, a relatively short AV delay is found to be optimal.

Congestive cardiac failure/dilated cardiomyopathy

Although a long AV delay (190–200 ms) was initially thought necessary for patients with reduced ejection fraction (<40%),[17] recent studies have documented a benefit from programming very short AV delays in patients with congestive heart failure due to idiopathic dilated cardiomyopathy.[28,45–51] Dual-chamber pacing with short AV delay has been proposed as a therapeutic alternative in patients with dilated cardiomyopathy and severe heart failure unresponsive to optimal medical therapy.[20,48–51] Hochleitner *et al.*[20,48] have reported an improvement of left ventricular function and symptoms in patients with dilated cardiomyopathy, by using DDD pacing with AV intervals of 100 ms. In some patients the beneficial effect lasted for several years. Similar improvement has recently been reported in patients with ischaemic heart disease.[50] Additional improvement in cardiac output has also been shown with the use of septal, short AV delay pacing.[64]

However, in a recent randomized study,[65] no improvement was noted in haemodynamic status shortly after pacemaker implantation or in clinical status and ejection fraction after long-term pacing. The absence of beneficial effects of AV-synchronous pacing with optimized AV delay in patients with severe heart failure was also demonstrated in another recent study.[66] Nishimura *et al.*[51] showed that dual-chamber pacing may improve acute haemodynamic variables, mainly by optimizing the timing of mechanical atrial and ventricular synchrony, but only in selected patients with dilated cardiomyopathy who have a prolonged PR interval. In those patients, functional mitral regurgitation may be so prolonged that it occupies up to 90% of the total RR interval, reducing ventricular filling time to less than 200 ms. Patients in whom there is already optimally timed mechanical atrial and ventricular synchrony may not benefit from dual-chamber pacing and they may experience haemodynamic deterioration with improper timing of atrial synchrony with dual-chamber pacing.

These results indicate that the issue remains unresolved, and routine use of permanent pacing with optimized AV delay as a primary treatment of congestive heart failure is not justified. In 10–15% of patients, usually those with prolonged PR interval and QRS duration >140 ms, DDD pacing with short AV delay may improve exercise capacity and is clinically justified.[75]

Hypertrophic cardiomyopathy

A number of recent studies[67-69] have documented that DDD pacing with a short AV interval may be an effective way to reduce the left ventricular outflow gradient and improve the clinical status in patients with hypertrophic cardiomyopathy. Fananapazir et al.[70] showed that this symptomatic and haemodynamic benefit often becomes more pronounced with time. The mechanism by which the gradient is decreased is unclear but seems to be related to a decreased septal motion, late activation at the base of the septum with right ventricular apical pacing or decreased left ventricular contractility. In order to achieve complete ventricular capture, which is required for successful therapy, optimization of the AV delay is necessary.[68,69,71] This is easily accomplished in patients with a PR interval between 120 and 180 ms, but when the PR interval is shorter, a very short AV delay (50–60 ms) is frequently required for complete ventricular capture.[72] This, however, may result in an increase of the gradient due to inadequate filling of the left ventricle from an ineffective atrial contraction. Prolonging the PR interval with drugs (beta-blockers, calcium antagonists) or via AV nodal modification by ablation can avoid the deleterious effect of a very short AV delay. In order to establish complete ventricular capture at all times, there should be separate programming of the paced and sensed AV delay and an automatic function to adapt the AV delay to increased heart rates.

Recently, Nishimura et al.[73] showed that the acute effect of pacing the right atrium and ventricle may be detrimental to both systolic and diastolic function of the left ventricle. Each of these haemodynamic alterations was evident at the optimal AV delay (defined as the longest interval with full ventricular activation by the pacemaker), but was of even greater magnitude at the shortest AV delay. Whether this detrimental effect translates into a clinical problem is uncertain since these observations were made in the cardiac catheterization laboratory under controlled conditions. In a multicentre study of 56 patients with hypertrophic cardiomyopathy, symptomatic improvement was detected after DDD pacing but no correlation between magnitude of gradient reduction and functional improvement could be established.[79]

At present, dual-chamber pacing with optimized AV delay looks beneficial for those patients with both marked obstruction to left ventricular outflow and severe symptoms of heart failure refractory to drug treatment. Pacing has no defined role in diminishing risk for sudden cardiac death, nor in relieving the symptoms of patients with the nonobstructive form of the disease.[74]

Methodology for Selection of the Optimal AV Delay

The ideal method to select the optimal AV delay for the individual patient has yet to be determined. The main approaches to this problem are measurement of interatrial conduction, and estimations of cardiac output or other metabolic indices at various AV intervals in order to determine the most beneficial value for a given situation. Several methods such as invasive measurement of cardiac output,[39] Doppler echocardiography,[9,33,36] radionuclide angiography,[19,30,40] cardiopulmonary exercise testing,[34,36,39] plethysmographic impedance[38] and plasma cAMP and atrial natriuretic peptide assays[44] have been used. Recently, Nishimura *et al.*[51] utilized the temporal relation of atrial and ventricular contraction for optimization of the AV delay in paced patients with dilated cardiomyopathy. High-fidelity pressure measurements from the left atrium and ventricle were obtained and the optimal AV delay was selected as the interval when the increase in LV pressure from the LV contraction would begin after the peak of the increase in left atrial pressure from atrial contraction but before atrial relaxation was complete.[51]

Although invasive haemodynamic assessment provides the most reliable measurements of cardiac output and intracardiac pressures, from the point of view of clinical practicality, Doppler echocardiography is probably the easiest and most cost-effective way to determine the optimal AV delay.[29,36] The methodology followed at our echo laboratories is the following. The cross-sectional area of the left ventricular outflow tract immediately before the aortic valve is measured at the long-axis parasternal view. At the four-chamber apical view, the Doppler signals of the transmitral flow and the ejection flow at the left ventricular outflow tracts are obtained. Cardiac output can thus be calculated from the velocity time integral of the Doppler signal according to the formula: $CO = VTI \times CSA \times HR$, where VTI is the velocity time integral, CSA the left ventricular outflow tract cross-sectional area and HR the heart rate. During atrial tracking or AV sequential pacing, the optimal AV delay is identified by determining the delay which allows a satisfactory recording of both the A and E waves with the A at the end of the P wave of the surface ECG and, in addition, achieves the highest values of the cardiac output (Figures 12.4 and 12.5). This procedure is cumbersome, however, and most often the resting AV delay is selected empirically.

Types of Algorithm in Modern Pacemakers

Two main types of algorithm have been used in modern pacemakers for automatic optimization and rate modulation of the AV delay.

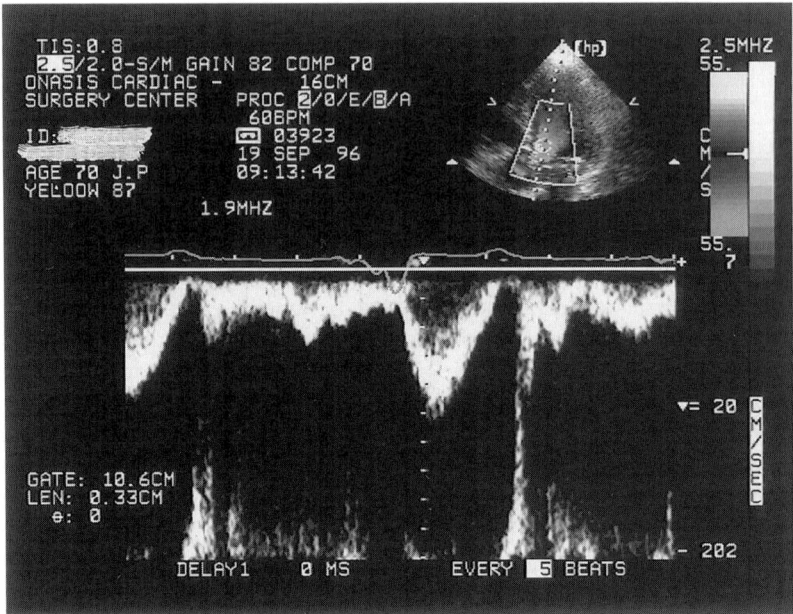

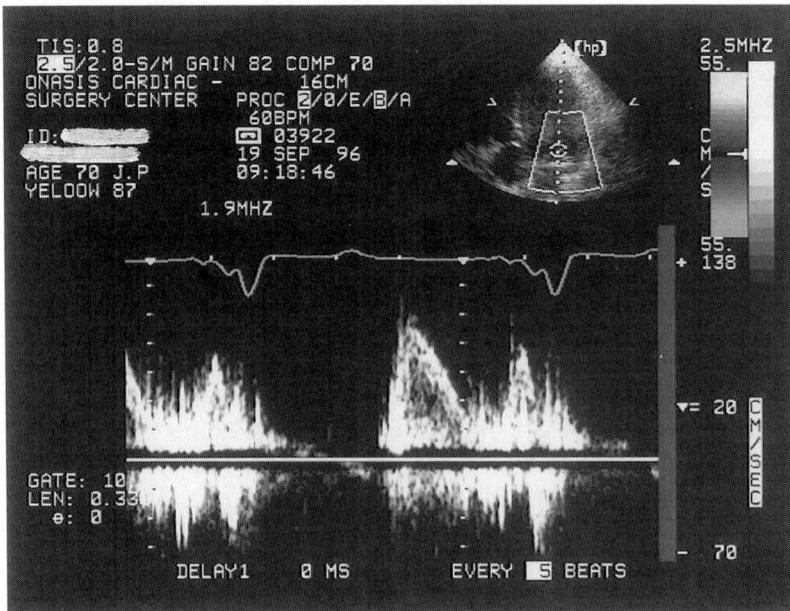

Figure 12.4 Atrial tracking at approximately 60 bpm and AV delays of 150 ms (*left panels*) and 250 ms (*right panels*). Note that with an AV delay of 250 ms, the Doppler cardiac output is higher than that with 150 ms.

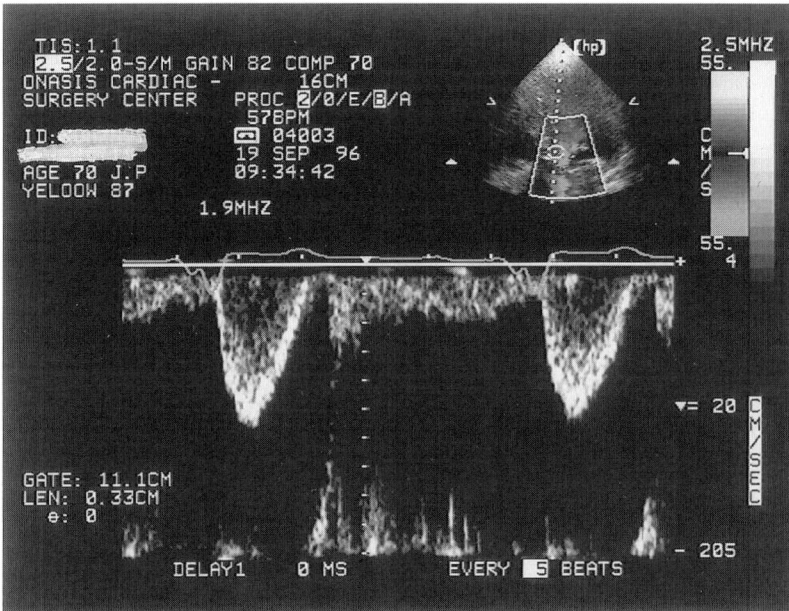

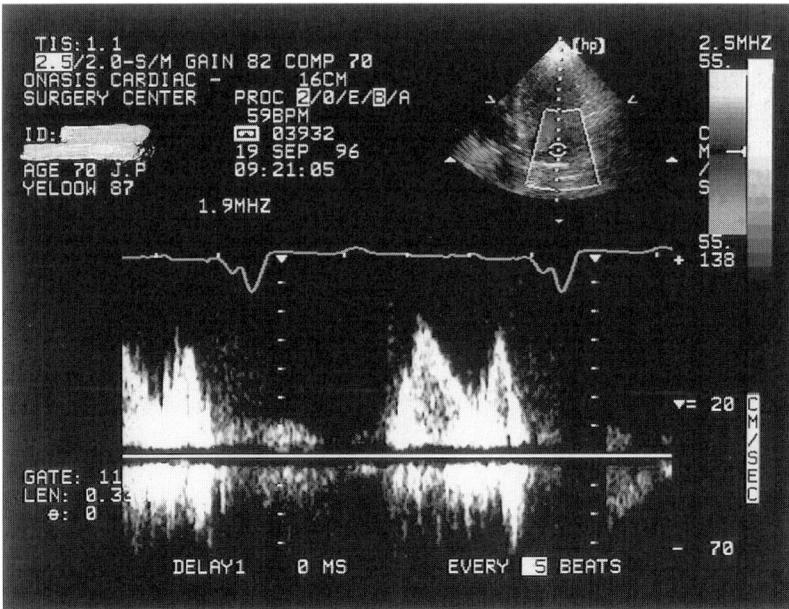

Figure 12.4 *Continued*

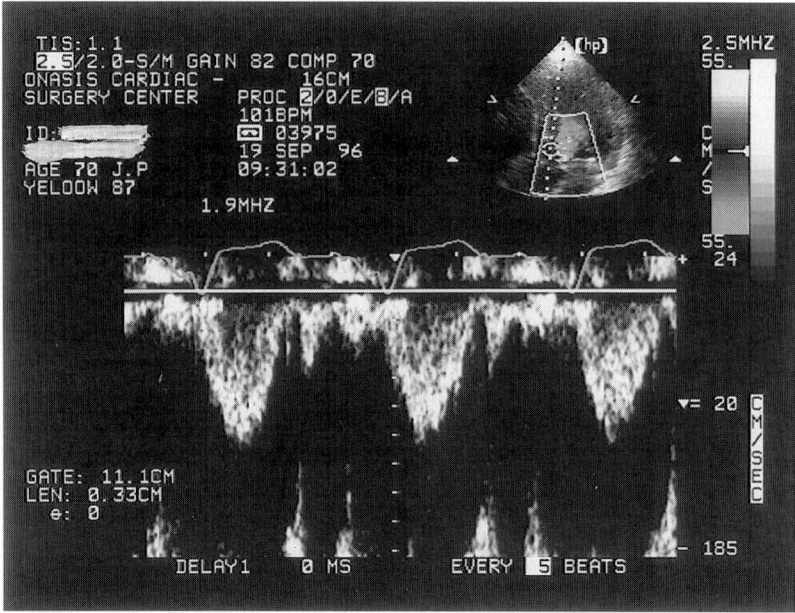

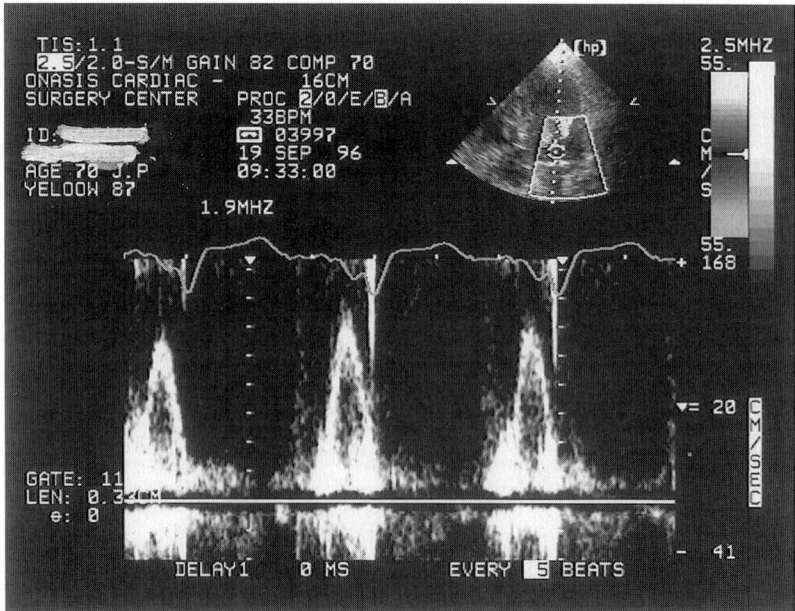

Figure 12.5 DDD pacing at 100 bpm and AV delays of 150 ms (*left panel*) and 250 ms (*right panel*). At this rate the cardiac output is higher with an AV delay of 150 ms.

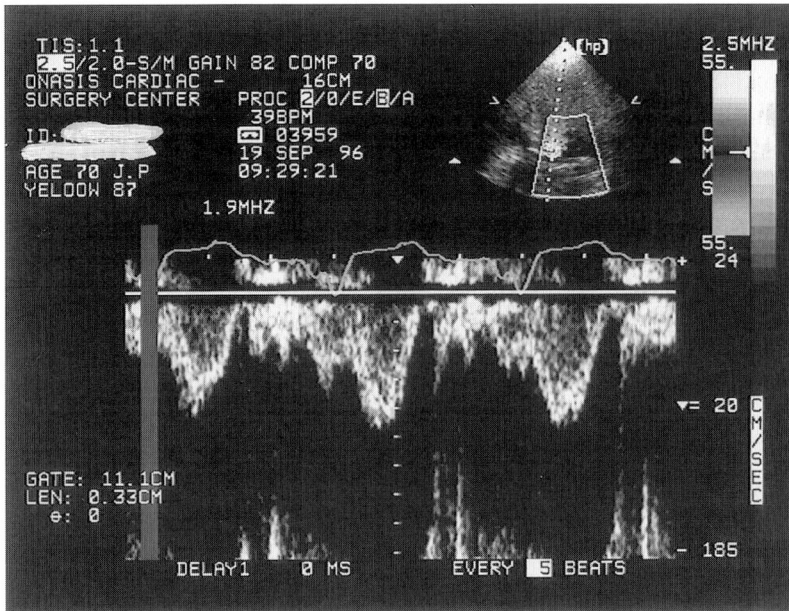

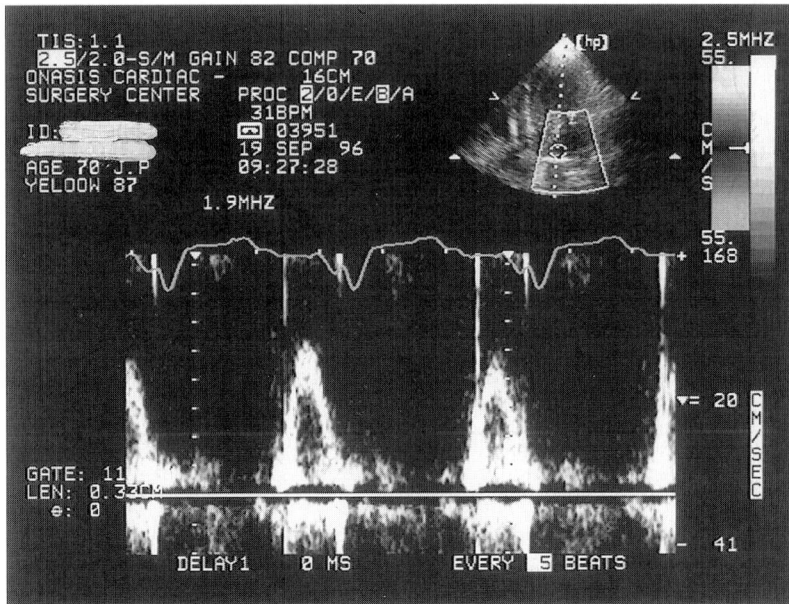

Figure 12.5 *Continued*

AV Delay Hysteresis

This helps to maintain a consistent interval between atrial and ventricular contractions whether AV sequential pacing or atrial tracking is used. Thus, the basic programmed AV interval is reduced by a fixed or programmable value when the unit switches from a paced atrial cycle to a sensed atrial cycle. Most of the devices have two different AV intervals: a 'sensed AV interval' and a 'paced AV interval', which can be programmed independently within large ranges from 30 to 300 ms, by 10–20 ms increments.

Automatic Rate-Adaptive AV Delay

Most modern DDD and DDD(R) pacemakers have an algorithm of automatic rate-adaptive AV delay, i.e. AV delay shortening with increased heart rate.

In the ELA Chorus^{TM} units the pacemaker computes the AV delay as a function of atrial rate. Two values are programmable: the basic rate AV delay, which is the AV delay used at the programmed basic rate, and the maximum rate AV delay, which is used at the programmed upper rate. Between minimum and maximum rates, the AV delay is determined by the pacemaker as a linear function of the paced atrial rate. In addition, these units have two other functions for modulation of the AV delay. *The fallback algorithm* is a feature aimed at preventing tracking of atrial arrhythmias. It shortens the AV delay following sensing of atrial ectopic beats and ensures a fixed AV delay of 31 ms combined with a limitation of the ventricular pacing rate to 120 bpm. The *DDD/AMC mode* (Automatic Mode Conversion^{TM}) switches the DDD unit to AAI mode as long as the atrial events are conducted normally to the ventricle; the pacemaker adjusts the basic and minimum AV delays as well as AV delay hysteresis according to the last eight registered PR intervals.

In the Siemens-Pacesetter pacemakers, the rate-responsive AV delay (RRAVD) may be programmed to three different delay curve levels: high, medium or low. These settings provide interval shortening of 3 ms/min, 2 ms/min and 1 ms/min, respectively. AV delay shortening occurs either at paced or tracked rates above 90 bpm and the minimum delay achievable is 31 ms.

In Intermedics models, the pacemaker adapts the AV delay to changes in the preceding atrial interval in an approximately 1:8 ratio (minimum change = 2.56 ms). Thus, for every 40 ms change in the atrial interval, the subsequent AV delay after a sensed event will change by 5 ms down to a minimum value which is calculated on the basis of the programmed pacing rate and remains above 75 ms.

In Medtronic units the paced AV interval is determined by the pacemaker according to the current sensor rate, whereas the sensed AV interval (i.e. the AV delay following a sensed atrial event) is determined according to the mean atrial rate. Minimum paced and sensed AV delays and the range of atrial rates in which the automatic AV delay function operates (start and stop rate) are programmable.

In CPI models the pacemaker automatically calculates the AV delay using the length of the previous VV cycle interval. Dynamic AV delay shortens at the percentage of the resting or maximum AV delay to the lower rate interval.

In Biotronic pacemakers optimization of the AV delay is feasible over five atrial rate ranges. AV delay decrements can be set to specific values or in accordance with predefined sets of parameters (low, medium and high).

In the previous generation of Vitatron units, the AV delay at various rates above the lower rate limit varied according to an exponential adaptation curve. This results in rapid shortening at lower heart rates but minor shortening at moderate and high rates. In newer models, a linear adaptation mode has been incorporated. There are two programmable options: median (i.e. AV shortening of 0.6 ms/min) and fast (0.9 ms/min). A difference of 40 ms is maintained between sensed and paced atrial events.

In the Telectronics DDD(R) pacemaker, the operating AV delay varies with changes in the metabolic indicated rate. At minimum rate, the operating AV delay will be the programmed AV delay. As the metabolic indicated rate increases, the operating AV delay shortens from the programmed AV delay by a degree proportional to one-sixteenth of the metabolic indicated rate. Thus, this unit uses the sensor rather than sensed or paced atrial events for modification of the AV delay.

Future Directions

It is obvious from the previous discussion that the term 'optimal AV delay' has a meaning only on an individual patient basis. Both the ideal resting value of the AV delay and, especially, its response to heart rate changes not only depends on the underlying atrial and ventricular disease, but also differs widely among individuals (Figure 12.6). A single algorithm for AV delay modification with heart rate in all patients, as provided by modern pacemakers, is therefore inadequate. Ideally, not only the resting AV delay but its response to exercise should also be individualized. Theoretically, supine bicycle exercise could be used and, provided that the Doppler signals are easily recordable in this setting, optimization of the AV delay should be achieved in the same way at different levels of exercise. These values could be used in order to construct an overall AV delay response curve which should determine the ideal AV delay at each level of physical exertion with its corresponding heart rate. The feasibility and clinical practicality of such an approach, however, may be limited. In addition, patterns of AV delay response are not currently programmable in most modern pacemakers.

The ideal pacemaker unit should be able to modify the AV delay not only according to pacing rate but also by measuring other metabolic indices or parameters reflecting ventricular contractility, outflow tract flow and end-diastolic pressure. Again, in patients with various types of heart disease individualization of the AV delay setting parameters should be necessary. Although from the physiological point of such an approach might be promising, its clinical value and cost-effectiveness have not been established.

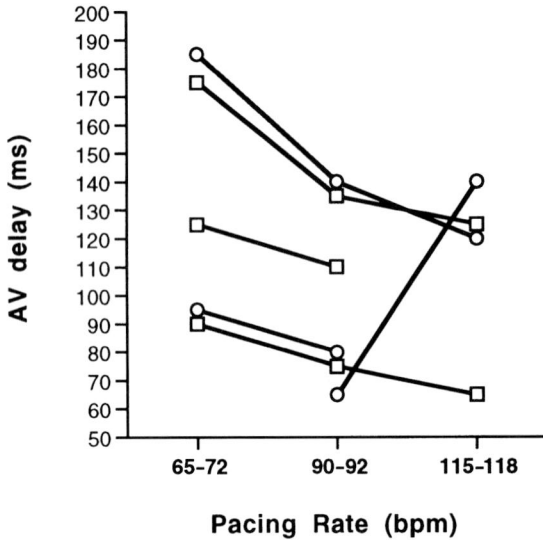

Figure 12.6 Optimal AV delays selected in individual patients with DDD pacemakers according to impedance plethysmography-derived stroke volume measurement. In one patient with severe cardiac dysfunction, the optimal AV delay was particularly short at low pacing rates, but increased values were found necessary in order to achieve an improved stroke volume at high pacing rates. (Data from Eugene et al.[38])

Conclusion

Optimizing AV delay intervals for paced and sensed atrial activity results in a significant increase of the resting cardiac output. Selection of an optimal AV delay is beneficial in certain types of atrial or ventricular disease, treated with dual-chamber pacing. During exercise, pacemakers with rate-adaptive shortening of the AV interval may offer better exercise performance, particularly in patients with a normal left ventricular function. However, the optimal AV delay as well as its response to metabolic demand, not only depends on the underlying atrial and ventricular disease but also differs among individuals. In clinical practice, no established method exists for the selection of an optimal AV delay and its adaptation to heart rate and physiological changes on an individual basis.

References

1. Karlof I. Hemodynamic effect of atrial triggered versus fixed rate pacing at rest and during exercise in complete heart block. *Acta Med Scand* 1975; **197**: 195–210.
2. Kruse I, Arnman K, Conradson B, Ryden L. A comparison of the acute and long-term hemodynamic effect of ventricular inhibited and atrial synchronous ventricular inhibited pacing. *Circulation* 1982; **65**: 846–55.
3. Leinbach RC, Chamberlain DA, Kastor JA, *et al.* A comparison of the hemodynamic effects of ventricular and sequential AV pacing in patients with heart block. *Am Heart J* 1969; **78**: 502.

4. Chamberlaine DA, Leinbach RC, Vassaux CE, *et al*. Sequential atrioventricular pacing in heart block complicating acute myocardial infarction. *N Engl J Med* 1970; **282**: 577.
5. Hartzler GO, Maloney ID, Curtis JJ, *et al*. Hemodynamic benefits of atrioventricular sequential after cardiac surgery. *Am J Cardiol* 1977; **40**: 232.
6. Sarnoff SJ, Gilmore JP, Mitchell JH. Influence of atrial contraction and relaxation on closure of mitral valve: observations on effects of autonomic nerve activity. *Circ Res* 1962; **11**: 26–35.
7. Braunwald E, Frahm CJ. Studies on Starling's law of the heart. IV: Observations on the hemodynamic functions of the left atrium in man. *Circulation* 1961; **24**: 633–42.
8. Naito M, Dreifus LS, David D, *et al*. Re-evaluation of the role of atrial systole to cardiac hemodynamics: evidence for pulmonary venous regurgitation during abnormal atrioventricular sequencing. *Am Heart J* 1983; **105**: 295–302.
9. Wish M, Fletcher RD, Gottdiener JS, *et al*. Importance of left atrial timing in the programming of dual-chamber pacemakers. *Am J Cardiol* 1987; **60**: 566–71.
10. Nitsch J, Seiderer M, Bull U, *et al*. Evaluation of left ventricular performance by radionuclide ventriculography in patients with atrioventricular versus ventricular demand pacemakers. *Am Heart J* 1984; **107**: 906–11.
11. Frielingsdorf J, Gerber A, Dur P, *et al*. Importance of an individually programmed atrioventricular delay at rest and on work capacity in patients with dual chamber pacemakers. *PACE* 1994; **17**: 37–45.
12. Pearson AC, Janosik DL, Redd RR, *et al*. Doppler echocardiographic assessment of the effect of varying atrioventricular delay and pacemaker mode on left ventricular filling. *Am Heart J* 1988; **115**: 611–21.
13. Von Bibra H, Wirtzfeld A, Hall R, Ulm K, Blomer H. Mitral valve closure and left ventricular filling time in patients with VDD pacemakers: assessment of the onset of left ventricular systole and the end of diastole. *Br Heart J* 1986; **55**: 355–63.
14. Ishikawa T, Kimura K, Nihei T, *et al*. Relationship between diastolic mitral regurgitation and PQ intervals or cardiac function in patients implanted with DDD pacemakers. *PACE* 1991; **14**: 1797–802.
15. Ishikawa T, Sumita S, Kimura K, *et al*. Critical PQ interval for the appearance of diastolic mitral regurgitation and optimal PQ interval in patients implanted with DDD pacemakers. *PACE* 1994; **17**: 1989–94.
16. Iwase M, Sotobata I, Yokata M, *et al*. Evaluation by pulsed Doppler echocardiography of the atrial contribution to left ventricular filling in patients with DDD pacemakers. *Am J Cardiol* 1986; **58**: 104–9.
17. Haskell RJ, French WJ. Optimum AV interval in dual chamber pacemakers. *PACE* 1986; **9**: 670–5.
18. Benchimol A, Duenas A, Liggett MS, *et al*. Contribution of atrial systole to the cardiac function at a fixed and at a variable ventricular rate. *Am J Cardiol* 1965; **16**: 11–21.
19. Videen JS, Huang SK, Bazgan ID, *et al*. Hemodynamic comparison of ventricular pacing, atrioventricular sequential pacing and atrial synchronous ventricular pacing using radionuclide ventriculography. *Am J Cardiol* 1986; **57**: 1305–8.
20. Hochleitner M, Hortnagl H, Ng CK, *et al*. Usefulness of physiologic dual-chamber pacing in drug-resistant idiopathic dilated cardiomyopathy. *Am J Cardiol* 1990; **66**: 198–202.
21. Labovitz AJ, Williams GA, Redd RM, *et al*. Noninvasive assessment of pacemaker hemodynamics by Doppler echocardiography: importance of left atrial size. *JACC* 1985; **6**: 196–200.
22. Janosic DL, Pearson AC, Buckingham TA, *et al*. The hemodynamic benefit of differential atrioventricular delay intervals for sensed and paced atrial events during physiologic pacing. *JACC* 1989; **14**: 499–507.
23. Pearson AC, Janosik DL, Redd RM, *et al*. Hemodynamic benefit of atrioventricular synchrony: prediction from baseline Doppler echocardiographic variables. *JACC* 1989; **13**: 1613–21.
24. Alt E, von Bibra H, Blomer H. Different beneficial AV intervals with DDD pacing after sensed or paced atrial events. *J Electrophysiol* 1987; **1**: 250–6.

25. Ritter P, Daubert C, Mabo P, et al. Haemodynamic benefit of a rate-adapted AV delay in dual chamber pacing. Eur Heart J 1989; 10: 637–46.
26. Atterhog JH, Loogna E. PR interval in relation to heart rate during exercise and the influence of posture and autonomic tone. J Electrocardiol 1977; 10: 331–6.
27. Luceri RM, Brownstein SL, Vardeman L. PR interval behaviour during exercise: implications for physiological pacemakers. PACE 1990; 13: 1719–23.
28. Daubert C, Ritter P, Mabo P, et al. Physiological relationship between atrioventricular interval and heart rate in healthy subjects: applications to dual chambers pacing. PACE 1986; 9: 1032–9.
29. Daubert C, Ritter P, Mabo P, Varin C, Leclercq C. AV delay optimization in DDD and DDDR pacing. In: Barold SS, Mugica J (eds), New Perspectives in Cardiac Pacing: 3. Futura, NY: 1993.
30. Leman RB, Kratz JM. Radionuclide evaluation of dual chamber pacing: comparison between variable AV intervals and ventricular pacing. PACE 1985; 8: 408–14.
31. Sulke AN, Chambers JB, Sowton E. The effect of atrioventricular delay programming in patients with DDDR pacemakers. Eur Heart J 1992; 13: 464–72.
32. Sheppard R, Ren JF, Ross J, et al. Doppler echocardiographic assessment of the hemodynamic benefits of rate adaptive AV delay during exercise in paced patients with complete heart block. PACE 1993; 16: 2157–67.
33. Lau CP, Wong CK, Leung WH, et al. Superior cardiac hemodynamics of atrioventricular synchrony over rate responsive pacing at submaximal exercise: observations in activity sensing DDDR pacemakers. PACE 1990; 13(II): 1832–7.
34. Haskell R, French WJ. Physiological importance of different atrioventricular intervals to improved exercise performance in patients with dual chamber pacemakers. Br Heart J 1989; 61: 46–51.
35. Ryden L, Karlsson O, Kristensson BE. The importance of different atrioventricular intervals for exercise capacity. PACE 1988; 11: 1051–62.
36. Mehta D, Gilmour S, Ward DE, et al. Optimal atrioventricular delay at rest and during exercise in patients with dual chamber pacemakers: a non-invasive assessment by continuous wave Doppler. Br Heart J 1989; 61: 161–6.
37. Wish M, Fletcher RD, Cohen A. Hemodynamics of AV synchrony and rate. J Electrophysiol 1989; 3: 170–5.
38. Eugene M, Lascault G, Frank R, et al. Assessment of the optimal atrioventricular delay in DDD paced patients by impedance plethysmography. Eur Heart J 1989; 3: 250–6.
39. Ritter P, Vai F, Bonnet JL, et al. Rate adaptive atrioventricular delay improves cardiopulmonary performance in patients implanted with a dual chamber pacemaker for complete heart block. Eur J CPE 1991; 1: 31–8.
40. Frielingsdorf J, Gerber AE, Dur P, Vuilliomenet A, Bertel O. Importance of an individually programmed atrioventricular delay at rest and on work capacity in patients with dual chamber pacemakers. PACE 1994; 17: 37–45.
41. Linde-Edelman C, Juhlin-Dannfert A, et al. The hemodynamic important of atrial systole: a function of the kinetic energy of blood flow? PACE 1992; 15: 1740–9.
42. Frielingsdorf J, Gerber AE, Hess OM. Importance of maintained atrio-ventricular synchrony in patients with pacemakers. Eur Heart J 1994; 15: 1431–40.
43. Barbieri D, Percoco GF, Toselli T, Guardigli G, Anasani L, Antonioli GE. AV delay and exercise stress tests: behaviour in normal subjects. PACE 1990; 13: 1724–7.
44. Theodorakis G, Kremastinos D, Markianos M, et al. c-AMP and ANP levels in VVI and DDD pacing with different AV delays during daily activity and exercise. PACE 1990; 13: 1773–8.
45. Dritsas A, Joshi J, Webb S, et al. Optimal atrioventricular interval during dual-chamber pacing: relation to underlying ventricular function (abstract). Eur Heart J 1993; 14 (suppl): 252.
46. Shefer A, Rozenman Y, David YB, et al. Left ventricular function during physiological cardiac pacing: relation to rate, pacing mode, and underlying myocardial disease. PACE 1987; 10: 315–25.
47. Frielingsdorf J, Dur P, Gerber AE, Vyilliomenet A, Bertel O. Physical work capacity with

rate responsive ventricular pacing (VVIR) versus dual chamber pacing (DDD) in patients with normal and dimished left ventricular function. *Int J Cardiol* 1995; **49**: 239–48.

48. Hochleitner M, Hortnagl H, Hortnagl H, Fridrich L, Gschnitzer F. Long-term efficacy of physiologic dual-chamber pacing in the treatment of end-stage idiopathic dilated cardiomyopathy. *Am J Cardiol* 1992; **70**: 1320–5.

49. Brecker SJD, Xiao HB, Sparrow J, Gibson DG. Effects of dual-chamber pacing with short AV delay in dilated cardiomyopathy. *Lancet* 1992; **340**: 1308–12.

50. Auricchio A, Sommariva L, Salo RW, Scafuri A, Chiareiello L. Improvement of cardiac function in patients with severe congestive heart failure and coronary artery disease by dual chamber pacing with shortened AV delay. *PACE* 1993; **16**: 2034–43.

51. Nishimura RA, Hayes DL, Holmes DR, Tajik AJ. Mechanism of hemodynamic improvement by dual-chamber pacing for severe left ventricular dysfunction: an acute Doppler and catheterization study. *JACC* 1995; **25**: 281–343.

52. Raichlen JS, Campbell FW, Edie RN, Josephson ME, Harken AH. The effect of the site of placement of temporary epicardial pacemakers on ventricular function in patients undergoing cardiac surgery. *Circulation* 1984; **70**: 118–23.

53. Heyndrick GR, Vilaine JP, Knight DR, Vatner SF. Effects of altered site of electrical activation on myocardial performance during inotropic stimulation. *Circulation* 1985; **71**: 1010–16.

54. Karpawich PP, Justice CD, Chang C-H, Gause CY, Kuhns LR. Septal ventricular pacing in the immature canine heart: a new perspective. *Am Heart J* 1991; **121**: 827–33.

55. Karpawich P, Chang C-H, Cavitt DL. Ventricular pacing-induced histopathology in the young with congenital heart block (abstract). *JACC* 1992; **19**: 326A.

56. Katritsis D, Camm AJ. AAI pacing: when is it indicated and how should it be performed? *Clin Cardiol* 1993; **16**: 339–43.

57. Barold SS. Repetitive reentrant and non-reentrant ventriculoatrial synchrony in dual chamber pacing. *Clin Cardiol* 1991; **14**: 754–63.

58. Hessen SE, Sheppard RC, Kutalek SP. Upper rate lockout: an unexpected feature of rate adaptive atrioventricular delay. *PACE* 1994; **17**: 103–7.

59. Barold SS. Ventricular- versus atrial-based lower rate timing in dual chamber pacemakers: does it really matter? *PACE* 1995; **18**: 83–96.

60. Katritsis D, Camm AJ. Chronotropic incompetence: a proposal for definition and diagnosis. *Br Heart J* 1993; **70**: 400–2.

61. Pieterse MGC, Den Dulk K, Van Gelder BM, Van Mechelen R, Wellens HJJ. Programming a long paced atrioventricular interval may be risky in DDDR pacing. *PACE* 1994; **17**: 252–7.

62. Mabo P, Pouillot C, Kermarrec A, Lelong B, Lebreton H, Daubert C. Lack of physiological adaptation of the atrioventricular interval to heart rate in patients chronically paced in the AAIR mode. *PACE* 1991; **14**: 2133–42.

63. Daubert C, Mabo Ph, Berder V, *et al.* Simultaneous dual atrium pacing in high degree interatrial blocks: hemodynamic results (abstract). *Circulation* 1991; **84**: II453.

64. Cowell R, Morris-Thurgood J, *et al.* Septal short atrioventricular delay pacing: additional hemodynamic improvement in heart failure. *PACE* 1994; **17**(II): 1980–3.

65. Gold MR, Feliciano Z, Gottlieb S, Fisher M. Dual-chamber pacing with a short atrioventricular delay in congestive heart failure: a randomized study. *JACC* 1995; **26**: 967–73.

66. Linde C, Gadler F, Edner M, *et al.* Results of atrioventricular synchronous pacing with optimized delay in patients with severe congestive heart failure. *Am J Cardiol* 1995; **75**: 919–23.

67. McDonald K, McWilliams E, O'Keeffe B, Maurer B. Functional assessment of patients treated with permanent dual chamber pacing as a primary treatment for hypertrophic cardiomyopathy. *Eur Heart J* 1988; **9**: 893–8.

68. Jeanrenaud X, Goy J-J, Kappenberger L. Effects of dual chamber pacing in hypertrophic obstructive cardiomyopathy. *Lancet* 1992; **339**: 1318–23.

69. Fananapazir L, Cannon RO, Tripodi D, Panza JA. Impact of dual-chamber permanent pacing in patients with obstructive hypertrophic cardiomyopathy with symptoms refractory to verapamil and β-adrenergic blocker therapy. *Circulation* 1992; **85**: 2149–61.

70. Fananapazir L, Epstein N, Curiel RV, Panza JA, Tripodi D, McAreavey D. Long-term results of dual-chamber (DDD) pacing in obstructive hypertrophic cardiomyopathy: evidence for progressive symptomatic and hemodynamic improvement and reduction of left ventricular hypertrophy. *Circulation* 1994; **90**: 2731–42.
71. Nishimura RA, Danielson GK. Dual chamber pacing for hypertrophic obstructive cardiomyopathy: has its time come? *Br Heart J* 1993; **70**: 301–3.
72. Gras D, De Place C, Leclercq C, Le Breton H, Mabo P, Daubert C. Key importance to individually optimize atrioventricular synchrony in obstructive hypertrophic cardiomyopathy treated by DDD-pacing (abstract). *Eur Heart J* 1994; **15** (suppl): 522.
73. Nishimura RA, Hayes DL, Ilstrup DM, *et al.* Effect of dual-chamber pacing on systolic and diastolic function in patients with hypertrophic cardiomyopathy: acute Doppler echocardiographic and catheterization hemodynamic study. *JACC* 1996; **27**: 421–30.
74. Cannon RO, Tripodi D, Dilsizian V, *et al.* Results of permanent dual-chamber pacing in symptomatic nonobstructive hypertrophic cardiomyopathy. *Am J Cardiol* 1994; **73**: 571–6.
75. Brecker SJD, Gibson DG. What is the role of pacing in dilated cardiomyopathy? *Eur Heart J* 1996; **17**: 819–24.
76. Symanski JD, Nishimura RA, Hayes DL, Tajik AJ. The effect of dual-chamber pacing on systolic and diastolic function in patients with hypertrophic cardiomyopathy: an acute Doppler/catheterization hemodynamic study (abstract). *Circulation* 1994; **90**: II654.
77. Betocchi S, Losi MA, Piscione F, *et al.* Atrio-ventricular pacing relieves obstruction but impairs diastolic function in hypertrophic cardiomyopathy (abstract). *JACC* 1994; **23** (suppl A): 11.
78. McDonald K, O'Sullivan JJ, King G, Conroy R, Maurer B. Dual chamber pacing improves left ventricular filling in patients with hypertrophic cardiomyopathy (abstract). *Eur Heart J* 1989; **10** (suppl): 401.
79. Slade AKB, Sadoul N, Shapiro L, *et al.* DDD pacing in hypertrophic cardiomyopathy: a multicentre clinical experience. *Heart* 1996; **75**: 44–9.
80. Frielingsdorf J, Desco T, Gerber AE, Bertel O. A comparison of quality-of-life in patients with dual chamber pacemakers and individually programmed atrioventricular delays. *PACE* 1996; **19**: 1147–54.
81. Kim YH, O'Nunain S, Trouton T, *et al.* Pseudopacemaker syndrome following inadvertent fast pathway ablation for atrioventricular nodal reentrant tachycardia. *J Cardiovasc Electrophysiol* 1993; **4**: 178–82.
82. Barold SS. Indications for permanent cardiac pacing in first degree AV block: class I, II or III? *PACE* 1996; **19**: 747–51.

13

Can New Pacing Sites Improve Haemodynamics?*

M. Rosenqvist

Since the introduction of permanent cardiac pacing some 40 years ago, the right ventricular apex has been the preferred site for stimulation. The main reason for choosing the apex is probably that it is usually easy to reach, provides good fixation and low capture thresholds.

Data derived from animal and human studies performed during the last decade have revealed, however, that ventricular stimulation might not be the most ideal. Not only does it cause an altered activation sequence, but it might also cause chronic myocardial changes over time.

In addition, several studies have been published showing that other ventricular pacing sites might be more beneficial, and that the optimal pacing site might be dependent on the condition of the underlying heart. The aim of this chapter is to review the possible value of alternative pacing sites, their feasibility and importance for cardiac performance.

Consequences of Right Ventricular Apical Stimulation

Activation Pattern

Normal cardiac contraction is characterized by preserved AV synchrony utilizing the intact conduction system and resulting in a narrow QRS complex and homogeneous and almost simultaneous activation of the left and right ventricles.

Stimulation from the right ventricular apex produces a prolongation of the QRS complex with a left bundle block configuration. This pattern of depolarization and repolarization creates asynchrony in left ventricular contraction with delayed activation of the left ventricle. Studies of regional motility using radionuclide phase imaging studies have shown that this abnormal contraction pattern is characterized by an alteration in septal movement during systole.[1,2]

* This study was supported by a grant from the Swedish Heart and Lung Foundation.

He *et al.*[3] showed that changes in the septum during right ventricular apical pacing were more pronounced at higher heart rates. That finding suggests that ventricular rate-responsive pacing might cause more profound changes than fixed-rate ventricular pacing.

The induction of dyssynchronous septal movement during apical stimulation has been found to be of value in patients with hypertrophic cardiomyopathies undergoing AV synchronous pacing with short AV delay. Gadler *et al.*[4] were able to show that apical pacing is of crucial importance for reducing left ventricular outflow tract obstruction in patients with hypertrophic cardiomyopathy. This effect was abolished when pacing was performed from the atrium or from the septum.

Wiggers, as long ago as 1925, demonstrated that activation of the cardiac muscle before excitation of the Purkinje system caused asynchrony in the contraction pattern and a deterioration in the resulting contraction force.[5] Studies in animals and in humans have shown that this change in the contraction pattern is associated with a deterioration in both global systolic and diastolic function.

Systolic Function

Askenazi *et al.*[6] studied patients during atrial and AV-synchronous stimulation and found that both positive and negative dp/dt significantly decreased during AV-synchronous pacing compared with atrial pacing. Since atrial pacing increased the peak systolic pressure, and the left ventricular end-diastolic pressure was similar, it was concluded that the differences were related to changes in afterload caused by asynchronous ventricular contraction. Similar observations have been made by others, in both human and animal studies.[7,8]

Boerth and Covell,[9] eliminating the influence of atrial contraction, showed that right ventricular stimulation produced an abnormal pattern of ventricular contraction which depressed global left ventricular function. Similar observations have been made in humans showing, in addition, that these differences persisted during exercise.[1,2]

Yamamoto *et al.*[10] used a tip manometer conductance catheter to construct pressure volume loops. They showed that the end-systolic elastance and the mechanical energy efficiency was higher during atrial than during AV-synchronous pacing owing to dyssynchronous ventricular contractions.

All the above studies were limited by the fact that they were performed in subjects with preserved AV conduction. Thus, the AV delay had to be programmed short enough to ensure complete ventricular capture. The relative advantage seen with atrial pacing might therefore have been compensated for by adjustment of the AV delay.[11] In another study by Rosenqvist *et al.*[12] this problem was dealt with by inducing complete heart block after atrial pacing. Myocardial function could subsequently be assessed at varying AV delays. Even in the presence of varying AV delays, atrial pacing resulted in a higher positive dp/dt, increased cardiac output and decreased left ventricular end-diastolic pressure. In that study, left ventricular systolic pressure remained unchanged, indicating an unaltered afterload, as noted by several other authors comparing atrial with AV-synchronous pacing.[13,14]

Betocchi *et al.*, who studied systolic and diastolic effects of atrial versus AV-synchronous pacing in patients, reported a similar trend towards decreased left ventricular diastolic pressure during atrial pacing.[14]

Thus, data in the literature consistently show that atrial stimulation improves contractility and reduces preload when compared with AV-synchronous pacing from the right ventricular apex.

Diastolic Function

Studies in animals suggest that abnormal ventricular activation causes an abnormal left ventricular relaxation, reflecting a diastolic dysfunction.[13,15,16] Bedotto *et al.*[17] studied the effect of asynchronous left ventricular relaxation in 25 patients referred for diagnostic cardiac catheterization. The patients were divided into those with abnormal and those with normal LV function. Relaxation was assessed by negative dp/dt and changes in the time constant of left ventricular relaxation. Right ventricular pacing caused a significant deterioration in LV diastolic function in patients with an abnormal LV function. Similar findings were reported by Betocchi *et al.* in patients with coronary artery disease.[14]

Rosenqvist *et al.*[12] assessed diastolic function during atrial pacing, followed by induction of complete heart block, and thereafter during AV-synchronous pacing with three different AV intervals. Atrial pacing was superior to AV-synchronous pacing with respect to negative dp/dt and cardiac output, indicating that the negative diastolic effects induced by apical pacing cannot be compensated for by optimizing the AV interval.

Cohn *et al.*[18] demonstrated that negative dp/dt is related both to the contractility of the ventricle and to the volume of the heart at the onset of relaxation. Thus, inotropic stimulation will directly increase the negative dp/dt. However, a decrease will also be the result of a reduction of left ventricular end-systolic volume. In accordance with these findings other investigators have shown that negative dp/dt is afterload-dependent, varying with LV systolic pressure.[19,20]

Thus, it remains to be established whether a deterioration in left ventricular relaxation during apical pacing is limited only to those with a depressed LV function.

Long-Term Effects

Some authors have studied the long-term effects of right ventricular apical pacing. Animal studies have shown histological evidence of the development of left ventricular myocardial disarray over time, when ventricular pacing was performed from the right ventricular apex.[21,22] In accord with these findings, Lee *et al.*[23] reported that right ventricular apical pacing produced an increase in myocardial catecholamine content and a mismatch in perfusion in dogs paced for 6 months from the right ventricular apex with and without AV-synchrony, compared with atrial pacing. These changes were seen in animals treated both with DDD and with ventricular pacing, but not in animals subjected to atrial pacing.

Data on the long-term effects of permanent cardiac pacing are scarce. Saxon *et al.*, in a retrospective analysis of a large group of patients with cardiac failure,[24] noted a higher incidence of haemodynamic deterioration among those with right ventricular apical stimulation. In retrospective case–control studies it was reported that AV-synchronous pacing, when compared with ventricular pacing, seemed to improve the prognosis among patients with congestive heart failure.[25,26]

Whether long-term pacing from the right ventricular apex could be deleterious in humans undergoing permanent cardiac pacing thus needs to be evaluated by prospective randomized trials.

Pacing From Alternative Sites

In view of the negative effects encountered with right ventricular apical pacing, it seems apt to explore whether pacing from alternative sites could limit these effects.

In patients with intact AV conduction (i.e. patients with sinus node disease) atrial stimulation preserving the normal activation pattern is a logical choice, thereby not only improving left ventricular haemodynamics but also providing beneficial effects in the long term.[27,28]

Recent studies of pacing in patients with paroxysmal atrial fibrillation, without other conduction disturbances, indicate that pacing from two different sites in the atrium might be the optimal pacing technique to prevent attacks of fibrillation. For a comprehensive review, see Chapter 3 in this book.

The problem becomes more difficult in the presence of depressed AV conduction, making atrial stimulation impossible or carrying an increased risk for impending high-grade AV block. In this situation it seems logical to explore alternative ventricular sites in order to optimize ventricular stimulation. Furthermore, it seems natural to explore sites close to the native conduction system to shorten the ventricular conduction time.

Experimental Studies

Vasallo *et al.*[29] demonstrated that pacing from the right ventricular mid-septum, or pacing from two ventricular sites simultaneously, was superior to conventional ventricular apical pacing. Kosowsky *et al.*[30] compared atrial synchronized His-bundle pacing with atrial synchronized apical right ventricular pacing and at three different AV intervals. LV function was consistently better during His-bundle pacing. These data suggest that pacing more closely to the natural Purkinje system might improve left ventricular function.

Rosenqvist *et al.*[12] studied the effect of proximal septal pacing, with the electrode fixed under the tricuspid leaflet, in animals with complete heart block at varying AV intervals (Figure 13.1). Independent of the programmed AV interval, septal pacing was associated with a higher positive and negative *dp/dt* compared with right ventricular apical pacing. In addition, the left ventricular activation time, as assessed

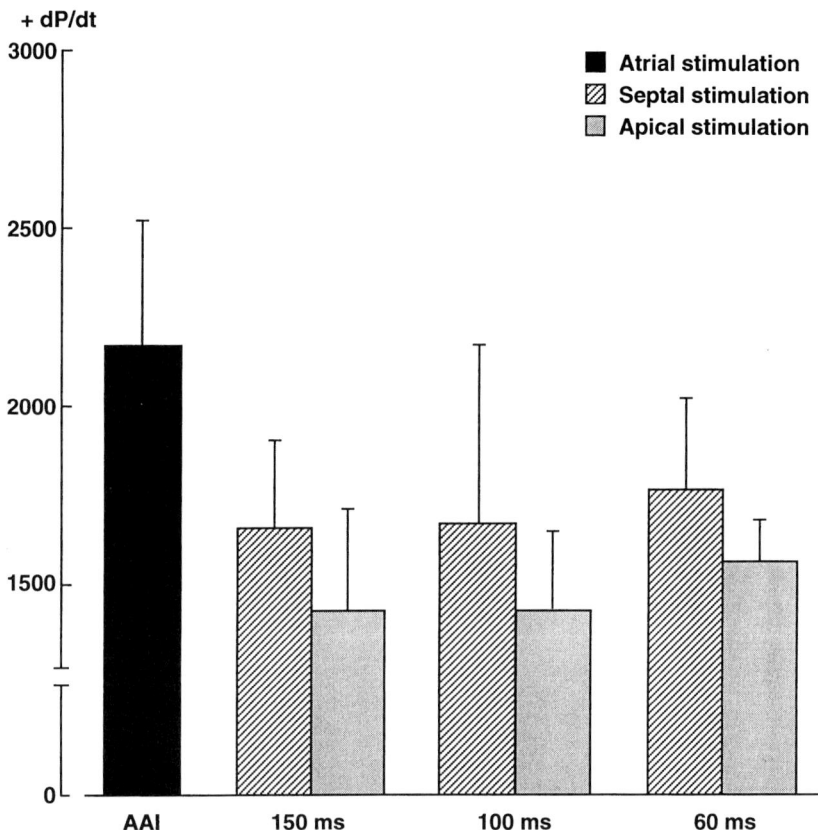

Figure 13.1 Positive *dP/dt* measurements from three dogs undergoing atrial, septal and apical pacing. Septal and apical pacing was performed in the DDD mode. Bars represent mean ± SD. (Reproduced with permission from reference 12)

by QRS width, was significantly decreased by an average of 25% during septal pacing (Figure 13.2), indicating a more rapid and less heterogeneous activation pattern.

Karpawich *et al*.[31] showed improved haemodynamic effects over the long term, in a chronic animal model using dog puppies, when pacing from the proximal septum as compared with that from the right ventricular apex. In addition these authors observed fewer signs of histological degeneration of the myocardium among dogs paced from the septum.

Studies in Humans

Single-lead pacing

Several groups have recently published evidence that pacing from alternative ventricular sites in humans might provide haemodynamic benefit. Cowell *et al*.[32]

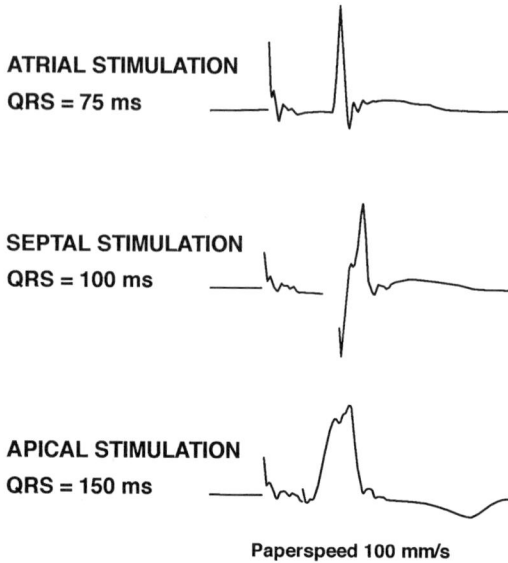

ATRIAL STIMULATION
QRS = 75 ms

SEPTAL STIMULATION
QRS = 100 ms

APICAL STIMULATION
QRS = 150 ms

Paperspeed 100 mm/s

Figure 13.2   ECG examples of changes in QRS width when pacing from the atrium, septum and apex. Note the intermediate QRS width when pacing from the septum. (Reproduced with permission from reference 12)

showed haemodynamic beneficial effects when pacing AV synchronously from the right ventricular septum as compared with the apex, in 15 patients with congestive heart failure with intact AV conduction and with an average LV ejection fraction of 33%. Cardiac output increased significantly by an average of 15% when stimulating from the septal region. No significant difference was seen when stimulating from the apex.

Deshmukh et al.[33] performed direct His-bundle pacing in four patients with congestive heart failure, using screw-in leads. The authors reported the same QRS configuration as during the intrinsic rhythm. After an average follow-up of 12 weeks, one lead was displaced, but in the remaining three patients the intrinsic QRS configuration was maintained. In a more recent report[34] the same authors described five patients with atrial fibrillation and depressed LV function who underwent AV junctional ablation followed by chronic His-bundle pacing with rate-responsive pacemakers, demonstrating that His-bundle pacing is feasible also in the presence of high-grade AV block. Giudici et al.[35] compared pacing from the right ventricular outflow tract with right ventricular apical pacing in a series of 58 patients requiring permanent pacing. Using transthoracic Doppler echocardiography they found a 20% average increase in cardiac output when pacing from the outflow tract. Surprisingly the improvement was most pronounced in male patients and was not correlated to a decrease in QRS width.

de Cock et al.[36] found a particular advantage for outflow tract pacing in patients with reduced cardiac output, whereas Kolettis et al.[37] in a similar study of patients with preserved normal left ventricular function found comparable haemodynamic effects independent of pacing from the apex or the outflow tract. Thus it remains to be established whether the positive effects reported for pacing from the outflow tract are limited to patients with a depressed LV function.

Two recent preliminary reports[38,39] studied the long-term (3–10 months) outcome of outflow tract pacing with respect to stimulation thresholds, R-wave signals and dislocation rates. There was no significant difference in outcome between the two pacing sites. Whether the beneficial haemodynamic effects observed during acute studies will persist over the long term remains to be established. At least two prospective studies are presently under way to evaluate the long-term effects of outflow tract pacing versus apical pacing.[40]

Biventricular pacing for heart failure

Recently, several groups have found evidence that biventricular stimulation can improve haemodynamics in patients with congestive heart failure. Foster *et al.*[41] studied 18 patients 12–36 hours after coronary bypass surgery by simultaneous stimulation from the right atrium and in epicardial anterior septal sites on the left and right ventricles. Biventricular pacing was compared with atrial pacing and single-site ventricular pacing. Simultaneous activation of the left and right ventricles was documented by isochronal epicardial mapping. During biventricular pacing the cardiac index increased and systemic vascular resistance decreased significantly, not only in comparison with monoventricular pacing but also with respect to atrial pacing.

Bakker *et al.*[42] reported six patients with end-stage congestive heart failure and left bundle branch block with an average ejection fraction of 16% who underwent pacing with two ventricular leads, one in the right ventricular apex and one epicardial left ventricular lead. Each patient had the AV delay fine-tuned and the optimal AV delay was programmed individually for each patient. Haemodynamic and functional changes were assessed after 3 months using peak oxygen uptake, anaerobic threshold and NYHA classification. The authors observed an average increase of more than 40% in both peak oxygen uptake and anaerobic threshold at follow-up. These changes were associated with a significant decrease in NYHA classification, from 4 to 2.5.

Cazeau *et al.*,[43] in a series of observations, have reported beneficial effects of biventricular pacing combining simulation from the right ventricular outflow tract and the left ventricle. Their observations indicate that the improved haemodynamic effect is related to a shortening of the ventricular activation sequence and contraction time. Preliminary data from eight patients undergoing chronic biventricular pacing are promising, but need to be confirmed in larger prospective studies. Chapter 1 of this book is a comprehensive review of pacing in congestive heart failure.

Conclusions

Right ventricular apical pacing seems to result acutely in a deterioration of both systolic and diastolic left ventricular function, in animals and humans. These changes are probably the result of an asynchronous LV activation pattern, inhibiting the septum from participating in the left ventricular contraction process.

There is experimental evidence that long-term ventricular pacing can result in structural changes over time. Whether such changes are prone to develop also in humans undergoing chronic pacing remains to be established.

Studies in both animals and humans have shown that it is feasible to stimulate from other sites, more close to the native conduction system than the right ventricular apex. These studies indicate that stimulation from the proximal septum and the right ventricular apex produces stable fixation and more efficient ventricular contraction.

In patients with severe congestive heart failure, pacing from more proximal sites and/or simultaneous stimulation of both ventricles seems to be of at least short-term benefit. However, large prospective studies are warranted to confirm these effects in a general population of congestive heart failure.

References

1. Rosenqvist M, Isaaz K, Botvinick E, *et al*. Relative importance of activation sequence compared to AV synchrony in left ventricular function. *Am J Cardiol* 1991; **67**: 148–56.
2. Leclercq C, Gras D, Le Helloco A, Nicol L, Mabo P, Daubert C. Hemodynamic importance of preserving the normal sequence of ventricular activation in permanent cardiac pacing. *Am Heart J* 1995; **129**: 1133–41.
3. He ZX, Darcourt J, Migneco B, Camous JP, Benoliel J, Bussiere F, Baudouy M, Morand P. Effect of pacing rate on regional left ventricular wall motion: assessment by quantitative analysis of equilibrium radionuclide angiography. *Int J Cardiac Imag* 1995; **11**: 193–9.
4. Gadler F, Linde C, Juhlin-Dannfeldt A, Ribeiro A, Rydén L. Influence of right ventricular pacing site on left ventricular outflow tract obstruction in patients with hypertrophic cardiomyopathy. *JACC* 1996; **27**: 1219–24.
5. Wiggers CJ. The muscle reactions of the mammalian ventricles to artificial surface stimuli. *Am J Physiol* 1925; **73**: 346–78.
6. Askenazi J, Alexander JH, Koenigsberg DI, *et al*. Alteration of left ventricular performance by left bundle branch block simulated with atrioventricular sequential pacing. *Am J Cardiol* 1984; **53**: 99–104.
7. Burkhoff D, Oikawa RY, Sagawa K. Influence of pacing site on canine left ventricular contraction. *Am J Physiol* 1986; **251**: H428–35.
8. Sheffer A, Rozenmann Y, Ben-David Y, *et al*. Left ventricular function during physiologic cardiac pacing: relation to pacing mode rate and underlying heart disease. *PACE* 1987; **10**: 315–25.
9. Boerth RC, Covell JW. Mechanical performance and efficiency of the left ventricle during ventricular stimulation. *Am J Physiol* 1971; **221**: 1686–91.
10. Yamamoto K, Kodama K, Masuyama H, *et al*. Role of atrial contraction and synchrony of ventricular contraction in the optimisation of ventriculoatrial contraction coupling in humans. *Br Heart J* 1992; **67**: 366–72.
11. Wish M, Fletcher RD, Gotdiener JS, *et al*. Importance of left atrial timing in the programming of dual chamber pacemakers. *Am J Cardiol* 1987; **60**: 566–71.
12. Rosenqvist M, Bergfeldt L, Haga Y, Rydén J, Öwall A, Rydén L. The effect of ventricular activation sequence on cardiac performance during pacing. *PACE* 1996; **19**: 1279–86.
13. Zile MR, Blaustein AS, Shimuzu G, *et al*. Right ventricular pacing reduces the rate of left ventricular relaxation and filling. *JACC* 1987; **10**: 702–9.

14. Betocchi S, Piscione F, Villari B, *et al*. Effects of induced asynchrony on left ventricular diastolic function in patients with coronary artery disease. *JACC* 1993; **21**: 1124–31.
15. Badke FR, Boinay P, Covell JW. Effects of ventricular pacing on regional ventricular performance in the dog. *Am J Physiol* 1980; **238**: H858–67.
16. Heyndrickx GR, Vantrimpont PJ, Rousseau MF, Pouleur H. Effects of asynchrony on myocardial relaxation at rest and during exercise in conscious dogs. *Am J Physiol* 1988; **254**: H817–22.
17. Bedotto JB, Grayburn PA, Black WH, *et al*. Alteration in left ventricular relaxation during atrioventricular pacing in humans. *JACC* 1990; **15**: 658–64.
18. Cohn PF, Liedtke AJ, Serup J, *et al*. Maximal rate of pressure fall (peak negative *dp/dt*) during ventricular relaxation. *Cardiovasc Res* 1972; **6**: 263–7.
19. Karliner JS, LeWinter MM, Mahler F, *et al*. Pharmacologic and hemodynamic influences on the rate of isovolumic left ventricular relaxation in the normal conscious dog. *J Clin Invest* 1977; **60**: 511–21.
20. Thompson DS, Wilmshurst P, Juul SM, *et al*. Pressure derived indices of left ventricular isovolumic relaxation in patients with hypertrophic cardiomyopathy. *Br Heart J* 1983; **49**: 259–67.
21. Adomian GE, Beazell J. Myofibrillar disarray produced in normal hearts by chronic electrical pacing. *Am Heart J* 1986; **112**: 79–83.
22. Karpawich PP, Justice CD, Chang CH, *et al*. Septal ventricular pacing in the immature canine heart: a new perspective. *Am Heart J* 1991; **121**: 827–33.
23. Lee M, Dae M, Langberg J, *et al*. Effects of chronic right ventricular apical pacing on left ventricular perfusion, innervation, function and histology. *JACC* 1994; **24**: 225–32.
24. Saxon LA, Stevenson WG, Middlekauf HR, *et al*. Increased risk of progressive hemodynamic deterioration in advanced heart failure patients requiring permanent pacemakers. *Am Heart J* 1993; **125**: 1306–10.
25. Alpert MA, Curtiss JJ, Sanfelippo JF, *et al*. Comparative survival after permanent ventricular and dual chamber pacing for patients with chronic high-degree atrioventricular block with and without preexistent congestive heart failure. *JACC* 1986; **7**: 925–32.
26. Linde-Edelstam C, Gullberg B, Nordlander R, *et al*. Longevity in patients with high degree atrioventricular block paced in the atrial synchronous or the fixed rate ventricular inhibited mode. *PACE* 1992; **15**: 304–13.
27. Rosenqvist M, Brandt J, Schüller H. Long-term treatment of sinus node disease: superiority of atrial stimulation. *Am Heart J* 1988; **116**: 16–22.
28. Andersen HR, Thuesen L, Bagge JP, *et al*. Prospective randomized trial of atrial versus ventricular pacing in sick-sinus syndrome. *Lancet* 1994; **344**: 1523.
29. Vasallo JA, Cassidy DM, Miller JM, Buxton AE, Marchlinski FE, Josephson ME. Left ventricular endocardial activation during right ventricular pacing: effect of underlying heart disease. *JACC* 1986; **7**: 1228–33.
30. Kosowsky BD, Scherlag BJ, Damato AN. Re-evaluation of the atrial contribution to ventricular function: study using His bundle pacing. *Am J Cardiol* 1968; **21**: 518–24.
31. Karpawich PP, Justice CD, Cavitt DL, *et al*. Developmental sequelae of fixed-rate ventricular pacing in the immature canine heart: an electrophysiologic, hemodynamic, and histopathologic evaluation. *Am Heart J* 1990; **119**: 1077–83.
32. Cowell R, Morris-Thurgood J, Ilsley C, Paul V. Septal short atrioventricular delay pacing: additional hemodynamic improvements in heart failure. *PACE* 1994; **17**(II): 1980–3.
33. Deshmukh P, Anderson KJ. Direct His bundle pacing: novel approach to permanent pacing in patients with severe left ventricular dysfunction and atrial fibrillation (abstract). *PACE* 1996; **19**(II): 700.
34. Deshmukh P, Golyan F, Anderson K, Zehr RD. AV nodal ablation in conjunction with direct His bundle pacing improves left ventricular function in patients with atrial fibrillation and cardiomyopathy (abstract). *Circulation* 1996; **94**: 119.
35. Giudici MC, Thornburg GA, Buck DL, Alldredge SG, Lewis JR, Coyne E, Bontu JRP, Sutton J. Permanent right ventricular outflow tract pacing improves cardiac output: comparison with apical placement in 58 patients. *PACE* 1994; **17**(II): 77.

36. de Cock C, Meyer A, Kamp O, Visser C. Hemodynamic benefit of right ventricular outflow tract pacing in patients with atrial fibrillation and slow ventricular response (abstract). *PACE* 1995; **18**(II): 847.
37. Kolettis TM, Theodorakis GN, Paraskevaiades I, Popov ZS, Kyriakides Livanis E, Kresmas-tionos DT. Left ventricular hemodynamics during short-term pacing from the apex versus the outflow tract of the right ventricle (abstract). *Eur Heart J* 1996; **17**: 485.
38. Kutarski A, Poleszak K, Baszak K. Right ventricular outflow tract is not worse than right ventricular apex site as a site of permanent ventricular pacing (abstract). *Eur Heart J* 1996; **17**: 484.
39. Staniewicz J, Swiateck G, Wilczck R, Lewicka-Nowak E. Permanent right ventricular outflow tract pacing: randomized comparison with right ventricular apex pacing (abstract). *Eur Heart J* 1996; **17**: 485.
40. Sutton R. Right ventricular outflow tract pacing. *Eur J CPE* 1996; **6**: 6–7.
41. Foster AH, Gold MR, McLaughlin JS. Acute hemodynamic effects of atrio-biventricular pacing in humans. *Ann Thorac Surg* 1995; **59**: 294–300.
42. Bakker P, Sen KC, de Jonge N, Klöpping C, Algra A, Robles de Medina E. Biventricular pacing improves functional capacity in patients with end stage congestive heart failure. *PACE* 1995; **18**: 825.
43. Cazeau S, Ritter P, Lazarus A, Gras D, Mugica J. Hemodynamic improvement provided by biventricular pacing in congestive heart failure: an acute study. *PACE* 1996; **19**: 568.

14

Is an 'Ideal' Sensor a Realistic Proposition?

S.-K. Leung and C.-P. Lau

Although the optimal rate adaptation in a pacemaker recipient may be different from that in a normal individual, it is assumed that sensors should mimic the behaviour of the healthy sinus node response to exercise and nonexercise needs. In addition, in patients with paroxysmal atrial tachycardias, the tracking of the sinus node during a paroxysm will not be possible and the use of a sensor to back up the sinus node is required. In this chapter, clinical and experimental sensors are reviewed to assess how realistic it is for a single sensor to match the ideal sinus node behaviour. The use of sensor combinations to overcome some of the shortcomings of a single artificial sensor will be addressed. Finally, a sensor can only be ideal if correctly programmed, and if it is able to change automatically according to the patient's clinical or physical status.

Classification of Sensors

Physiological Classification

Sensors for rate-adaptive pacing can be classified according to the physiological 'level' they detect.[1] A primary sensor is one which detects the changes that determine the normal sinus response to physiological needs. These include the sensing of circulating catecholamines and neural activities. Although these may be the most ideal indicators for a rate-adaptive system, technical realization has yet to be achieved. The majority of rate-adaptive sensors proposed belong to the secondary sensors: they detect the internal changes consequent upon exercise. Some, such as the sensing of the QT interval, respiratory changes, average atrial rate, central venous temperature, venous blood pH, stroke volume, the pre-ejection interval, and right ventricular pressure, have been realized in either clinical or investigational units. These sensors respond at a variable speed from the onset of exercise and have variable proportionality to workload. A third group of sensors, the tertiary sensors, detect external changes as a result of exercise. An example is the sensing of body movement. As expected, there is only a loose relationship between workload and sensor changes for this group. The use of the 24-hour clock to vary the lower rate can be considered as a tertiary sensor.

Technical Classification

An alternative method is to group the available sensors according to the technical methods used for sensing (Table 14.1). Sensors derived from a common technical principle share a similar hardware requirement and sensor stability, and similar drawbacks and limitations. *Impedance* is a measure of electrical resistance and is derived by measuring the resistivity from an injected electric current across a tissue. The simplicity of design has made it suitable for use in implanted pacing electrodes, either with a standard pacing electrode or with specialized multi-electrode catheters. The arrangement generally involves injection of subthreshold pulses from an electrode pair (source current), and recording of the changes in impedance using a receiving electrode pair. This has been used to detect changes in respiratory parameters, and to reflect the right ventricular stroke volume and the pre-ejection period. As the baseline impedance is different between individuals and within an individual from time to time, such devices do not measure the absolute level of impedance but only the changes over a preceding baseline. In general, a moving average is used to establish a baseline and an 'adaptive' period is required to achieve this before the sensor can be activated. As subthreshold stimuli need to be injected for impedance measurement, the sensor is energy expensive although the overall battery drain is in the order of several months of the pacemaker's longevity. As the pacemaker box is usually used as an electrode for either sourcing or recording the impedance current, motion of the pacemaker box (e.g. arm movement) can significantly affect the

Table 14.1 Technical classification of sensors

Methods	Derived parameters	Physiological variables
Body movement	Vibration Acceleration	Reflects body movement as indirect indicator of exercise
Impedance sensing	Respiratory parameters	Respiratory rate Minute Ventilation™
	Haemodynamic parameters	Stroke volume Pre-ejection period Right ventricular ejection time
Ventricular evoked response	Evoked QT interval Ventricular depolarization gradient	QT interval reflects autonomic activity QRS area reflects autonomic activity
Special sensors on pacing electrode	Physical parameters	Central venous temperature Right ventricular pressure and its derivatives (dp/dt) Average atrial rate Right atrial pressure
	Biochemical parameters	Mixed venous pH Mixed venous oxygen saturation

impedance measurement and the sensor indicated rate response.[2-4] Similarly, exogenous electrical interference such as diathermy may lead to erroneous sensing.[5] An *evoked ventricular electrogram* results from a suprathreshold pacing stimulus. This paced ventricular complex has a characteristic waveform from which the QT interval and the vector integrated R-wave area (the so-called ventricular depolarization gradient or paced depolarization integral, PDI) can be derived from a conventional unipolar pacing electrode. Both parameters are sensitive to changes in heart rate and the autonomic nervous system. As a large polarization effect occurs after a pacing impulse, a special pulse waveform and post-pulse compensation are needed to eliminate this effect to allow accurate determination of these parameters. At present, these parameters can only be derived from a unipolar ventricular stimulus. In the presence of intrinsic conduction, the system has to overdrive the ventricle to estimate the parameter, and fusion beats can sometimes cause confusion. These parameters cannot be derived from the atrial level. As the QT interval is also rate-dependent, sensor-driven rate adaptation due to QT shortening may lead to further QT shortening, resulting in positive feedback tachycardia.[6] Thus a special algorithmic correction is required to measure the rate-independent QT shortening due to autonomic nervous activities.

The most widely used physical principle for detecting exercise is through the recording of body movement and acceleration forces. As vibrations accompany dynamic physical activities, such vibrations can be detected using sensors located at the level of the pacemaker casing. Minimal or no energy expenditure is required for such a system and, as the sensor does not need to have contact with the body fluid, it is usually stable over time. Another advantage is that all the hardware is within the pacemaker case, it does not depend on the electrode arrangement and can be used with standard unipolar and bipolar pacing electrodes. This makes it ideal for combining with other sensors and for pacemaker upgrading. It is used often as a 'backup' sensor when a new sensor is being investigated. As a group, body movement has only a loose relationship with workload. Therefore, the sensor-indicated rate has low proportionality, and physical activities that do not involve body movement will not be detected by these sensors.

The last group of sensors involves detection of various physical and chemical parameters and generally requires a dedicated sensor incorporated onto a pacing lead. These dedicated sensors allow chemical compositions of the bloodstream or intracardiac haemodynamics to be measured, and may result in a more 'physiological' sensor system. However, the long-term stability of these sensors is questionable. They are also energy expensive. These sensors have only a limited application in the field of rate-adaptive pacing, but may open the possibility for ambulatory monitoring of the intracardiac environment using an implanted device.

Characteristics of an Ideal Sensor

An ideal sensor to replace the atrium as an indicator for rate response should be capable of simulating the sinus response during physiological changes.[7] It should be characterized by a *proportional* (or accurate) response to the level of exertion, and an adequate rate response must occur at an adequate *speed*. In many individuals, the sinus rate will increase prior to exercise as a result of the anticipatory response. With both supine and upright isotonic exercise, sinus rate and cardiac output increase within 10 seconds of the onset of exercise.[8–10] Both cardiac output and sinus rate increase exponentially, with a half-time that ranges from 10 to 45 seconds, the rate of rise being proportional to the intensity of work[8] and linearly related to the oxygen uptake. At the termination of upright exercise there is a delay of approximately 5–10 seconds before cardiac output starts to decrease, followed by an exponential fall with a half-time of 25–60 seconds.[11] An ideal sensor and its instrumentation should exhibit these rate kinetics.

The need for exercise is but one of the many physiological requirements for a variation in heart rate. An ideal sensor should also be *sensitive* enough to detect both exercise and nonexercise needs, such as isometric exercise which results in an increase in cardiac output and heart rate,[12] upright posture which results in a higher sinus rate, and other influences induced by physiological manoeuvres like the Valsalva, baroreceptor reflexes, anxiety reactions and diurnal variation. The ability to decrease the pacing rate during sleep is not only physiological, it also lowers battery consumption. The sensor should also be *specific* enough not to be affected by interference from nonphysiological changes. The chronotropic response obtained with a rate-adaptive pacing system is ultimately dependent on the algorithm or logic used to relate changes in the sensed parameter into changes in pacing rate. In addition, optimal programming can dramatically affect the final rate modulation.

Although a sensor for physiological needs may possess these qualities, it must also be technically compatible in an implantable system without the need for a special lead, remain stable over time, and require minimum power consumption.

Activity Sensing (Table 14.2)

Physical Principles

The detection of body movement indicates dynamic exercise and may be used as a measure of activity level. The physical forces involved have been studied in detail using three-dimensional accelerometers.[13,14] In these studies, accelerometers were attached to the pacemaker case, which usually slants slightly backward in the normal implant position. During walking, the axis along the surface of the pacemaker is associated with the highest acceleration force, followed by the anteroposterior axis of the pacemaker, and the lateral axis only detects sideways 'swaying' movement rather than walking. As the top side of an implanted pacemaker is not constant, only the anteroposterior axis is used in practice. The frequency content of acceleration forces occurring during daily activities is predominantly in the low frequency range (<4 Hz), whereas external vibrations such as those occurring during travelling in a motor vehicle are above 10 Hz. The strength of the integrated acceleration signal bears a closer relationship to different speeds and gradients of walking than does just counting acceleration pulses with each walking step. To further refine the distinction between different forms of activity such as cycling and stair-climbing, newer signal-

Table 14.2 Current activity sensing pacemakers

Sensor	Algorithm	Examples	Manufacturers
Piezoelectric crystal	Activity signals counting	Activitrax™ Legend™ Thera™	Medtronic Inc., Minneapolis, MN, USA
	Integration algorithm	Sensolog™ Synchrony™ Triology™ DR+	Siemens-Elema Pacesetters, Solna, Sweden
Accelerometers	Linear rate-response curve	Excel™ Vigor™	Cardiac Pacemakers Inc., St Paul, MN, USA
	Triphasic rate-response curve	Relay™ Dash™ Marathon™	Intermedics Inc., Freeport, TX, USA
Mercury ball	Detects gravitational acceleration	Swing™ 100	Sorin Biomedica, Saluggia, Italy
Magnetic ball	Electrical signal generated by movement of magnetic ball	Sensorithm™ 2045	Siemens-Elma Pacesetters, Solna, Sweden

processing methods involving the interaction of threshold, slopes and morphology of acceleration forces have been tested in *in vitro* models.[15]

Sensor and Algorithms

Body vibrations and accelerations are detected by a sensor in the pacemaker casing which converts the strength of mechanical forces into calibrated electrical signals. The clinically available activity-sensing pacemakers use either a piezoelectric crystal or an accelerometer (Figure 14.1). A piezoelectric crystal emits a small electric current when it is deformed, and thus converts motion energy into electrical energy. In the piezoelectric activity-sensing pacemaker, the crystal is bonded to the inside of the pacemaker casing that faces the pectoral muscle, and correct orientation of the sensor is important during implantation. As the sensor is coupled to varying body mass of the patient, individual variations in signal strength are significant. On the other hand, an accelerometer is attached to the electronic circuitboard instead of the pacemaker case. This arrangement allows the detection of true acceleration forces in the lower frequency range and is independent of the orientation of the implanted pacemaker.

In one version of the piezoelectric pacemaker (Legend™, Medtronic Inc., Minneapolis, MN, USA), body activity is detected by counting the activity signals that exceed a predetermined programmable threshold, and the number of counts occurring within a given time can be related to an increase in pacing rate by a series of programmable responses with a linear relationship between activity counts and pacing rate. The activity threshold determines the degree of activity required to elicit a pacing rate response, whereas the rate-response slope converts activity counts above the threshold into a pacing rate.[16] Programmable rate onset and rate decay curves are available.

Piezoelectric   Accelerometer   Gravitational   Inductive

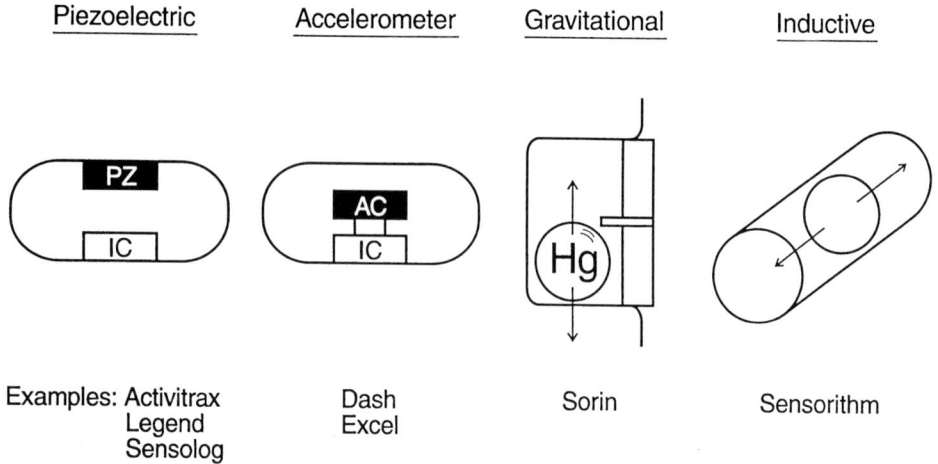

Examples: Activitrax   Dash   Sorin   Sensorithm
Legend   Excel
Sensolog

Figure 14.1 Schematic of activity-sensing pacemakers. A piezoelectric crystal (PZ) is attached to the inside of one surface of the pacemaker case (which faces the muscle) to detect transmitted vibrations during exercise. In an accelerometer (AC)-based activity-sensing device, the accelerometer is attached to the electronic integrated circuitboard (IC) to detect accelerations. In the gravitational sensor, a mercury ball (Hg) rolls over a disc with switches to give an index of body activity as well as an indication of the posture of the body. The inductive activity sensor consists of a magnetic ball moving freely inside a plastic elliptical housing surrounded by two copper-wire coils. Activity is detected by electrical signals generated by the movement of the magnetic ball.

Another model (Sensolog^{TM}, Siemens-Elema Pacesetters, Solna, Sweden) uses an algorithm which involves an integration of vibration signals that exceed a preselected threshold. In bench-testing, the vibration signal-integration algorithm produces a rate response proportional to the level of external forces applied, while the vibration-counting algorithm responds in an on–off fashion, with the maximum rate achieved once the external force exceeds a certain level.[17] However, the rate responses of the two algorithm types in patients are very similar.[18] The signal-integration algorithm is more responsive to arm exercise, has somewhat higher sensitivity to pressure,[18] and is more dependent on the nature of the footwear the patient uses compared with the vibration-counting algorithm.

In accelerometer-based activity-sensing pacemakers, the levels of acceleration in the low-frequency range (<4 Hz) are integrated to derive an integrated signal. Signals are linked to a linear or a triphasic rate/acceleration curve. In a triphasic curve, a relatively steep slope is used at low and high levels of exercise for rapid rate increases and recovery, with an intermediate gentle slope to allow for a relatively stable rate change during ordinary daily activities. The rate response of the accelerometer-based activity-sensing pacemaker had been shown to be proportional to the workload during treadmill exercise and the intrinsic heart rate in healthy volunteers and pacemaker patients.[19–21] In a comparison between an acceleration-sensor pacemaker (Relay^{TM}, Intermedics Inc., Freeport, TX, USA) and a piezoelectric-sensor rate-adaptive pacemaker (Legend^{TM}, Medtronic Inc., Minneapolis, MN, USA), the acceleration sensor gave a better approximation to the sinus rate and better rate specificity to workload on exercise tests,[20,22] higher rate responses to jogging and standing, and less susceptibility to interference by direct pressure and external forces applied on the pacemaker.[23]

Other Activity-Sensing Principles

Using the tilt switch principle, a gravitational acceleration sensor uses a mercury ball rolling over a disc with switches, and the rate of opening and closing of these switches by the mercury gives an index of body activity.[24] Furthermore, the position of the mercury ball can detect vertical movements of the centre of gravity and gives an indication of the posture of the body, so this sensor may be a good indicator of postural changes. In practice, there may be difficulty in maintaining a stable position of the implanted pacemaker in the pocket, so that it may not be possible to keep the 'top' of the disc in a constant position for posture detection. The gravitational sensor is used in the Sorin Swing™ 100 (Sorin Biomedica, Saluggia, Italy) single-chamber rate-adaptive system. The movements of the mercury droplet evoked by displacement of the centre of gravity enable the system to detect variations of gravimetric acceleration. Signals with frequencies lower than 5 Hz will increase the pacing rate according to the programmed slope. Signals with a frequency higher than 5 Hz will increase the pacing rate to the 'noise protection' rate, i.e. 10 bpm faster than the programmed basic rate. In healthy volunteers, the rate response of Swing™ 100 was shown to be correlated to the sinus rate at the early stages of treadmill exercise and discontinuous treadmill exercise tests.[25] A multicentre study with Holter monitoring and treadmill exercise tests showed reliable rate increase during daily activities and treadmill exercise tests,[26] and the sensor was immune to physical interference.

Another new rate-adaptive pacemaker, Sensorithm™ 2045 (Siemens-Elema Pacesetters, Solna, Sweden), controls its pacing rate response by an inductive activity sensor mounted on a printed circuitboard inside the pulse generator. The sensor consists of a magnetic ball moving freely in three dimensions inside a plastic elliptical housing which is surrounded by two copper-wire coils. When the ball is moving, electrical signals are generated. The processed sensor signal is then used to change the pacing rate in response to the patient's activity according to the programmed reaction times, slopes and recovery times. The sensor does not respond to pressure applied on the pulse generator.[27] This sensor increased the exercise time, walking distance and maximum oxygen uptake during exercise tests comparing it with the VVI mode.[27] However, in another report, it was found that the sensor overpaced in the early stage of exercise and the proportionality of rate response during linear increasing metabolic workload was still unsatisfactory.[27]

Advantages of Activity Sensing

The main advantage of activity sensing is the rapidity at which a rate response can be achieved.[28,29] The reliability and stability of the sensor are important reasons for its extensive use. Clinical benefits have been extensively documented. Compared with the VVI mode, activity-initiated rate-adaptive pacing enhances exercise capacity,[30] maximum oxygen consumption, and anaerobic threshold.[31,32] Symptoms such as physical intolerance and breathlessness are also reduced in the rate-adaptive mode compared with VVI pacing.[33,34]

Departure from Ideal Behaviour

The main disadvantage of activity sensing is the low proportionality to the level of workload.[30,35,36] Body movement is dependent on the way in which an activity is performed rather than on the work intensity. The magnitude of rate increase during arm exercise and cycle ergometry is inadequate. An activity sensor is limited in its ability to achieve the programmed upper rate with exertion, or mount an excessive rate acceleration during ordinary daily activities. Ascending stairs gives a lower acceleration signal compared with descending stairs.[37–39] Although newer signal-processing methods are suggested to improve the activity-sensing rate response, a recent comparative analysis of the signal-processing methods (i.e. the 1–4 Hz bandpass filter versus the 15 Hz bandpass filter and the threshold-crossing and integration algorithms) being used by the available motion-based rate-responsive pacemakers found that the advantages and disadvantages of each filter and algorithm combination depended upon the type of activity and exercise.[40]

Furthermore, at the end of exercise, vibration ceases immediately and an arbitrary rate decay curve has to be implemented which bears no relation to the incurred metabolic debt. In addition, an activity sensor has low sensitivity. Nonexercise requirements such as anxiety reactions cannot be detected using this principle. Activity-sensing pacemakers are also unresponsive to isometric exercise and autonomic manoeuvres (e.g. Valsalva manoeuvre).[36] Specificity of rate response is also an issue. For example, environmental vibrations such as those occurring during various forms of transport may inadvertently trigger the pacemaker,[41] especially if the higher frequency range is used for acceleration sensing. Direct pressure on the piezoelectric crystal (e.g. with the patient lying on the pacemaker side) may lead to an excessive rate response.

Minute Ventilation Sensing (Table 14.3)

Physiological Principles

Within the aerobic threshold, minute ventilation increases linearly with the workload and oxygen consumption.[42,43] Thus, by measuring the change in minute ventilation during exercise, a rate response closely related to oxygen consumption can be derived for muscular exercise. Recently, it was reported that the relationship between heart rate and minute ventilation is not linear but logarithmic, with an initial steep rise followed by a decrease in slope during higher levels of work.[44,45] This is due to the effect of increased ventilatory drive above the anaerobic threshold to compensate for the increase in blood lactate and carbon dioxide production that results from anaerobic glycolysis and lactic acidosis at higher exercise intensities.[46] Hence, main-

Table 14.3 Current minute-ventilation sensing pacemakers[a]

Algorithm	Examples	Manufacturers
Linear rate-response curve	Meta™ I, II Meta™ DDDR Chorus™ RM	Telectronics, Englewood, CO, USA ELA Medical, Montrouge, France
Biphasic linear response curve	Meta™ III Tempo™ D, DR	Telectronics, Englewood, CO, USA

[a] Minute Ventilation is a trademark of Telectronics Rhythm Management Systems.

taining the linear heart rate to minute ventilation slope beyond the anaerobic threshold to peak exercise, the pacemaker may produce a significant overpacing effect above the anaerobic threshold.

Sensor and Algorithm

Minute ventilation is measured using a tripolar configuration for impedance sensing with the pacemaker case as the common reference electrode. In one model (Meta™ MV, Telectronics, Englewood, CO, USA), low-amplitude current pulses (1 mA lasting for 15 μs) are injected at the ring electrode at every 50 ms interval and sensed between the distal electrode and the pacemaker case of a standard pacing lead (Figure 14.2).

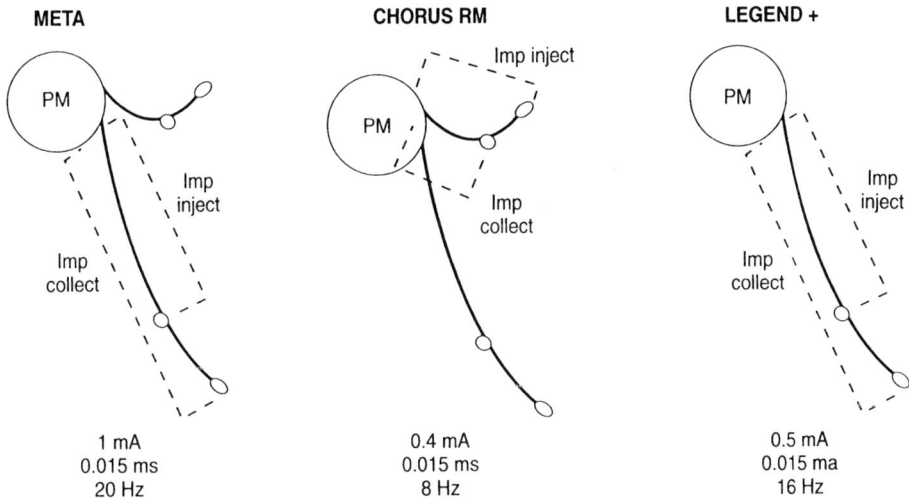

META

CHORUS RM

LEGEND +

1 mA
0.015 ms
20 Hz

0.4 mA
0.015 ms
8 Hz

0.5 mA
0.015 ma
16 Hz

Figure 14.2 Schematic of minute-ventilation (MV)-sensing pacemakers. Impedance measurements are derived from small alternating currents injected between the electrode pair situated between the pacemaker casing and one electrode. The resultant current is received by the same electrode pair (in a bipolar arrangement) or by another pair (tripolar). Transthoracic impedance increases with inspiration, decreases with expiration, and its amplitude varies with the tidal volume. The respiratory rate can be derived from the impedance reversal during a respiratory cycle. From these impedance changes, the change in the minute ventilation can be measured.

Transthoracic impedance increases with inspiration, decreases with expiration, and its amplitude varies with the tidal volume. Impedance reversal during a respiratory cycle also enables the respiratory rate to be derived. When this system was first introduced, a curvilinear rate-adaptive slope was used with an initial slow phase, followed by a steep rise. This was subsequently modified to a linear and finally a hyperbolic slope. Other types of minute ventilation sensing pacemakers have been introduced with slightly different electrode arrangements for impedance measurement.

Advantages of Minute Ventilation

Minute volume is an indirect but reliable marker of metabolic demands and the rate response is proportional to the level of exertion.[38] The pacing rate is highly correlated with the sinus response.[47,48] When respiratory gas exchange was measured, the pacing rate was shown to be significantly correlated with oxygen consumption, minute ventilation, respiratory quotient, tidal volume, and respiratory rate.[49,50] Compared with VVI pacing, minute-ventilation-driven VVI(R) pacing increased exercise capacity by 33%,[49] and maximum oxygen consumption and cardiac output are significantly better.[51] Improvement in symptoms was also documented in the VVI(R) mode.[49] Minute ventilation has good long-term stability, and programming of the sensor is relatively simple. In addition, detection of the physiological variation in the minute ventilation can be used to reduce the pacing rate during sleep.[52]

Departure from Ideal Behaviour

The speed of rate response of the first-generation minute ventilation sensor (Meta™ MV, Telectronics) was slow and had a delay of 30–45 seconds.[47,53] This was due partly to the minute-ventilation averaging algorithm used and the curvilinear rate-adaptive curve, resulting in a slow increase of rate at the onset but reaching the maximum rate earlier during exercise compared with the sinus rate.[38,50] The pacing rate might also remain high after exercise for 1–2 min prior to returning gradually to the baseline.[47] A more linear slope and programmable speed of onset of rate response is available in the new generation of minute-ventilation sensing pacemakers (Meta™ III 1206, Telectronics). In addition, onset of rate response can be enhanced by the use of a rate augmentation factor which enables a more aggressive linear slope at low levels of workload up to 50% of the maximum programmed rate. This new algorithm has been shown to significantly improve the initial heart rate response, rate response during exercise and the peak heart rate achieved.[54] However, because of these changes, fluctuations in the paced heart rate were observed with the minute-ventilation sensor during low workloads.[48] Respiration is also potentially influenced by phonation and coughing, which have no relevance to cardiac output. Reported influences include attenuation in rate response during phonation,[51] and an inappropriate tachycardia has been reported in a patient with advanced heart failure and the rapid breathing phase of Cheyne–Stokes dyspnoea.[55] In addition, the minute-ventilation sensing pacemaker is also sensitive to motion artefacts,[53] commonly induced by upper limb movement which affects impedance. Finally, the impedance sensor necessarily increases the power drain of the pacemaker.

Ventricular Paced QT Interval

Physiological Principle

The ventricular paced QT interval varies with heart rate and shortens during exercise and isoprenaline infusion and is independent of the presence or absence of AV synchronization.[56–58] Thus, when adjusted for the QT changes due to rate changes, the detection of QT shortening is a method of sensing sympathetic activity.[57] As the magnitude of the QT interval is different between sensed and paced beats, the endocardial T wave is always sensed after a paced beat since the amplitude of the spontaneous T wave is relatively small compared with that of the paced T wave. As the end of the T wave is difficult to define electronically, it is taken to be the maximum negative deflection of the first derivative of the T wave (i.e. the downslope of the QT).

Sensor and Algorithm

Sensing of the QT interval is only possible with a unipolar ventricular pacing stimulus (Figure 14.3). In the early QT pacemakers, a linear relationship between the QT interval and the heart rate was assumed and the slope of the rate response had to be programmed. An estimation of the QT shortening attributed to rate change alone had to be determined by pacing at two rates (i.e. 70 bpm and 100 bpm) at rest. The pacing rate response during exercise was subsequently determined by the rate-adjusted QT shortening which represents the change due to an increased sympathetic activity after correcting for the change in QT interval as a result of rate change.

There are a number of limitations in the slope adjustment in this early QT sensing pacemaker, such as delay in the onset of the rate response and post-exercise tachycardia which are related to the assumption of a linear relationship between the change in the QT interval and the heart rate.[57] It was subsequently shown that this relationship was best expressed as an exponential formula in a canine model and in humans.[59–62] The use of a curvilinear rate-response curve with a higher slope at the onset of exercise together with an automatic slope-adaptation algorithm has significantly reduced the delay in onset of rate response during exercise.[61] In patients with native rhythm, the pacemaker spontaneously shortens its escape interval intermittently until a capture beat results to effect QT measurement.

Advantages of QT Sensing

The rate response of the QT sensing pacemaker is proportional to workload and a smooth and progressive rate response occurred during graded treadmill exercise.[63,64] In an early study, it was shown that QT-driven VVI(R) pacing led to a 45% increase in

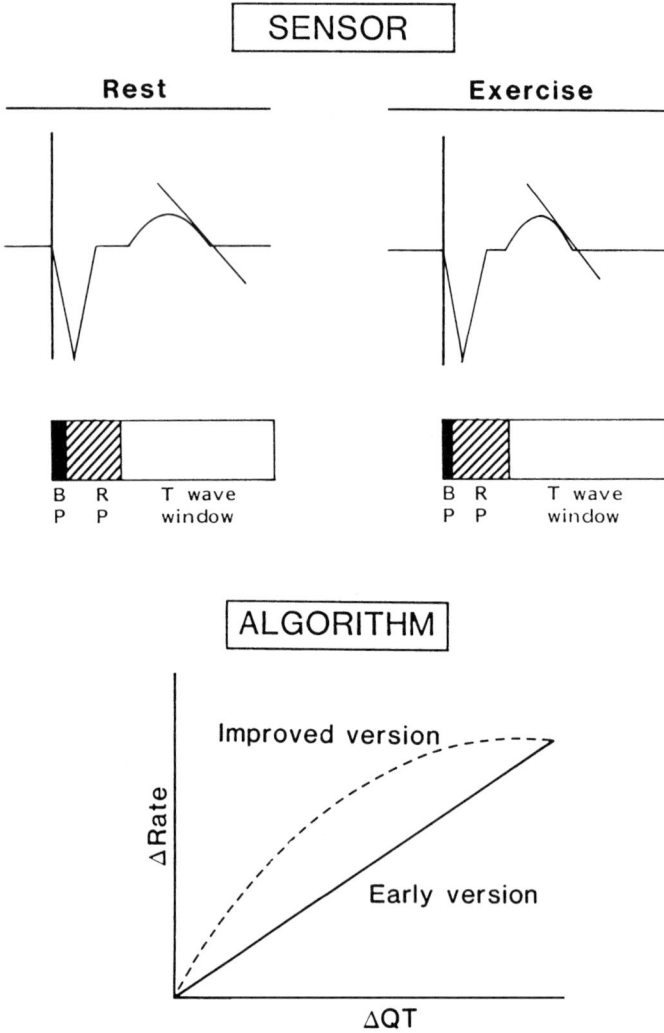

Figure 14.3 Sensing of the ventricular paced QT interval. The intracardiac T wave is measured from the pacing spike to the maximum negative derivative of the T wave. If this occurs within a T-wave sensing window, rate adaptation will occur. A linear slope was used in the early QT sensing pacemakers but this has been replaced by a curvilinear slope in the newer series. BP = blanking period, RP = refractory period. (Reproduced from reference 152 with permission)

cardiac output and 57% increase in exercise duration compared with conventional VVI pacing.[64] Exercise performance was also comparable to that achieved during VAT pacing with the same attained upper rate.[65] Besides responding to exercise, the QT sensing pacemaker responds to emotional stresses.[66] Diurnal variation of the QT interval is a well-recognized phenomenon, with the QT interval lengthening during sleep.[67–69] This property of the QT interval may be used to physiologically vary the lower rate during night-time pacing. The ability to use conventional electrodes for pacing and sensing is another advantage of the QT sensor.

Departure from Ideal Behaviour

There were a number of problems with slope adjustment in the early QT sensing pacemakers. When adequately programmed to respond to ordinary activities like walking, delay in onset of rate response to brief activities was still observed.[63] The speed of response could be improved by setting a higher slope. However, this may result in pacing rate oscillation between the lower and upper rate with small changes of the QT interval.[6] A positive feedback loop is established in this situation: the QT interval shortens as a result of an increase in rate, which then leads to further rate-dependent shortening of the QT duration, resulting in a further increase in rate. Although an improvement in exercise duration over VVI pacing was shown,[65] the chronotropic response differed significantly from patient to patient and in the same patient from one occasion to another. Some of the above-mentioned limitations of the QT sensing pacemaker were attributed to the assumption of a linear relationship in the change in QT interval and the heart rate in the early QT sensing pacemakers.[57] Although the new curvilinear QT sensing algorithm has significantly improved the speed of rate response,[61] the speed of rate response is still too slow during brief periods of exercise, with the maximum heart rate often being attained only after exercise. This may be in part related to the observed delay between the onset of exercise and the increase in norepinephrine level to which the QT interval principally responds.[70]

A response to nonexercise-induced catecholamine changes is said to be a desirable feature of the QT sensing principle. However, this increase in rate is unpredictable and sometimes minor emotional changes can lead to excessive tachycardia.[6,70] In an occasional patient, the QT interval may not shorten during exercise, despite a normal catecholamine response and a normal response to isoprenaline infusion.[71,72] As the QT interval is responsive to nonexercise-related stress, the rate response can be significantly affected during myocardial ischaemia and cardioactive medications. For example, during acute inferior myocardial infarction, the pacing rate of the QT sensing pacemaker may vary according to the infarct-induced autonomic changes, resulting in either inappropriate rate reduction or tachycardia.[73,74]

Sensing of the endocardial T wave can be affected by local polarization resulting from the pacing stimulus, occurring at a frequency of 26%.[75] This has been significantly improved, however, by using a low polarization electrode and special waveform for post-pulse compensation: in a study of 1500 electrodes, satisfactory T wave sensing was found in 94.1% of patients.[76] Although significantly correlated with the paced QT interval, spontaneous QRS complexes have low predictive value for the paced QRS morphology, and thus intermittent pacing will be necessary to ensure correct QT detection in patients with high intrinsic heart rates. Because of these limitations, a QT interval sensor is seldom used as a stand-alone sensor but rather in combination with an activity sensor.

Are 'New Physiological' Sensors the Ideal?

Innovative sensors have been developed with the aim of overcoming the departure from ideal behaviours of the conventional types. Most of these sensors require special pacing electrodes, some of which have been examined in investigational models.

Central Venous Oxygen Saturation (SvO_2)

Physical activities increase cardiac output, and oxygen extraction from the blood and a widening of the tissue arteriovenous oxygen difference occurs if the cardiac output does not match the requirements of increased tissue oxygen consumption.[77] The changes in SvO_2 rapidly reflect the metabolic need in response to exercise and the relationship between heart rate and SvO_2 is not affected by physical fitness or cardiac disease.[77-79] Hence, a SvO_2 sensing pacing system can theoretically adjust the pacing rate to achieve an optimal SvO_2, establishing a semiclosed loop rate-adaptive system. The SvO_2 sensor utilizes one or two light-emitting diodes incorporated proximally to the pace/sense electrode, and the emitted light is reflected by the red cells and received by a phototransistor at the site of the diode. As the change in SvO_2 will affect the intensity of light absorption, SvO_2 can then be determined.

The preliminary clinical experience with implanted SvO_2 sensors showed a rate response proportional to exercise level.[80-82] In one study, the rate response of a SvO_2 sensor (Oxyelite, Medtronic Inc., Minneapolis, MN, USA) was compared with a conventional piezoelectric activity sensor during activities of everyday living and nonexercise-related physiological changes, and the SvO_2 sensor showed a better proportionality in rate response, which occurred at a comparable speed of response[81,83] (Figure 14.4).

SvO_2 is not linearly related to the workload, the majority of the drop in SvO_2 occurring in the first minute of exercise with minimal further decrease with increased workload. The main limitation is the requirement of a special pacing lead and the stability of the sensor. For example, in one study, two out of eight devices were not functional over a short period of 6 months.[83] Fluctuation of the SvO_2 level also required repeated reprogramming[77,81] and can lead to improper pacing rates.[78]

Right Ventricular Pressure and its First Derivative

The first derivative of the right ventricular pressure (dp/dt) is influenced by the contractile state of the heart, the ventricular filling pressure and the heart rate, there being a positive correlation between maximum dp/dt and the sinus rate in normal subjects.[84] Thus, the change in the maximum value of dp/dt is a sensitive indicator of the change in left ventricular contractility and is directly proportional to change in sympathetic tone.[85,86] Right ventricular pressure can be detected by a hermetically sealed pressure sensor containing a piezoelectric crystal and electronic circuitry incorporated into an insulated bipolar lead. The piezoelectric crystal transduces the right ventricular pressure signal into an analogue electrical signal and maximum dp/dt is derived in the pacemaker circuitry.

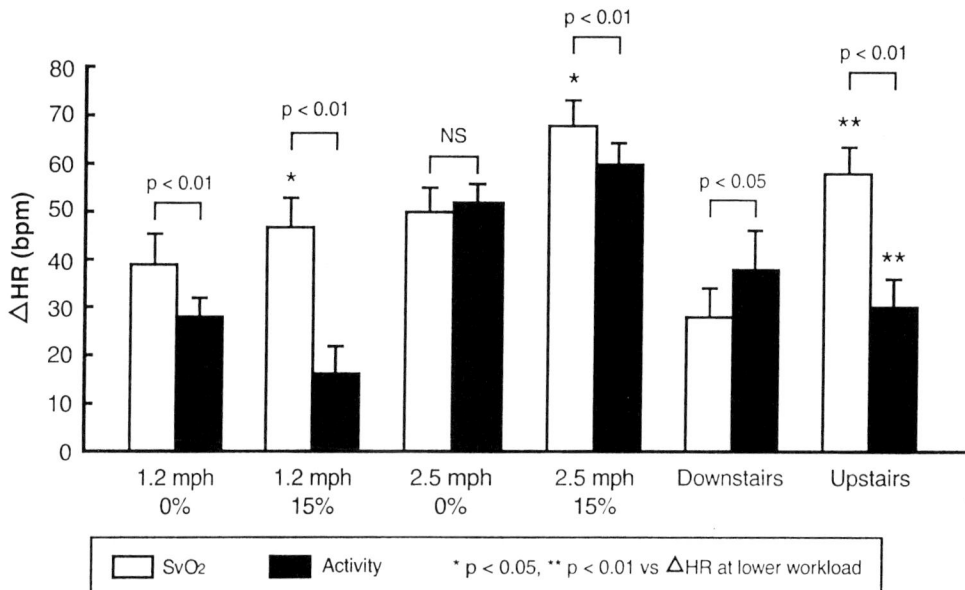

Figure 14.4 Changes in heart rate (ΔHR) during walking and stair-climbing. The central venous saturation (SvO$_2$) driven rate was higher when the patients walked at a faster speed ($p < 0.01$ for 1.2 and 2.5 mph) and at a higher gradient, and the heart rate was higher on ascending stairs. The activity-driven rate responded only to an increase in speed of the treadmill ($p < 0.01$ for 1.2 and 2.5 mph) but not to an increase in gradient, and the pacing rate was slower on ascending stairs. (Reproduced from reference 83 with permission)

The advantages of the dp/dt sensing principle are its good proportionality to workload, its sensitivity to nonexercise requirements, and its ability to noninvasively obtain intracardiac haemodynamics. In a limited number of investigational implants (Deltatrax[TM], Medtronic Inc., Minneapolis, MN, USA), the pacing rate was reported to correlate well with estimated oxygen consumption during exercise ($r = 0.93 \pm 0.04$).[53,87,88] The increase in pacing rate paralleled the heart rate that was expected from the metabolic reserve during treadmill testing in the VVI(R) mode.[53] Exercise time was significantly prolonged in the VVI(R) mode compared with the VVI mode during paired exercise testing.[89] The speed of rate response was rapid and the recovery rate decay after exercise was physiological.[53,88] There was, however, considerable variability in the chronotropic response during the early phase of exercise.

This sensor is limited by a technical problem with electrical insulation and by fibrin coating, and sensor function is affected when it becomes buried within the cardiac trabeculae.[90] Dp/dt is elevated by an increase in heart rate which may potentially lead to a positive feedback. A paradoxical decrease in pacing rate during upright tilt and standing position and a marked increase in pacing rate with a change in posture were also observed.[53,87] In patients with paroxysmal or chronic atrial arrhythmia, the effect of random timing of atrial contractions may generate variable dp/dt. Also, rate response can be affected by the occurrence of right ventricular dysfunction. Although it has been shown that right ventricular dp/dt was rather insensitive to acute right ventricular ischaemic changes in patients with normal sinus rhythm,[91] the effect of heart failure and negative inotropic drugs on dp/dt have not yet been systematically studied. The sensor also requires relatively high energy consumption.

Central Venous Temperature

In normal individuals, heat produced during exercise correlates directly with the total metabolic rate in the absence of endocrine disturbances. Accurate measurement of central venous temperature variation with a thermistor can predict heart rate response during exercise. The main advantage of using central venous temperature as a sensor for rate-adaptive pacing is its proportionality to moderate and heavy workloads and its sensitivity to changes such as fever and diurnal variation.[92]

There are, however, many limitations of this principle of rate-adaptive pacing. The overall speed of rate response is slow.[90] A special pacing electrode with a thermistor is required, and a failure of insulation (especially at the lead–connector interface) has been reported in all temperature-sensing leads from all manufacturers.[93,94] The temperature system is not sensitive to the range of workloads that are encountered during ordinary daily activities. Central venous temperature shows wide inter- and intra-individual variability, depending on the presence of an initial temperature drop at the beginning of exercise (the 'dip response'), the status of cardiac function, and metabolic state.[93,95,96] Central venous temperature can also be affected by several external or internal parameters not related to physical activities: vasodilatation, emotion, environmental changes in temperature, consuming cold drinks, hot baths, fever. A blunted rate response occurred during exercise with increased heat dissipation such as during swimming.

pH Sensing

An increase in tissue metabolism during exercise results in the production of carbon dioxide, which leads to a fall in the pH of venous blood. The pH drops more in patients with inadequate cardiac output due to chronotropic incompetence than that in normal individuals.[97] pH was sensed by an iridium/iridium-oxide ring at the atrial level of a conventional ventricular lead, with the pacemaker casing serving as the reference electrode (silver/silver-chloride later replaced by iridium/iridium-oxide). Initial experience demonstrated questionable long-term stability and reliability of the sensor.[98]

Cardiac Contractility

Cardiac contractility is sensitive to the circulating catecholamines, and can be used to respond to both exercise and nonexercise requirements. These include measuring the stroke volume, pre-ejection interval and right ventricular contractility.

Stroke volume

Stroke volume tends to remain constant during continuous exercise, and so a sensor aims to maintain a constant stroke volume during exercise.[8,99] Impedance is the simplest method for determining stroke volume, whereby impedance variations measured between the pacemaker case and electrodes within the right ventricle correlate with changes in RV volume.[100,101]

Theoretically, stroke volume is a rapidly responding parameter and may be a useful indicator for determining an appropriate rate recovery after exercise.[84,102–104] However, in one model (Precept™, Cardiac Pacemakers Inc., St Paul, MN, USA), owing to the algorithm and circuitry employed, there was a delay of 2 min before an exercise rate response occurred. Owing to the difference in geometry between the right and left ventricles, the correlation between impedance-based and actual stroke volume is only moderately good. In addition, this method detects only relative changes in stroke volume rather than the absolute stroke volume. Sensing of stroke volume by the impedance method is susceptible to the influence of respiratory changes, catheter movement, changes in posture and preload; and a varying AV interval relationship and intrinsic conduction.

Pre-ejection interval

The systolic pre-ejection interval (PEI) is defined as the time from electrical systole to ventricular ejection during which isovolumetric contraction of the ventricle takes place. The PEI shortens in response to an increase in stroke volume or end-diastolic volume, and sympathetic responses such as those occurring during exercise and emotional stress.[103–105] A decrease in PEI value indicates metabolic stress and results in a pacing rate increase. A tripolar lead was used in an investigational model (Precept™, Cardiac Pacemakers Inc., St Paul, MN, USA). The PEI system was sensitive to both exercise and nonexercise requirements, and its response was shown to be proportional to workload with a linear and constant rate response pattern during both exercise and recovery.[106]

Measurement of the PEI is affected by factors other than the sympathetic tone, such as preload, the right ventricular function, the timing of the atrial contraction and the posture of the individual. For example, sensor-driven tachycardia can result from postural-related sensor activation. Although this has been suggested to be a useful marker or prodrome of vasovagal syndrome, in practice, the pacemaker-induced tachycardia required either inactivation of the sensor or reprogramming to a suboptimal rate-adaptive slope.[107] The PEI also substantially varied with alternating sensed/paced events, intermittent bundle branch block and fusion beat.[107] The use of the special tripolar lead is another limitation of this sensor.

Autonomic nervous system controlled closed-loop cardiac pacing

In patients with chronotropic incompetence, the inotropic state of the heart remains intact and can be used as an indicator for rate response. Using a short-duration 4 kHz square-wave conductance signal at a constant current of $40\,\mu A$ injected through the tip of a unipolar electrode following a paced or sensed complex, a conductance curve can be obtained which reflects autonomic nervous system activities. This parameter, termed the 'ventricular inotropic parameter', can be used to adjust the pacing rate.[108]

In a multicentre study of 105 patients who received a prototype of this ANS-controlled pacemaker (Neos-PEP[TM], Biotronik, Berlin, Germany), during bicycle ergometry exercises and Holter recordings the pacing system functioned satisfactorily in 93% of patients.[109] However, proper programming of the pacemaker system was difficult in 7% of patients who had low exercise capacity and/or intermittent AV block. The long-term stability and the influence of medications (especially negative inotropic agents) on this sensor need further studies.

Ventricular Depolarization Gradient

A pacing stimulus on the ventricular myocardium produces a depolarization (followed by repolarization) and 'distortion' of the pacing stimulus waveform. In a normal individual, the magnitude of the gradient of the vector integral of the paced QRS, the so-called 'ventricular depolarization gradient', decreases with exercise, stress and emotion during fixed-rate ventricular pacing, and increases with an increase in pacing rate.[110] Balancing the effects of circulating catecholamines and the increase in pacing rate, the depolarization gradient remains relatively unchanged during exercise and various forms of stress in the intact normal heart, and a theoretical closed-loop rate-adaptive negative feedback system can be achieved.[110] This system requires only a standard bipolar electrode with no special electric current (Prism[TM] CL, Telectronics, Englewood, CO, USA).

In the ventricular depolarization gradient-sensing pacemaker, a rapid onset of rate response to exercise occurred within 10 seconds of exercise with a high correlation ($r = 0.91$) between the recorded pacing rate and the intrinsic P-wave rate and a significant response to isometric exercises and mental stress.[111,112] However, this sensor showed wide individual variability and only a moderate proportionality of rate response.[111] The early prototype was not developed beyond a VVI(R) version, and even then it was functional in a small number of patients. The gradient decreases on passive upright tilt but increases in the supine posture, resulting in tachycardia, and a paradoxical effect also occurs with the use of beta-blockade.[111,113,114]

Peak Endocardial Acceleration

The contractile state of the heart can be identified by the maximum velocity of shortening of unloaded myocardial contractile elements, and this can be done with a catheter-tip accelerometer in the ventricle. The contractility state can be assessed indirectly from the 'peak endocardial acceleration', which can be derived from the endocardial vibration measured by the accelerometer in the right ventricle during the isovolumetric phase.

A micro-accelerometer placed on the tip of a normal endocardial pacing lead has been developed by Sorin Biomedica (Italy) as a new physiological sensor for rate-adaptive pacing. This consists of an acceleration sensor built into an undeformable capsule located on the tip of a standard unipolar ventricular pacing lead placed in the right ventricle so as to be sensitive to its acceleration and insensitive to the pressure of blood and myocardium. The system has a frequency response up to 1 kHz and a sensitivity of 5 mV/G (1 G = 9.8 m/s). In preliminary experience in sheep using an external system and an implantable radiotelemetry system, the peak endocardial acceleration was not affected by heart rate but was significantly increased by emotional stress, exercise stress tests and natural inotropic stimulation.[115] It followed the changes in left ventricular dp/dt^{max}. Similar results were obtained in patients being tested during electrophysiological studies using an external system, and the change in peak endocardial acceleration were found to be linearly related to the right ventricular dp/dt.[115,116] These myocardial vibrations are not affected by ischaemia in the area in which the sensor is fixed.[117]

Limitations of this sensor system include the unknown relative contributions of valvular movement and change in preload to the myocardial vibrations, and the measured peak endocardial acceleration is uncertain. The system requires a dedicated lead with questionable long-term reliability and stability, although the initial study on sheep showed acceptable medium-term results.[115] Lastly, the effects of preload on the peak endocardial acceleration have not been studied.

Sensor Combinations

The limitations of currently available sensors imply that none is suitable for every patient under all circumstances. As the sinus node behaviour is the result of multiple stimulatory or inhibitory reflexes, in replacing the failing sinus node with a pacing rate simulating the physiological heart rate, multiple inputs have to be taken into account. Therefore, further technical improvements cannot be limited to refinement or development of single-sensor systems, but must inevitably lead to a combination of complementary systems.

The 'clinical' sensors are mainly limited because a fast-responding sensor is not proportional, whereas a proportional sensor is relatively slow (Table 14.4). In addition, an activity sensor is relatively insensitive to nonexercise stress, is nonspecific and liable to external interference.

Table 14.4 Relative advantages of clinical sensors

	Speed	Proportionality	Specificity	Sensitivity
Activity	H	L	L	L
Minute ventilation	M	H	M	L
QT	L	M	H	M

H= high, L= low, M = moderate.

Table 14.5 Aspects of sensor combinations

	Speed of response	Proportionality	Sensitivity	Specificity	Sensors for non-rate-adaptive control
	Activity	Minute ventilation QT	Dirunal variation: 24-hour clock	Sensor cross-checking: minute ventilation and activity	*Automatic mode switching*
Combinations			Emotional response: QT	QT and activity	*Automatic threshold detection*
					? Minimize myocardial oxygen consumption

Dual-sensor pacemaker technology has now been available for several years, using a multitude of different sensor combinations. The combinations aim to create a sensor system which best simulates the sinus node response in normal individuals by combining the strong points and eliminating the weak points of each sensor (Table 14.5). Sensor combinations aim at improving the speed of rate response, proportionality to workload, sensitivity to physiological changes induced by exercise and nonexercise requirements and specificity in rate adaptation (Figure 14.5). A sensor more specific to exercise can be used to prevent false-positive rate acceleration by a more sensitive, yet relatively nonspecific, sensor. In the absence of the specific sensor indicating exercise, the response of the other sensor can be either nullified or restrained to a limited level or duration. In addition, an appropriate rate recovery can shorten the repayment of oxygen debt and promote lactate clearance.[102] Therefore, it is necessary to incorporate sensors which have more proportionality for this part of the exercise cycle.

Sensors and Algorithms

A multisensor pacemaker combines the best features of two or more sensors in an appropriate fashion, based on their chronotropic response characteristics as well as the technical ease of combination. Preferably, the combined sensors should be compatible with a standard unipolar or bipolar pacing lead, and implantable with ease at the time of a pacemaker change. A number of possible sensor combinations have been suggested (Table 14.6), but only three clinical sensors have been used successfully in combinations (activity, minute ventilation and QT) although a number of investigational units have also evolved. Because of its simplicity and reliability, an activity sensor is used in all sensor combinations.

The sensor combinations can be additive, blending or cross-checking (Figure 14.6). In the additive form, the inputs from two sensors are compared and the faster rate is chosen. A differential combination (blending) combines the inputs of two sensors,

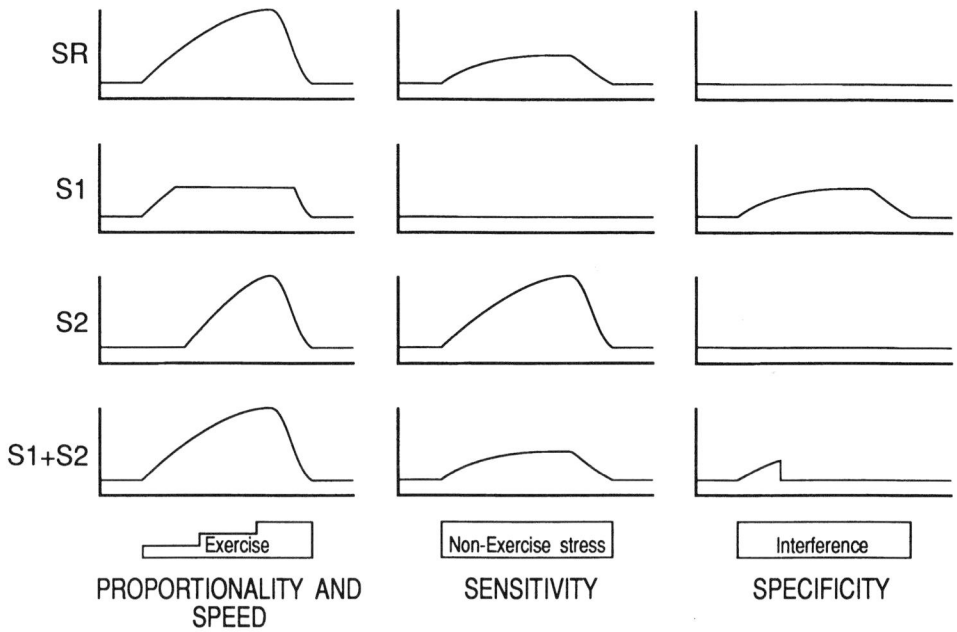

Figure 14.5 Algorithms for sensor combinations to achieve either better proportionality and speed of response, or sensitivity, or specificity. The graphs from top to bottom depict the responses of the sinus node (SR), sensor 1 (S1), sensor 2 (S2) and the combined rate profile for S1 and S2. SR shows ideal proportionality, speed of rate response, and freedom from interference. S1 is a rapidly responding sensor although it is neither proportional nor sensitive and is susceptible to interference. S2 is a proportional and sensitive sensor although it has a slow response. It is also specific to exercise. Note the improved ability of the combined-sensor approach in simulating the sinus rate under different conditions. (Reproduced from reference 152 with permission)

either as a fixed ratio or different upper rates (e.g. fast-reacting sensor determines the initial exercise rate response while a proportional sensor determines the later stages of exercise). Finally, a more specific sensor may be used to cross-check with a nonspecific sensor to avoid false rate acceleration. In this instrumentation, the rate adaptation of a

Table 14.6 Sensor combinations proposed and/or implemented

Sensor combination	Pacemakers	Manufacturers

Activity
  + minute ventilation
	Legend Plus™ VVIR
	DX2™ DDDR
		Medtronic Inc., Minneapolis, MN,
		  USA

Activity
  + QT
	Topaz™ VVIR
	Diamond™ DDDR
		Vitatron Medical BV, Dieren,
		  The Netherlands

Minute ventilation
  + ventricular depolarization gradient
	Sentri™ VVIR (not beyond
	  prototype)
		Telectronics, Englewood, CO, USA

Stroke volume
  + systolic pre-ejection period
	Precept™ VR DDDR
	  (model 1100)[a]
		Cardiac Pacemakers Inc.,
		  Minneapolis, MN, USA

Activity
  + central venous oxygen saturation
	Oxyelite™ DDDR
	  (model 8007)[a]
		Medtronic Inc., Minneapolis, MN,
		  USA

[a] Sensors separately instrumented.

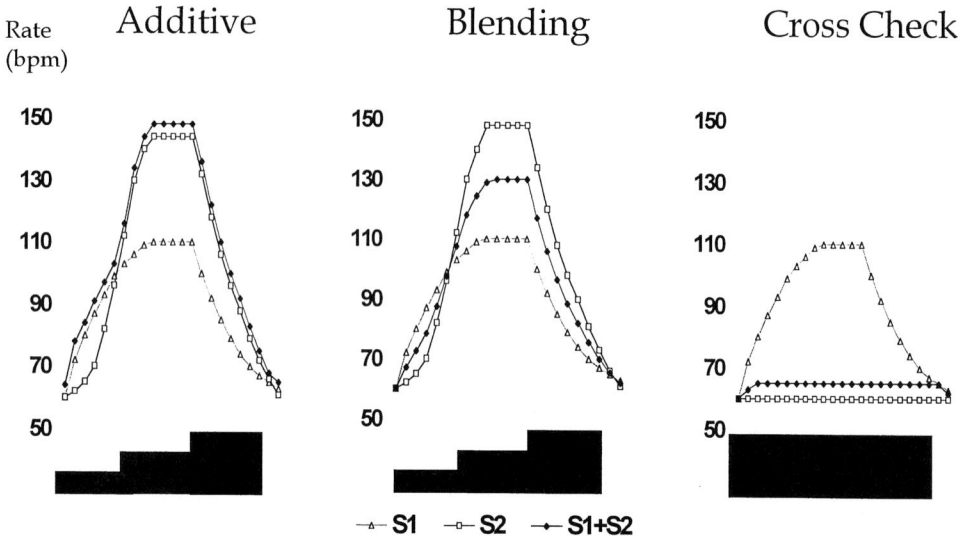

Figure 14.6 Algorithms to combine sensors. In the additive form, the faster rate from sensor 1 (S1) or sensor 2 (S2) is chosen. In the differential input, the sensor rate responses from S1 and S2 are blended to give an intermediate rate. In sensor cross-checking, the more specific sensor S2 has cross-checked the less specific but faster sensor S1 when S2 does not indicate the presence of exercise.

less-specific sensor is only allowed for a restricted magnitude and duration of rate adaptation. In the absence of the other sensor(s) indicating exercise, a diagnosis of false-positive rate acceleration with the first sensor is made, and the pacing rate will return to the baseline so that prolonged high-rate pacing will be avoided. Such sensor cross-checking can be reciprocal between the two sensors or applied only to a less-specific sensor by a more-specific one.

Dual-Sensor Rate-Adaptive Pacemakers

QT and Activity (Table 14.7)

Principles

The main limitation of the QT-sensing principle is the relatively slow speed of onset of rate response and the susceptibility of the QT interval to drugs and ischaemia.[63] On the other hand, it is a proportional sensor which is also sensitive to nonexercise requirements. Its combination with an activity sensor thus significantly improves the speed of onset of rate response. The Topaz™ and Diamond™ pacemakers (models 515 and 800, Vitatron Medical BV, Dieren, The Netherlands) are dual-sensor single- and dual-chamber pacemakers using this combination. A piezoelectric sensor is used for activity sensing. The algorithms of sensor combinations are both blending and cross-checking. Activity and QT inputs can be variously programmed: activity < QT,

Table 14.7 The QT and activity combination

Hardware	
QT	Unipolar evoked ventricular QT interval
Activity	Piezoelectric crystal
Mode	VVI(R) (Topaz™) or DDD(R) (Diamond™)
Software	
Blending	QT and activity in programmable proportions
Cross-checking	QT to limit duration of activity response if exercise not confirmed
Automaticity	Measures QT interval and activity input in relation to lower and upper rates

activity = QT and activity > QT, at ratios of 30:70, 50:50 and 70:30 respectively. To avoid false acceleration of the activity sensor, the pacemaker allows an activity rate response for only a short duration unless confirmed by changes in the QT sensor (sensor cross-checking).

Advantages

Blending of QT and activity sensors produces a quick rate response at exercise onset, a more proportional rate response during the latter part of the exercise and during the recovery period.[118] The fast rate-adaptive response during the first stage of exercise is due primarily to the activity-sensing, with a high correlation between the activity sensor counts and the mean pacing rate ($r = 0.94$); whereas the QT sensor predominates during the latter stages of exercise, with a low correlation between activity sensor counts to pacing rate ($r = 0.14$).[118] A multicentre study of 79 patients using the Topaz™ showed that exercise in the dual-sensor mode produced a more gradual rate response than exercise in the activity mode alone. The rate profile during treadmill exercise testing resulting from dual-sensor pacing was improved over single-sensor pacing.[119,120] In one study, continuous recording and comparison of combined sensor and sinus rates during daily life activities and standardized exercise testing were performed in 12 patients, and a close correlation between the dual-sensor indicated rate and the sinus rate during daily life activities and treadmill exercise was observed (see below).[121] Furthermore, an inappropriately high rate response from the activity sensor due to external vibrations could be limited by sensor blending and cross-checking.[122] Automatic rate adaptation has been shown to be feasible[123] (see below).

Departure from ideal behaviour

The sensor rate response during more vigorous daily activities is still suboptimal.[121] A study using an earlier model combining QT and activity sensing programmed at the nominal settings showed the rate response to emotional stress to be inadequate.[118] With a sensitive activity-sensor setting, activity counts may be registered at rest when the QT sensor is inactive. This may result in the cross-checking of the activity sensor by the QT sensor at rest, and when an exercise begins this cross-checking can delay the speed of the dual-sensor rate response[124] (Figure 14.7). Despite the use of automatic

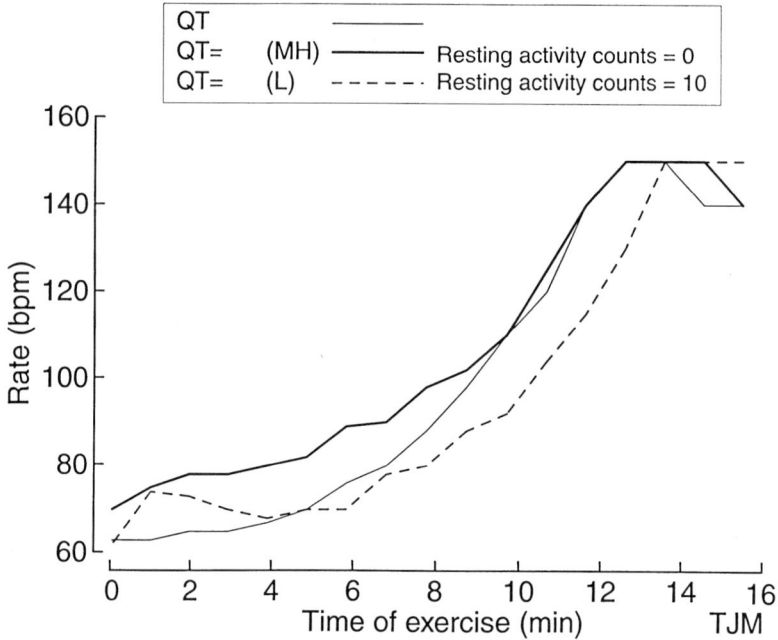

Figure 14.7   Rate response profiles of a patient in the QT-only and in the combined QT activity dual-sensor mode, with the activity sensor threshold optimally programmed to medium-high (QT = ACT [MH]) and to highest sensitive setting (low threshold, QT = ACT [L]). A significant delay was observed during exercise in the QT-only mode, which was improved in the QT = ACT [MH] mode. Despite a more sensitive activity setting in the QT = ACT [L] VVI(R) mode, the pacing rate decreased after an initial transient increase, and the rate increase lagged behind those of the QT-only and QT = ACT [L] VVI(R) modes. This was due to cross-checking of the activity sensor as the resting activity count was significantly raised, and the combined sensor responds only when the QT sensor detects exercise. (Reproduced from reference 124 with permission)

rate adaptation, the activity threshold and the relative contributions of each sensor need to be programmed, and this increases the complexity of programming.

Minute Ventilation and Activity (Table 14.8)

Principles

Minute ventilation (MV) has high proportionality but only a medium speed of rate response and is also potentially influenced by conditions which may not have direct relevance to cardiac output.[47,51,53,55] A piezoelectric activity sensor has been combined with an MV sensor to improve the initial response time, while allowing a proportional rate response to higher workload.

In the Legend Plus[TM] VVI(R) pacemaker (model 8446, Medtronic Inc., Minneapolis, MN, USA), an 'additive' sensor combination algorithm is used. A sensor indicated rate for each sensor is calculated and the faster one determines the pacemaker rate.

Table 14.8 Activity and minute ventilation combinations

	Legend Plus™	DX2™
Hardware		
Activity	Piezoelectric crystal	Piezoelectric crystal
Minute ventilation	Subthreshold impedance from ventricular lead	Subthreshold impedance from either atrial or ventricular leads
Mode	VVI(R) only	DDD(R)
Software		
Algorithm	Additive: 'faster win', but activity upper rate limited to 100 bpm	Blending of activity and minute ventilation, but activity upper rate limited by an interim ADL rate[a] Cross-checking between activity and minute ventilation sensor
Automatic adaptation	NA[a]	Rate profile adaptation using target rate histogram

[a] ADL = activity of daily living; NA = not available.

The rate response settings for each subsystem are determined by using a 3-min walking test: impedance values and activity counts are recorded and the recommended activity and MV rate response settings are calculated and displayed on the programmer.

A more sophisticated sensor combination algorithm is used in the DX2™ (model 7970 from the same manufacturer). The pacing rate in this investigational model is determined by automatic and nonprogrammable 'blending' of activity and MV contributions, using daily activities as a guide. Both sensors in the DX2™ contribute to the sensor-indicated rate between the lower and an interim rate limit, the so-called 'activity-of-daily-living (ADL) rate'.[125] The influence of the activity sensor diminishes and that of the MV sensor increases as the integrated sensor-indicated rate moves towards the ADL rate, and thereafter rate adaptation is driven completely by the MV sensor[126] (Figure 14.8). The activity sensor also will cross-check against high MV-sensor driven pacing rates. Sensor cross-checking against the MV sensor is effected if the activity sensor counts are low; the MV driven rate will then be limited in magnitude and duration. This minimizes the influence of nonphysiological minute ventilation signals associated with upper body motion such as arm movement, or hyperventilation.[126]

Advantages

During treadmill exercise and stair-climbing, the combined sensor mode in the Legend Plus™ was shown to be more proportional to low and high workload activities than the activity–VVI(R) sensor mode, but it was similar to the MV–VVI(R) mode.[127,128] A faster rate response with a shorter delay time, time to 50% of rate response and time to 90% of rate response in the DX2™ pacemaker was reported, compared with the MV sensor, at submaximal exercise and activities of daily living; although the rate kinetics of the activity sensor and dual-sensor were similar.[126] The average maximal sensor rates were significantly higher for the dual-sensor mode,

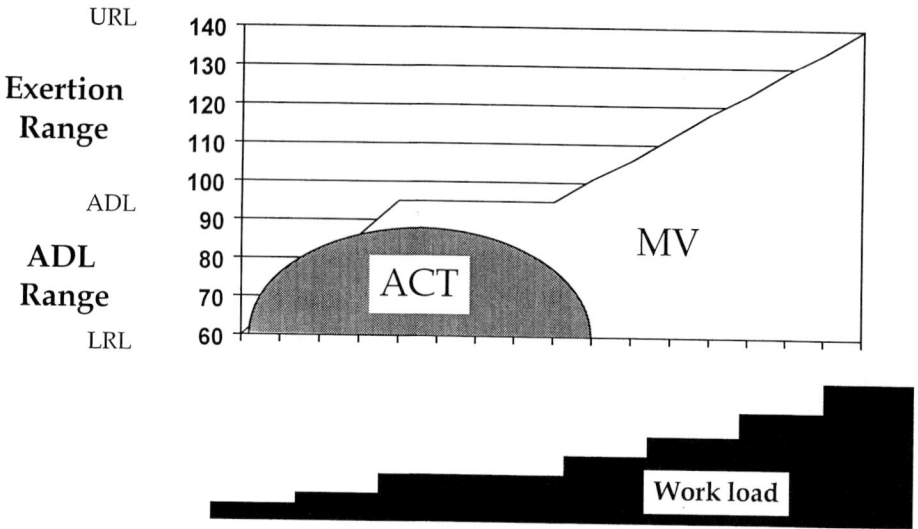

Figure 14.8 Sensor integration algorithm utilized by the DX2™ combined minute-ventilation (MV) and activity (ACT) pacemaker. Activity contributes to the integrated sensor-indicated rate between the lower rate (LRL) and activities-of-daily-living (ADL) rate. The influence shifts towards the MV sensor until the ADL rate is achieved; thereafter the MV sensor determines the upper rate (URL) response. (Reproduced from reference 126 with permission)

compared with either activity and MV modes, during daily activities (Figure 14.9). The rate response setting can be optimized automatically by matching the patient's personal sensor rate profile to a nominal target rate histogram (see below).

Departure from ideal behaviour

Neither the MV sensor, the activity sensor nor their combination respond well to nonexercise needs such as postural changes, the Valsalva manoeuvre, baroceptor reflexes and emotional stress. Use of the 'additive' sensor combination algorithm with no sensor cross-checking in the Legend Plus™ renders the pacemaker susceptible to interference effects from environmental vibrations and direct pressure on the activity sensor, as well as to interference on the minute ventilation sensor such as from arm-swinging. To a certain extent, these false-positive responses are minimized in the newer DX2™ with sensor cross-checking.

Advantages and Problems of Combining Sensors (Table 14.9)

The use of multiple sensors to detect body requirements will improve the system's responsiveness in terms of speed, proportionality, sensitivity and specificity. In addition, there are advantages in having an additional sensor for rate-adaptive pacing should one sensor fail, either technically or if the patient's cardiac status changes. An example is the use of antiarrhythmic medications that interact with the

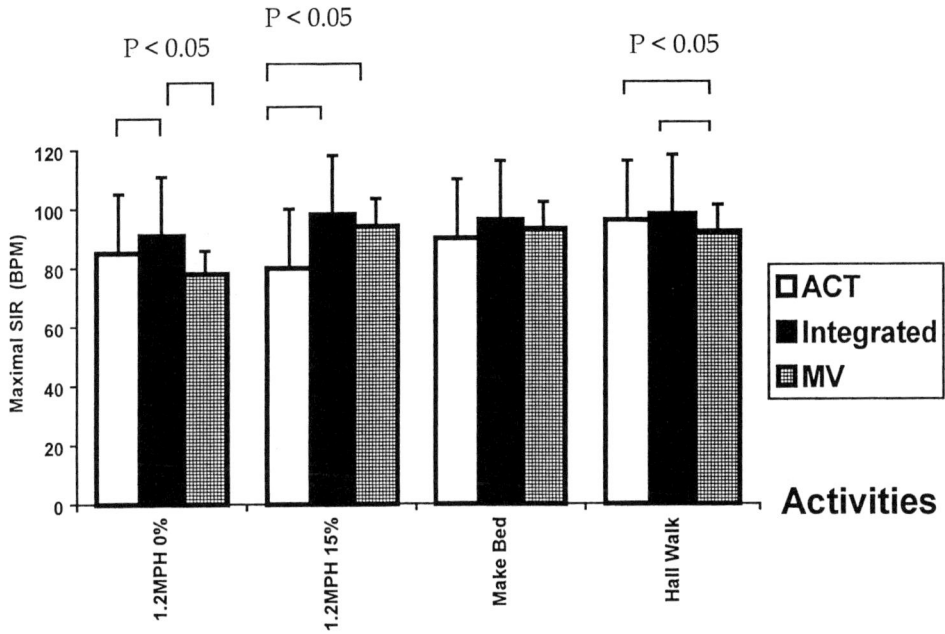

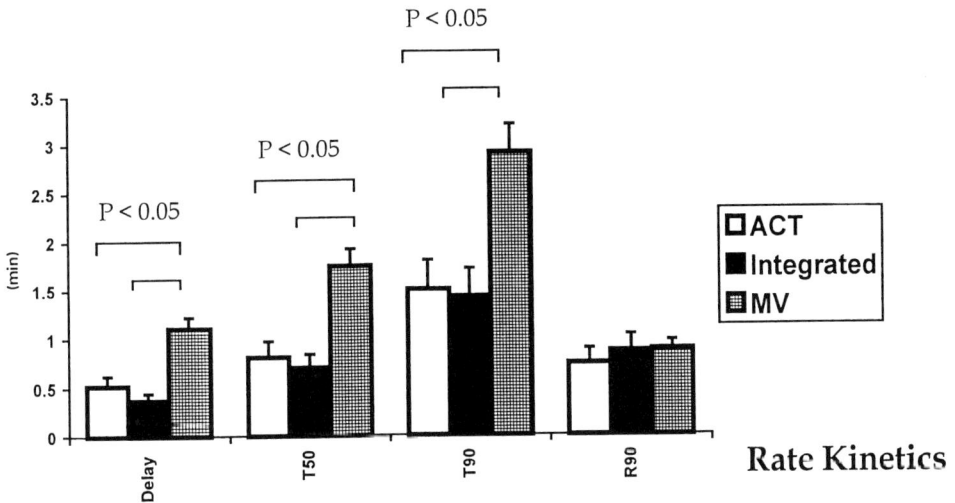

Figure 14.9 *Top:* Comparison of the average maximal sensor-indicated rate (SIR) during submaximal exercise and activities of daily living (ADL). The integrated minute-ventilation and activity (MV + ACT) mode gave a better average SIR during the submaximal exercise and hall walking compared with the MV and ACT sensor modes. *Bottom:* Comparison of the delay time, time to reach 50% (T50) and 90% (T90) of the maximal increase in pacing rate during exercise and time for the pacing rate to decrease by 90% (R90) during hall walking. MV resulted in the longest delay time, T50 and T90, compared with the ACT and integrated sensor modes. 1.2 mph 0% = submaximal exercise at 1.2 miles per hour at 0% gradient; 1.2 mph 15% = submaximal exercise at 1.2 miles per hour at 15% gradient. (Reproduced from reference 126 with permission)

Table 14.9 Advantages and potential problems with multisensor rate-adaptive pacing

	Multisensor pacing	Single-sensor pacing
Advantages		
Combination of merits of different sensors	Improvement in speed, proportionality and sensitivity	Better algorithm to improve sensor response
Improved specificity	Sensor cross-checking	Not possible
Sensor for backup rate adaptation	One sensor may replace the other sensor if it fails, or a change in a patient's condition precludes the use of one sensor	Not possible
Sensor controls parameters other than rate	Multiple sensors may be needed to control other pacing parameters	
Potential problems		
Increased cost	Multisensor devices may be more expensive	
Increased battery drain	Energy consumption is increased with two sensors; this may be reduced with the use of low-energy pacing electrodes or automatic pacing output control	Less energy expensive
Complexity of programming	A prioritization of multiple sensor inputs has to be made	
	Sensors have to be individually programmed	
	Automaticity may reduce the need for programming	
Clinical superiority	Clinical advantages of multi-sensor versus single-sensor pacing remain to be confirmed	Clinical superiority over fixed-rate devices demonstrated

QT sensor. Finally, multiple sensors will be required to control parameters other than rate.

Most of the problems with using sensor combinations have now been overcome. Increasing battery consumption and the bigger pulse generator size have been cited, but these issues are likely to be solved with technical improvements and low-energy pacing leads. Arbitration between sensors in a cross-checking algorithm can sometimes be a problem and impairment of rate response may be observed from undesirable cross-checking.[124] However, problems of programming complexity such as these are now addressed with automaticity. The remaining issue is to demonstrate a clinical difference between the single- and multiple-sensor pacing modalities.

Automaticity

An appropriate rate-control algorithm or careful programming can overcome some intrinsic limitations of many sensors. In contrast, inappropriate programming of a pacing system can distort the chronotropic response of an otherwise ideal sensor. For the physician, programming a rate-adaptive sensor is often time-consuming. It may involve multiple exercise testing, especially if a more objective sensor adjustment using exercise parameters is used. The use of a dual-sensor may more than double this effort. There is no simple standard to which a setting for one sensor can be adjusted, and often the sensor is programmed to achieve a rough output based on the physician's 'assessment' of the patient's overall physical state and activity level. Apart from the initial inconvenience of multiple programming, the actual requirements of the patient may change over time, and may require adjustments to be made when the physician is not available. Thus, a self-adjusting sensor is not only for the clinician's convenience, but a clinical need. Automaticity might be achieved using a closed-loop sensor, semi-automatic adjustment, or autoprogramming.

Automatic Lower and Upper Rate Adjustment

The optimum lower pacing rate can be adjusted with the aim of achieving the minimal atrial rate in patients who have complete atrioventricular block.[129] It is clinically useful to programme a lower pacing rate that is physiologically appropriate for the hours of sleep. A reduced resting heart rate also improves the longevity of the pulse generator.

The variability of the lower and upper rate parameters is best addressed using automatic programming. The simplest approach is to use a 24-hour clock to reduce the lower rate during sleep (Figure 14.10), but this becomes difficult when a subject changes his or her sleeping hours or travels to a different time zone. Certain sensors exhibit diurnal variation characteristics and are exploited to vary the diurnal rate. For example, daily activity and heart rate trends show a relatively high variation in activity signals when awake and active, and low variability during sleep. Measuring the variation of the activity signal (activity variance) by an activity sensor, the pacemaker can automatically adjust the lower rate during profound rest and sleep.[130] Similarly, a period of reduced impedance changes is used to define sleep and reduces the resting heart rate in an MV-sensing pacemaker.[52] Such diurnal variation is theoretically possible for temperature-sensing and QT-sensing devices.

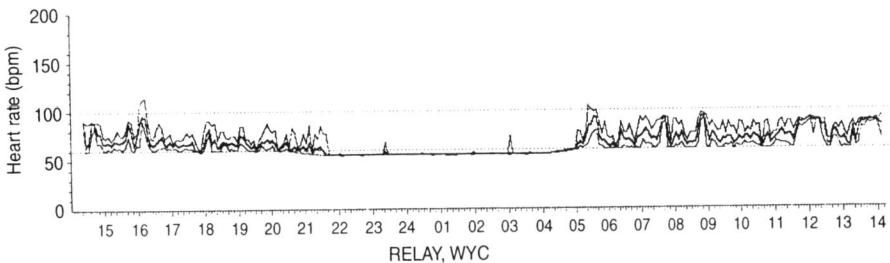

Figure 14.10 Holter recording of a patient with an accelerometer-based DDD(R) pacemaker capable of varying the lower rate according to an inbuilt 24-hour clock. Note the decrease of resting rate to 55 bpm during sleeping hours. Rate response according to the sensor can still be effected at the sleep rate, except that the sensor-indicated rate begins at a lower resting rate.

The patient's age, physical fitness, activity level and the presence of structural heart disease should be taken into account when choosing the maximum sensor-driven rate.[131,132] The percentage improvement in maximum exercise capacity has been shown to be linearly related to the maximum heart rate achieved,[133] but the proportion of time spent by these patients with heart rates near the upper rate limit must also be considered.[132,134] The typical pacemaker recipient achieves a rate of 150 bpm for less than 0.5% of the day, and there is no difference in the exercise capacity in patients with an upper rate limit of 125 bpm and 150 bpm during walking tests.[135,136] There is as yet no algorithm to automatically address the upper rate limit. The nominal setting of 120–130 bpm for most rate-adaptive devices may be too low, and may significantly affect the sensor response during ordinary daily activities.[137] An attempt to maintain the rate profile at the daily activity level is seen in the new-generation minute-ventilation pacemaker (Tempo™ D, DR, Telectronics, Englewood, CO, USA) in which the rate-adaptive slope is determined from the age-predicted anaerobic threshold level rather than being chosen by the physician.

Open- and Close-Loop Rate-Adaptive Pacing Systems

A rate-adaptive system can operate as either a closed or an open loop. In a completely closed-loop system a detected physiological change is used to effect a rate change, which in turn effects a negative feedback change on the physiological parameter, so that the physiological variation responsible for the rate change will return to the baseline condition. The balance of output and input should eliminate programming of the rate response setting, and *theoretically* the lower and upper rate can be self-adjusting. Any subsequent changes in the patient's cardiovascular condition should not require programming adjustment because the system should automatically try to correct the parameter to which it is sensitive.

A theoretical closed-loop negative-feedback control was originally proposed with the detection of central mixed venous oxygen saturation.[77] However, apart from the instability of the oxygen saturation sensor, rate-adaptive adjustment was still necessary to control the speed at which rate adaptation occurred and to offset the variable baseline oxygen saturation. Another sensor originally thought to work as a closed loop was that based on the ventricular depolarization gradient,[110] but again this was proved unstable for clinical use.[83]

Semi-automatic Programming

Many rate-adaptive pacemakers automatically determine the sensor output during a given workload and suggest the sensor threshold or slope settings that will provide a prescribed pacing rate. In the Sensolog™ and Synchrony™ activity-sensing pacemakers (Siemens-Elema Pacesetters, Solna, Sweden), sensor data are collected during casual and brisk walking to define two levels of exercise workload. The appropriate rate-adaptive parameters are then derived automatically to achieve the desired heart rate response.[138–140] In the accelerometer-based pacemakers (Relay™, Dash™ and

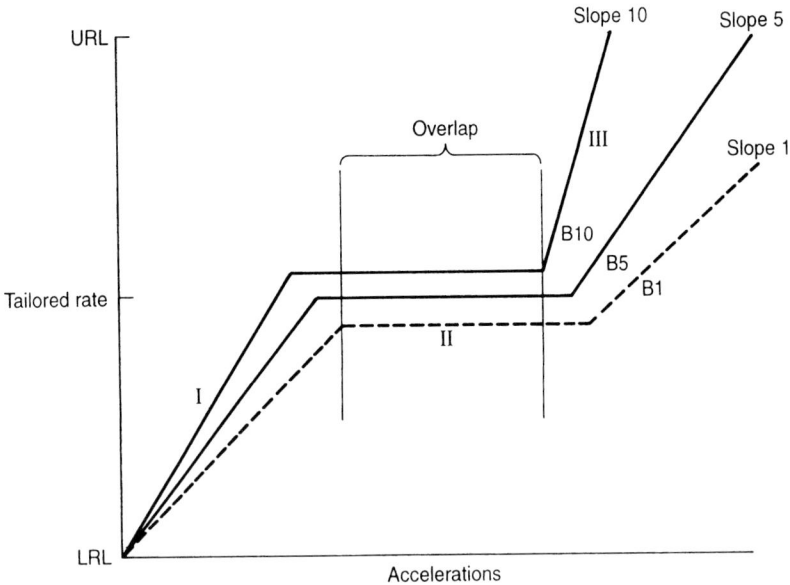

Figure 14.11 Triphasic rate response curves of an accelerometer-based activity-sensing DDD(R) pacemaker. Phases I and III represent low and high levels of accelerations, respectively, and are related to a steeper slope of rate change. Phase II represents ordinary activities at which the change in rate is small. The transition between phases II and III is termed the 'break-point', which remained relatively constant at different slope values. Thus, there is substantial overlap in rate changes during ordinary level of acceleration despite the use of a different slope. B1, B5 and B10 = break-points at slopes 1, 5 and 10, respectively; LRL = lower rate limit, URL = upper rate limit. (Reproduced from reference 23 with permission)

Marathon™, Intermedics Inc., Freeport, TX, USA), acceleration data are collected during a 1–3 min exercise test and automatically coupled to a programmable rate response, a feature known as 'tailor to patient' (Figure 14.11). This is useful in achieving an appropriate rate response that is sufficient for most patients during daily activities. However, the rate-adaptive slope uses a triphasic curve which has a more aggressive slope at the lower and higher levels of exercise; a formal exercise test may still be needed to assess the rate response characteristics at the higher workloads. In the minute-ventilation-sensing pacemaker (Meta™ MV, Meta™ DDDR and Tempo™ DR, Telectronics, Englewood, CO, USA), the rate response slope or the recommended rate response factor is determined automatically by matching the maximum pacing rate and the peak impedance value at peak exercise when subjecting the patient to an exercise. The recommended rate response factor can then be obtained from the programmer.[49]

Autoprogramming

There are currently two methods of automatic programming for open-loop sensors: one using a 'self-learning' algorithm, the other using a 'population norm' approach.

Self-learning rate response algorithms

In the combined QT- and activity-sensing pacemakers, the QT and activity slopes at the upper and lower rate limits are automatically adjusted by a daily learning process. The pacemaker monitors the dynamics of the QT interval and activity counts and continuously updates its maximum and minimum sensor values.[123] The self-learning process adjusts the rate response slope at the upper rate and lower rate limits respectively (Figure 14.12). Each time the pacemaker reaches the upper rate limit, it continues to monitor the QT interval and the activity counts. If further shortening of the QT interval or increase in activity counts is observed while pacing at the upper rate limit, this indicates the upper rate limit has been reached too soon and the rate response slope at the upper rate is automatically decreased by one step, which will give a more gradual approach to the upper rate limit. On the other hand, if the upper rate limit has not been reached for more than 8 days, this slope is automatically increased by one step. Similarly, the QT interval is measured regularly at the lower

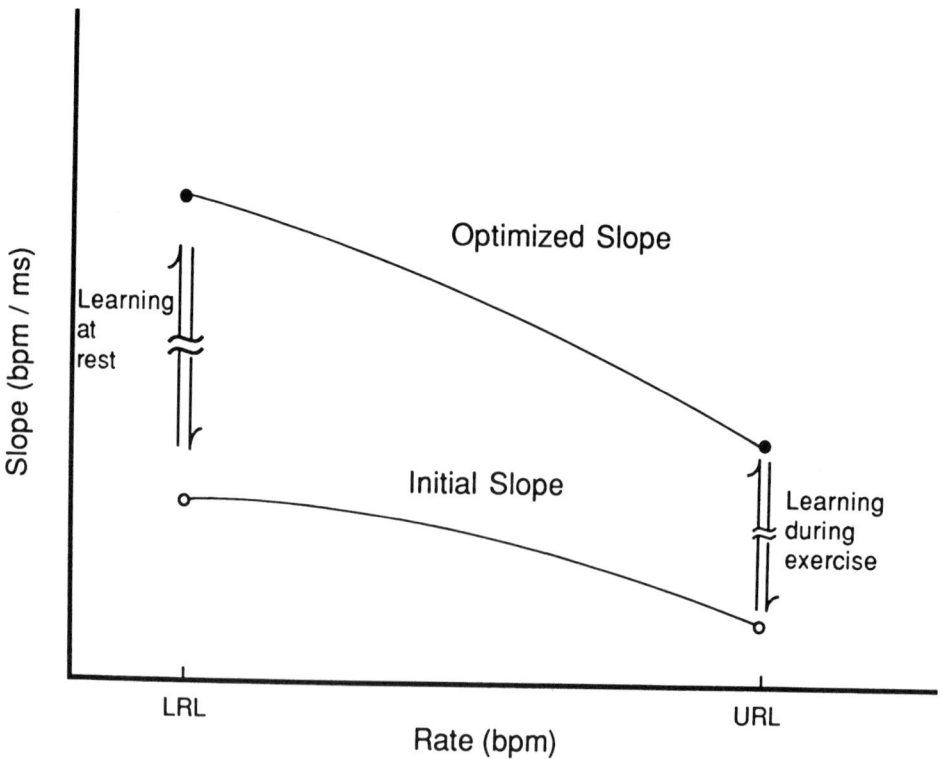

Figure 14.12 Automatic adjustment of the QT rate-response slope. At the lower rate limit (LRL), the QT/rate relationship is assessed once every night, and the slope is adjusted automatically one step in the direction of change. During maximum exercise at the upper rate limit (URL), if further QT shortening occurs, the slope declining factor will be advanced one step further so that the URL will be attained later in a repeat exercise. Conversely, if the upper rate is not attained in 8 days, the slope declining factor will be reduced by one step. (Reproduced from reference 152 with permission)

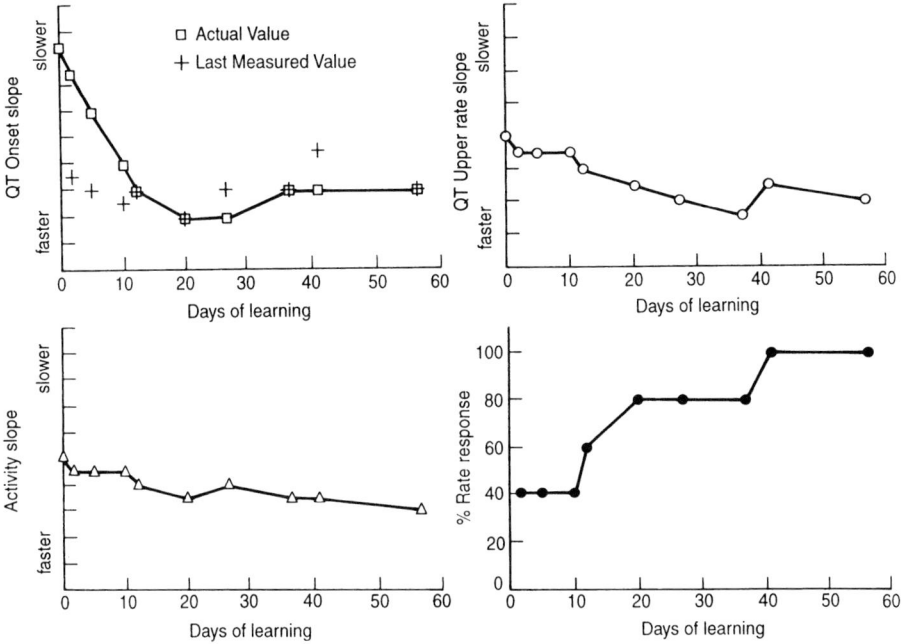

Figure 14.13 Rate-response slopes and percentage rate responses as a function of the daily learning time for a representative patient with a combined QT/activity dual-sensor VVI(R) pacemaker. The slopes are on a relative scale indicating a 'faster' or more responsive side and a 'slower' or less responsive side. *Top left:* QT onset slope reached the measured optimum level in 8–11 days. *Top right:* QT upper rate slope showed forward regulation from 14 to 40 days, then backward regulation started indicating that the upper rate was reached on that date, or more likely before. *Bottom left:* Activity slope demonstrated forward regulation during periods ranging from 14 to 56 days. *Bottom right:* Holter recording showed the rate response increased to 100% of the rate range at 6 weeks after implantation. (Reproduced from reference 123 with permission)

rate interval, with the patient presumably at rest. If the QT interval continues to lengthen at rest, this suggests the lower rate limit is reached too soon, and the slope for the lower rate limit is decreased.

Changes of the QT and activity slopes from factory settings have been reported.[123] Most of the changes occurred within the first 2 weeks and were stabilized at 6 weeks (Figure 14.13). Starting at a lower rate of 60 or 70 bpm, the combined sensors reached the programmed maximum rate of 110 or 120 bpm at 2–5 weeks (mean 19 days).

The clinical efficacy of self-learning automatic programming has been compared with the normal sinus node.[121] The normal sinus rate and the combined activity and QT sensor-indicated rate in 12 patients with complete heart block and normal sinus node function. During exercise, the combined sensor-indicated rate were highly correlated with the sinus rate ($r = 0.96$, $p < 0.001$). In addition, the difference in the sinus rate and sensor-indicated rate was within 4 bpm during exercise and 8 bpm during daily activities (Figure 14.14). A prospective comparative study of the efficacy of self-learning versus manual programming was conducted in nine patients with

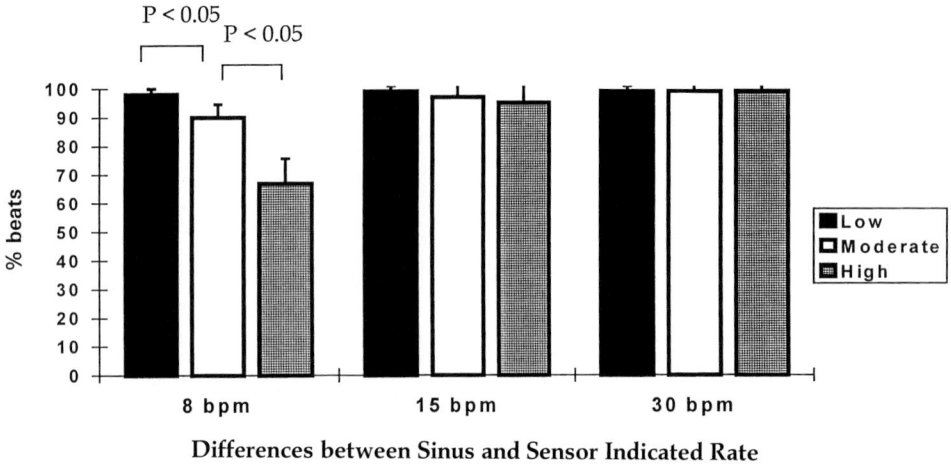

Figure 14.14 Sensor–sinus difference in 12 patients during daily activities, classified according to magnitude of difference (8, 15 or 30 bpm) and levels of activities: low (L), moderate (M) and high (H). Most of the sensor-indicated rates were within 8 bpm of the sinus rate, especially at low levels of daily

complete heart block and normal sinus node function who received a combined activity and QT DDD(R) pacemaker (model 800, Diamond™, Vitatron BV, Dieren, The Netherlands). Patients underwent treadmill exercise and 12 activities of daily living in the VDD mode. Sensor-indicated rates during these activities as derived from automatic programming and from manual optimization using a submaximal treadmill exercise were compared. The sensor rate determined by either method was close to sinus rhythm, although the rate response profile and rate kinetics can further be improved by manual optimization.[141]

The main limitation of this self-learning approach is that it assumes that every patient will be exerted up to the programmed upper rate during their activities of daily living, at least once in 8 days. However, in practice, for those patients who perform maximum exertion infrequently or who are confined to bed, the automatic optimization may over adjust the rate response slope, resulting in an inappropriately fast packing rate when the patient resumes usual daily activities.

Principles of the population norm approach

A characteristic rate distribution over 24 hours occurs in a normal individual, depending on sex, age, activity and fitness level.[131,132] Heart rate profiles were recorded by 48-hour ambulatory ECG monitoring in groups of normal subjects during regular daily activities and during seven upper and lower extremity exercises. It was found that the daily heart rate behaviour was submaximal in nature, with transient heart rate increases which exceeded 55% of the heart rate reserve.[132] The less-fit subjects had more increases in heart rate and utilized greater heart rate reserve during activities of daily living than did the average and fit subjects, and patients aged over 65 had longer durations of heart rate increases to greater than 110 bpm.[131,142] Based on these data, a 'nominal' histogram was derived reflecting the normal rate profile for the population with various levels of physical fitness as determined by age, sex and activity, and this was used to adjust the desired distribution of pacing rate.

AutoSlope™ adjustment by distribution of heart rate reserve

The heart rate in normal subjects varies between the resting and the age-predicted maximal heart rate. Overall, the heart rate of most individuals exceeds the 23rd percentile of the heart rate reserve for only 1% of the time. In the Triology™ DR + activity-sensing pacemaker (Siemens Pacesetter Inc., Sylmar, CA, USA), the pacemaker's microprocessor maintains a 7-day histogram of the sensor level and automatically adjusts the sensor slope once every 7 days such that 99% of the sensor activity is within the initial 23% of the heart rate reserve (Figure 14.15). The maximum adjustment is limited to two slopes and the slope changes are not made if the patient is inactive (as defined by absence of activity-sensor activities). AutoSlope™ offsets from −1 to +3 are available for fine adjustment of sensor response in individual patients. Positive offsets increase and a negative offset decreases the functional slope.

In 93 patients implanted with the Triology™ DR+ pacemaker, the sensor-indicated rate during brisk walking after automatic slope adaptation was compared with the desired sensor rate selected by the physician. The AutoSlope™ facility provided the desired sensor rate in 82.1% of the evaluation and in 75.6% of patients.[134] The rate modulation provided by the autoslope was appropriate in 83.1% of evaluation and 76.3% of patients at chronic follow-up. Despite the automatic slope adaptation, approximately 50% of the patients required further programming of the slope offset to fine-tune the sensor rate response. In this study, the desired sensor rate and the

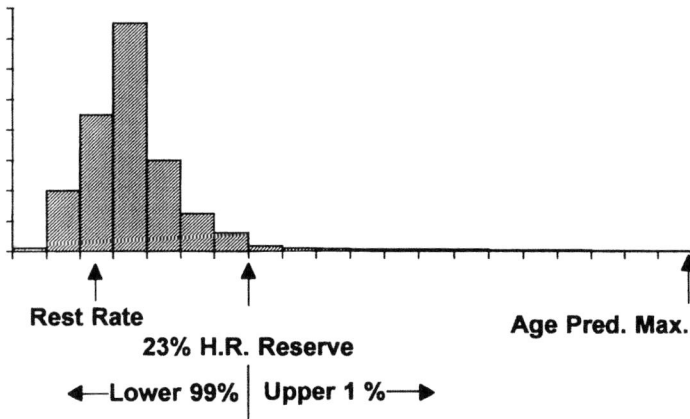

Figure 14.15 The distribution of heart rate frequency on which was based the automatic rate-adaptive algorithm of the Triology™ DR+. The sensor is automatically adjusted so that a rate response to occupy 23% heart rate (HR) reserve is attained. (Reproduced from reference 134 with permission)

appropriateness of the rate modulation were decided subjectively at the discretion of the physician rather than evaluated objectively.

Rate profile optimization by target rate histogram

Based on the 'nominal' target rate histogram, a device which automatically adjusts the sensor setting to match this histogram has been developed (model 7970, DX2™, Medtronic Inc., Minneapolis, MN, USA). The DX2™ is a combined activity and minute-ventilation-sensing DDD(R) pacemaker. In addition to sensor autoprogramming, the device initiates implant detection through the detection of lead impedance (Figure 14.16) and lead polarity recognition.[143,144] After confirming stable lead impedance over 6 hours, the device will automatically switch to the DDD(R) mode, and the baseline minute ventilation is automatically measured.[126,145] An optimal heart rate profile based on the patient's activity level and frequency of exercise is programmed as the 'target rate histogram' (Figure 14.17). This template is used to adjust the submaximal rate response during both daily activities and more vigorous exercise. Once each day, the pacemaker evaluates the percentage of time spent pacing in both the submaximal and maximal rate ranges by comparing the sensor rate profile against the target rate histogram. From this comparison, the pacemaker automatically controls how rapidly the sensor-indicated rate increases and decreases in these ranges.

The reliability of implant management in providing automatic detection of lead polarity and sensor initiation has been reported[143] (Figure 14.18). The efficacy of

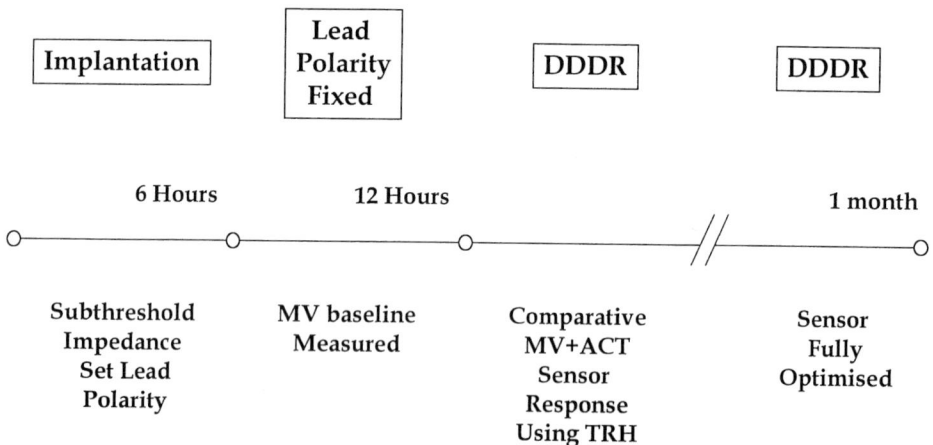

Implantation	Lead Polarity Fixed	DDDR	DDDR

6 Hours	12 Hours		1 month

Subthreshold Impedance Set Lead Polarity	MV baseline Measured	Comparative MV+ACT Sensor Response Using TRH	Sensor Fully Optimised

Figure 14.16 Automatic implant-detection and sensor-initiation algorithm utilized by the DX2™ combined minute-ventilation and activity DDD(R) pacemaker. The first step is to detect lead implantation itself by continuous subthreshold current injection and impedance measurement by the pacemaker atrial and ventricular ports in the unipolar and bipolar fashion. This allows detection of implant and lead configuration and the lead polarity will be set automatically. After stable lead impedance has been measured for 6 hours, the MV and ACT sensors are initialized automatically, and operating baselines for the MV and ACT sensors are determined automatically by collecting MV and ACT sensor data while pacing at the programmed lower rate. After an additional 6 hours, the pacemaker automatically begins dual-sensor DDD(R) pacing. (Reproduced from reference 151 with permission)

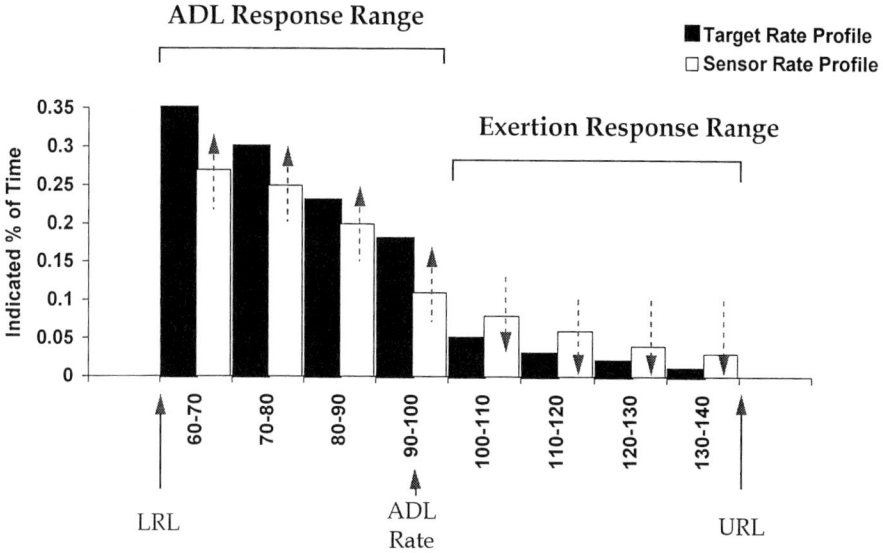

Figure 14.17 Illustration of the sensor-rate profile matched against a target-rate profile. The ADL range are moderate pacing rates between the lower rate (LRL) and the ADL rate. The exertion rates are rates from the ADL rate to the upper sensor rate (URL). By comparing the sensor-rate profile against the target-rate profile once each day, the pacemaker automatically controls how rapidly the sensor-indicated rate increases and decreases in these ranges. (Reproduced from reference 151 with permission)

automatic optimization of the rate response was compared with manual programming in a prospective study of seven patients who received this device, by measuring the rate kinetics during activities of daily living and in maximal and submaximal treadmill exercise. The rate changes derived by automatic programming and by manual adjustment were compared. After automatic rate profile optimization the pacing rate during hall walking increased from 78 ± 3 bpm at predischarge to 90 ± 5 bpm at 2 weeks and 98 ± 3 bpm at 3 months follow-up (Figure 14.19). Pacing rate during maximal treadmill exercise increased from 89 ± 6 bpm to 115 ± 5 bpm at 3 months after implantation, with a significant increase in exercise duration from 7.2 ± 1 min to 9.6 ± 2 min. The accuracy of automatic programming versus manual programming was reassessed at 1 month: during maximal exercise, submaximal exercise and activities of daily living, the average maximal pacing rates attained and the speed of rate response did not differ significantly between the two methods of programming.[145]

The main limitation of the population-norm approach is that an individualized standard still has to be programmed for each individual patient, and data from a wider patient population is necessary to ascertain the safety of this approach. An inherent risk of using a histogram is the uncertainty that a rate response has occurred at the appropriate time, as only the rate *distribution* rather than the rate *profile* is used as the template. In addition, the onset and recovery patterns which are important sensor rate-response characteristics are not addressed by the histogram approach.

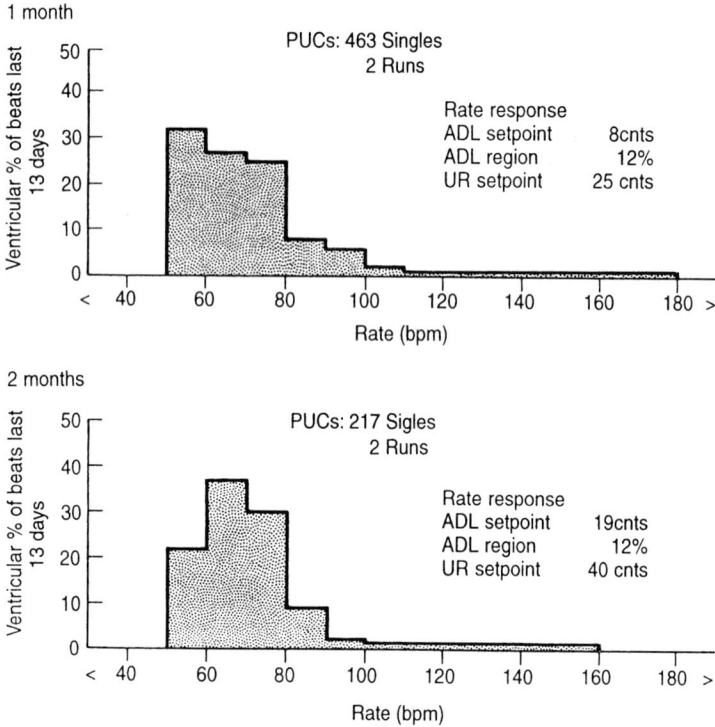

Figure 14.18 Representative long-term rate histograms obtained from one patient at 1 month (*top panel*) and 2 months (*bottom panel*) follow-up after automatic optimization by the target-rate histogram. One month after implantation, the rate histogram showed a high percentage of time pacing at the lower rate. After 2 months of continuous optimization, the pacing rate distribution shifted towards the higher rate ranges.

Is Ideal Behaviour Necessary?

This question can be addressed in terms of the accuracy of rate adaptation, physiological benefit and clinical benefit.[146]

Accuracy of Rate Adaptation

The proportionality aspect of single sensors has been discussed. It is generally observed that a fast sensor is likely to be less proportional than a slower 'physiological' sensor, and so arises the need for sensor combinations. Dual-sensor systems show a more accurate rate response, especially in comparison with an activity sensor alone. In one study, in the combined activity and MV sensor mode the correlation between pacing rate and the externally measured oxygen uptake on treadmill testing and bicycle testing were $r = 0.837$ and 0.733 respectively, compared with $r = 0.62$ and 0.643 for the activity sensor alone.[128] There was no significant difference when compared with the MV sensor mode. In another study, combined QT and activity pacemakers,

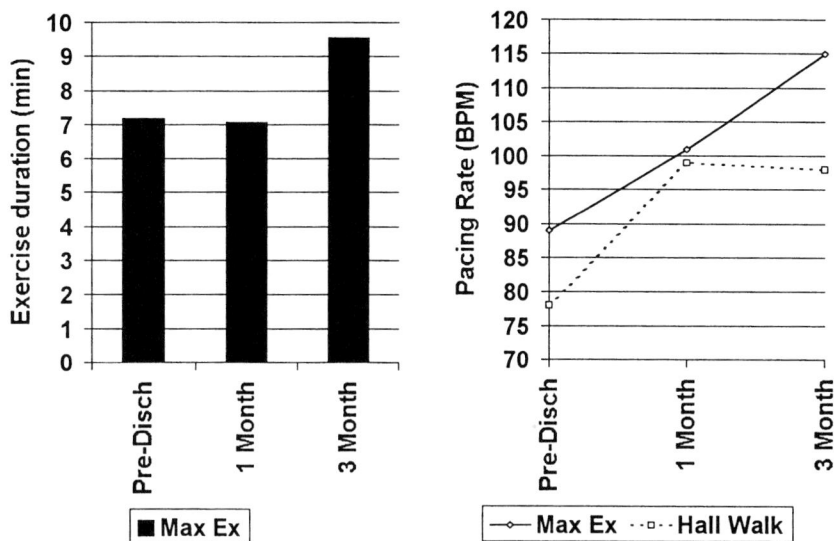

Figure 14.19 *Left panel:* Changes in the exercise duration during maximum exercise with implant duration. There is an increase in exercise duration at 3 months compared with predischarged exercise test with automatic rate optimization. The exercise duration at 1 month did not differ significantly from the predischarged exercise. *Right panel:* Changes in sensor-rate response to hall walking and maximal treadmill exercise with duration of implant. Whereas the daily activity range has optimized by 1 month, continuous adaptation of the sensor to achieve a higher rate response occurred up to 3 months after implantation. (Reproduced from reference 151 with permission)

the activity sensor 'overpaced', the QT sensor underpaced and the combination did significantly better than the individual sensors.[120,147] The impact of automaticity on the fine-tuning of sensor(s) remains to be addressed. Thus, as far as proportionality and speed of rate response are concerned, the current sensor combinations are an improvement over single-sensor pacing.

Physiological Benefits

Accurate rate adaptation may lead to better cardiopulmonary physiology. At higher levels of exertion, the ability to increase rate is the most important determinant of cardiac output and exercise capacity. In pooled data, a positive linear correlation between improvement of exercise capacity and heart rate was observed.[133] Since exercise capacity is a relatively insensitive measure of functional benefit,[148] the total exercise duration and maximal exercise workload generally do not differ between the dual- and single-sensor rate-adaptive modes.[120,147,149] Thus, the use of more sensitive and perhaps multiple indicators, such as cardiac output and respiratory gas exchanges, may be necessary to unmask mode differences. The recent application of oxygen kinetics to measure oxygen deficit at the onset of exercise may be an alternative indicator of an appropriate speed of rate response. In a combined minute ventilation and activity VVI(R) pacemaker, the heart-rate/oxygen-consumption

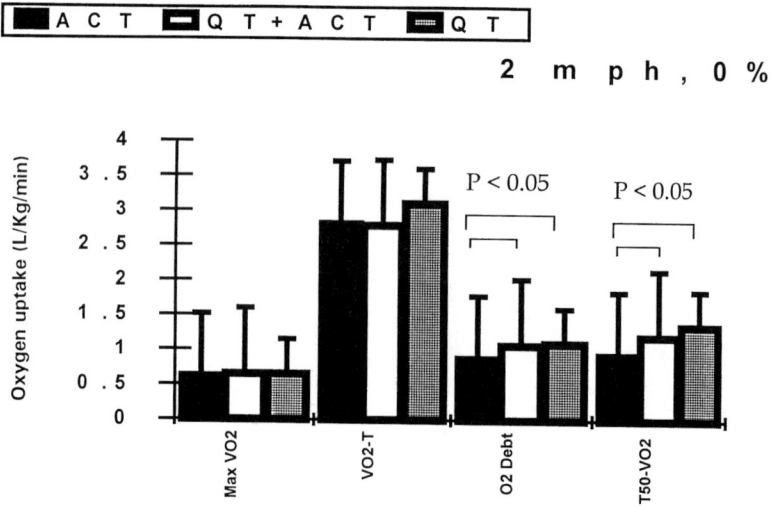

Figure 14.20   Oxygen kinetics in various VVI(R) sensor modes during constant submaximal exercise. The activity sensor, being the fastest in response, incurs the minimum oxygen debt and time to achieve 50% of the maximal oxygen uptake (T50-$\dot{V}O_2$). There is no statistically significant difference in oxygen debt and T50-$\dot{V}O_2$ between the combined sensor mode and the QT sensor mode. The steady-state oxygen uptake ($\dot{V}O_2^{max}$) and the total oxygen uptake ($\dot{V}O_2$-T) were similar between the three sensor modes. (Reproduced from reference 120 with permission)

relationship was significantly better than with activity sensing alone, although the response was similar to that of minute ventilation.[127] Anaerobic threshold and maximum exercise performance were similar in the single-sensor modes and dual-sensor mode.

In one study of combined QT and activity pacemakers, the activity sensor improved oxygen uptake kinetics compared with the QT sensor, and the dual-sensor device functioned at an intermediate level[120] (Figure 14.20). However, despite a marked difference in the pacing rate responses, it was not well reflected in the maximal oxygen uptake, the total exercise duration and the anaerobic threshold. A similar finding was reported from the addition of activity to an MV sensor.[125] It seems that sensor combinations using an activity sensor to give a quick initial response significantly improves oxygen transport during activities of daily living in patients with rate-adaptive pacemakers.

In a recent study of eight patients, performances of single-sensor and combined QT/activity sensor VVI(R) modes during submaximal and maximal treadmill exercise were compared using exercise cardiac output by the carbon-dioxide rebreathing method.[147] Comparing the pacing rate response based on the change in metabolic workload, the activity sensor 'overpaced', the QT sensor 'underpaced' and the dual sensor achieved the best approximation to normal. The increase in cardiac output at 1 min after the onset of exercise was higher in the activity and dual-sensor modes than in the QT sensor mode (Figure 14.21). The 'underpaced' QT sensor mode utilizes the contractility reserve to compensate for the slower rate increase with a compensatory increase in stroke volume during submaximal exercise. The more rapid rate-dependent increase in cardiac output at the beginning of exercise in

Exercise CO   **Exercise HR**

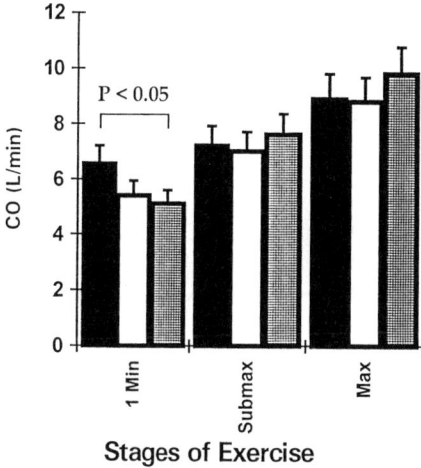

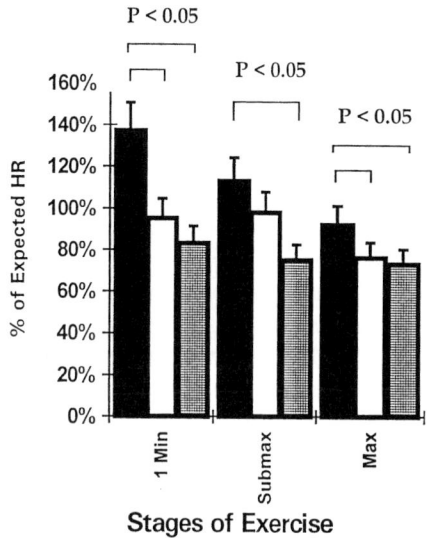

Figure 14.21 *Right panel:* Exercise HR response in the ACT, QT + ACT and QT VVI(R) modes expressed as a percentage of the HR predicted according to the metabolic workload. Overpacing is defined as actual HR $\geqslant 120\%$ of the expected HR and underpacing $\leqslant 80\%$ of each quartile of exercise. The ACT sensor overpaced especially in the first minute of exercise, whereas the QT sensor underpaced throughout exercise. The QT + ACT sensor give a rate response close to the expected rate. *Left panel:* Exercise cardiac output in the ACT, QT + ACT and QT VVI(R) modes. The ACT VVI(R) mode gave a significantly higher CO at 1 min after the exercise began compared with the QT-VVI(R) mode. The QT + ACT VVI(R) mode resulted in an intermediate response. There was no statistically significant difference in the CO between the three sensor modes at the submaximal and maximal exercise. (Reproduced from reference 147 with permission)

the dual-sensor pacing mode may be related to the physiological changes associated with the better heart rate to workload relationship.

Clinical Outcome

The ultimate goal of pacemaker therapy is to improve symptoms and quality-of-life measures, and these have been used to compare pacing modes. A within-patient, randomized, double-blind crossover study was done in 10 patients using a combined activity/MV sensing VVI(R) pacemaker for high-grade AV block with chronic, persistent or paroxysmal atrial fibrillation. These patients performed 2 weeks of out-of-hospital activity in the activity-only, MV-only and dual-sensor VVI(R) and VVI modes.[149] Patients were assessed (a) on their perceived general well-being on an analogue scale, (b) on a specific-activities functional status questionnaire and (c) by standardized daily activity protocols and graded treadmill testing. Their subjective perception of exercise capacity and functional status was significantly lower in the VVI mode than in the VVI(R) mode. However, there was no clear advantage of dual-sensor VVI(R) pacing over activity-sensor pacing: 4 out of the 10 patients preferred the activity VVI(R) mode, 3 preferred the dual-sensor mode and 3 had no preference. Furthermore, 3 patients found dual-sensor VVI(R) least acceptable, 3 found minute ventilation least acceptable and 1 found both dual-sensor and MV sensor pacing unacceptable. There was no significant difference in objective performance between the three VVI(R) modes. These not unexpected results suggest that there are no major differences between sensors and their combinations in gross clinical terms. However, the number of patients was small and so the study could not be expected to reveal anything other than major differences, which would be important in the longer term. Also, the difficulty of doing multiple comparisons and the order of pacing modes studied are limitations that restrict the value of the results.

Lukl et al.[150] assessed the quality of life with regard to cardiovascular symptoms, physical activity, psychosocial and emotional functioning and self-perceived health during DDD and dual-sensor VVI(R) pacing. Significant improvement during DDD pacing was demonstrated in all subgroups of patients (sick sinus syndrome, chronotropically competent and incompetent patients and patients with high-grade AV block). Their overall result was that DDD pacing offered better quality of life than dual-sensor VVI(R) pacing, so the latter could not compensate for the lack of AV synchrony. The only objective benefit so far reported was by Cowell et al.,[122] who described a patient who had an inappropriately high rate response from an activity sensor owing to vibrations during car travel, which caused angina in this patient with coronary artery disease. Angina pectoris was prevented appropriately in the VVI(R) dual-sensor mode by sensor cross-checking.

Conclusion

Because of their simplicity and proven clinical superiority in improving cardiac output and exercise capacity, compared with fixed-rate ventricular pacing, single implantable sensors are widely used in clinical practice. However, despite the large number of single sensors that have been proposed or used, none is ideal. The normal sinus node is controlled by multiple inputs to achieve its rate during exercise and various nonexercise physiological changes. Thus, it is impossible for a single sensor to cater completely for these physiological requirements and to provide ideal rate characteristics under all circumstances. Dual-sensor pacemaker technology aims to combine the strong points and eliminate the weak points of each sensor used in combination, so as to create a system which best simulates the sinus node response. This approach may further enhance the prospects for a rate-adaptive pacing system.

Although sensor combinations are feasible, appear to be reliable and provide a better rate profile and cardiovascular physiology than a single-sensor system, their clinical benefits need further confirmation in randomized studies. At present a multisensor pacemaker should be considered simply as one that gives a better rate response without being ideal. Automatic pacemaker programming and rate response adjustment make multisensor devices more convenient, but the safety and efficacy of the currently available rate adaptation algorithms need to be studied further.

References

1. Rickards AF, Donaldson RM. Rate-responsive pacing. *Clin Prog Pacing Electrophysiol* 1983; **1**: 12–19.
2. Sahakian AV, Tompkins WJ, Webster JG. Electrode motion artifacts in electrical impedance pneumography. *IEEE Trans Bio Med Eng* 1985; **32**: 448–51.
3. Webb SC, Lewis LM, Morris-Thurgood JA, *et al.* Respiratory-dependent pacing: a dual response from a single sensor. *PACE* 1988; **11**: 730–5.
4. Lau CP, Ritche D, Butrous GS, *et al.* Rate modulation by arm movements of the respiratory dependent rate responsive pacemaker. *PACE* 1988; **11**: 744–52.
5. Van Hemel NM, Hamerlijnck RPHM, Pronk KJ, *et al.* Upper limit ventricular stimulation in respiratory rate responsive pacing due to electrocautery. *PACE* 1989; **12**: 1720–3.
6. Winter UJ, Behrenbeck DW, Candelon B, *et al.* Problems with the slope adjustment and rate adaptation in rate responsive pacemakers: oscillation phenomena and sudden rate jumps. In: Behrenbeck DW, Sowton E, Fontine G, Winter UJ (eds), *Cardiac Pacemakers.* Damstadt: Steinkopf Verlag, 1985: 107–12.
7. Gillette P. Critical analysis of sensors for physiological responsive pacing. *PACE* 1984; **7**: 1263–6.
8. Loeppky JA, Greene ER, Hoekenga DE *et al.* Beat-by-beat stroke volume assessment by pulsed Doppler in upright and supine exercise. *J Appl Physiol* 1981; **50**: 1173–82.
9. Miyamoto Y. Transient changes in ventilation and cardiac output at the start and end of exercise. *Jpn J Physiol* 1981; **31**: 153–68.
10 Higginbotham MB, Morris KG, William RS, *et al.* Regulation of stroke volume during submaximal and maximal upright exercise in normal man. *Circ Res* 1986; **58**: 281–91.
11. Cardus D, Spensor WA. Recovery time of heart frequency in healthy men: its relations to age and physical condition. *Arch Phys Med* 1967; **48**: 71–7.
12. Longhurst JC, Kelley AR, Gonyea WJ, *et al.* Cardiovascular responses to static exercise in distance runners and weight lifters. *J Appl Physiol* 1980; **49**: 676–83.
13. Lau CP, Stott JR, Toff WD, *et al.* Selective vibration sensing: a new concept for activity-sensing rate responsive pacing. *PACE* 1988; **11**: 1299–309.
14. Alt E, Matula M, Theres H, *et al.* The basis for activity controlled rate variable cardiac pacemakers: an analysis of mechanical forces on the human body induced by exercise and environment. *PACE* 1989; **12**: 1667–80.
15. Schmidt M, Ammer R, Evans F, *et al.* Improved accelerometer-based rate adaptive pacing by means of second-generation signal processing. *PACE* 1996; **19**: 1698–703.
16. McAlister HF, Soberman J, Klementowicz P, *et al.* Treadmill assessment of an activity-modulated pacemaker: the importance of individual programming. *PACE* 1989; **12**: 486–501.
17. Strangl K, Wirtzfeld A, Lochschmidt O, *et al.* Physical movement sensitive pacing: comparison of two activity-triggered pacing system. *PACE* 1989; **12**: 102–10.
18. Lau CP, Tse WS, Camm AJ. Clinical experience with Sensolog 703: a new activity sensing rate responsive pacemaker. *PACE* 1988; **11**: 1444–55.
19. Charles RG, Heemels JP, Westrum BL, *et al.* Accelerometer-based adaptive-rate pacing: a multicenter study. *PACE* 1993; **16**: 418–25.
20. Bacharach DW, Hilden TS, Millerhagen JO, *et al.* Activity-based pacing: comparison of a device using an accelerometer versus a piezoelectric crystal. *PACE* 1992; **15**: 188–96.
21. Borst U, Siekmeyer G, Maisch B, *et al.* A new motion responsive pacemaker: first clinical experience with an acceleration sensor pacemaker. *PACE* 1992; **15**: 1809–14.
22. Alt E, Matula M, Holzer K. Behavior of different activity-based pacemakers during treadmill exercise testing with variable slopes: a comparison of three activity-based pacing systems. *PACE* 1994; **17**: 1761–70.
23. Lau CP, Tai YT, Fong PC, *et al.* Clinical experience with an accelerometer based activity sensing DDDR pacemaker using an accelerometer sensor. *PACE* 1992; **15**: 334–43.
24. Alt E, Matula M, Thilo R, *et al.* A new mechanical sensor for detecting body activity and posture, suitable for rate responsive pacing. *PACE* 1988; **11**: 1875–81.

25. Soussou AI, Helmy MG, Guindy RR, *et al.* A new acceleration driven pacemaker. Rate modulation versus normal sinus rhythm: comparison during treadmill exercise. *PACE* 1992; **15**: 1804–8.
26. Bongiorni MG, Soldati E, Arena G, *et al.* Multicenter clinical evaluation of a new SSIR pacemaker. *PACE* 1992; **15**: 1798–803.
27. Faerestrand S, Ohm OJ. Clinical study of a new activity sensor for rate adaptive pacing controlled by electrical signals generated by the kinetic energy of a moving magnetic ball. *PACE* 1994; **17**: 1944–9.
28. Hatano K, Kato R, Hayashi H, *et al.* Usefulness of rate responsive atrial pacing in patients with sick sinus syndrome. *PACE* 1989; **12**: 16–24.
29. Metha D, Lau CP, Ward DE, *et al.* Comparative evaluation of chronotropic response of QT-sensing and activity-sensing rate responsive pacemakers. *PACE* 1988; **11**: 1405–12.
30. Lau CP, Tse WS, Camm AJ. Clinical experience with Sensolog 703: a new activity sensing rate responsive pacemaker. *PACE* 1988; **11**: 1444–55.
31. Benditt DG, Mianulli M, Fetter J, *et al.* Single-chamber cardiac pacing with activity-initiated chronotropic response: evaluation by cardiopulmonary testing. *Circulation* 1987; **75**: 184–91.
32. Smedgard P, Kristensson BE, Kruse I, *et al.* Rate-responsive pacing by means of activity sensing versus single rate ventricular pacing: a double-blind cross-over study. *PACE* 1987; **10**: 902–15.
33. Lindemans FW, Rankin IR, Murtaugh R, *et al.* Clinical experience with an activity sensing pacemaker. *PACE* 1986; **9**: 978–86.
34. Lipkin DP, Buller N, Frenneaux M, *et al.* Randomized crossover trial of rate responsive Activitrax and conventional fixed rate ventricular pacing. *Br Heart J* 1987; **58**: 613–16.
35. Kubisch K, Peters W, Childakis I, *et al.* Clinical experience with the rate responsive pacemaker Sensolog 703. *PACE* 1988; **11**: 1829–33.
36. Lau CP, Mehtha D, Toff W, *et al.* Limitations of rate response of activity-sensing rate-responsive pacing to different forms of activity. *PACE* 1988; **11**: 141–50.
37. Candinas RA, Gloor HO, Amann FW, *et al.* Activity sensing rate responsive versus conventional fixed rate pacing: a comparison of rate behavior and patient well-being during routine daily exercise. *PACE* 1991; **14**: 204–13.
38. Lau CP, Wong CK, Leung WH, *et al.* A comparative evaluation of minute ventilation sensing and activity sensing adaptive-rate pacemakers during daily activities. *PACE* 1989; **12**: 1514–21.
39. Matula M, Schlegl M, Alt E. Activity controlled cardiac pacemakers during stair walking: a comparison of accelerometer with vibration guided devices and with sinus rate. *PACE* 1996; **19**: 1036–41.
40. Greenhut SE, Shreve EA, Lau CP. A comparative analysis of signal processing methods for motion-based rate responsive pacing. *PACE* 1996; **19**: 1230–47.
41. Lamas GA, Keefe JM. The effects of equitation (horseback riding) on a motion responsive DDDR pacemaker. *PACE* 1990; **13**: 1371–3.
42. Astrand I. Aerobic work capacity in men and women with special reference to age. *Acta Physiol Scand* 1960; **169** (suppl): 15.
43. Astrand PO, Saltin B. Maximal oxygen uptake and heart rate in various types of muscular activity. *J Appl Physiol* 1961; **16**: 977–81.
44. Lewalter T, Jung W, MacCarter D, *et al.* Heart rate during exercise: what is the optimal goal of rate adaptive pacemaker therapy? *Am Heart J* 1994; **127**: 1026–30.
45. Treese N, MacCarter DJ, Akbulut O, *et al.* Ventilation and heart rate response during exercise in normals: relevance for rate variable pacing. *PACE* 1993; **16**: 1693–700.
46. Wasserman K, Hansen JE, Sue DY, *et al.* Principles of exercise testing and interpretation. Philadelphia: Lea & Febiger, 1987; 3–26.
47. Mond H, Strathmore N, Kertes P, *et al.* Rate responsive pacing using a minute ventilation sensor. *PACE* 1988; **11**: 1866–74.
48. Candinas R, Eugster W, MacCarter D, *et al.* Does rate modulation with a minute

ventilation pacemaker simulate the intrinsic heart rate response observed during representative patient daily activities. *Eur J CPE* 1944; **2**: 89–95.

49. Lau CP, Antoniou A, Ward DE, *et al*. Initial clinical experience with a minute ventilation sensing rate modulated pacemaker: improvements in exercise capacity and symptomatology. *PACE* 1988; **11**: 1815–22.
50. Kay GN, Bubien RS, Epstein AE, *et al*. Rate-modulated cardiac pacing based on transthoracic measurements of minute ventilation: correlation with exercise gas exchange. *JACC* 1989; **14**: 1283–9.
51. Lau CP, Antoniou A, Ward DE, *et al*. Reliability of minute ventilation as a parameter for rate responsive pacing. *PACE* 1989; **12**: 321–30.
52. Morris-Thurgood J, Chiang CM, Rochelle J, *et al*. A rate responsive pacemaker that physiologically reduces pacing rates at rest. *PACE* 1994; **17**: 1928–32.
53. Lau CP, Butrous GS, Ward DE, *et al*. Comparison of exercise performance of six rate-adaptive right ventricular cardiac pacemakers. *Am J Cardiol* 1989; **63**: 833–8.
54. Slade AKB, Pee S, Jones S, *et al*. New algorithms to increase the initial rate response in a minute volume rate adaptive pacemaker. *PACE* 1994; **17**: 1960–5.
55. Scanu P, Guilleman D, Grollier G, *et al*. Inappropriate rate response of the minute ventilation rate responsive pacemaker in a patient with Cheyne–Stokes dyspnea (letter). *PACE* 1989; **12**: 1963.
56. Bazett HC. An analysis of the time relationship of electrocardiograms. *Heart* 1920; **7**: 353–70.
57. Rickards AF, Normal J. Relation between QT interval and heart rate: new design of physiologically adaptive cardiac pacemaker. *Br Heart J* 1981; **45**: 56–61.
58. Hedman A, Nordlander R, Pehrsson SK. Changes in QT and QTa intervals at rest and during exercise with different modes of cardiac pacing. *PACE* 1985; **8**: 825–31.
59. Sarma JSM, Sarma RJ, Bilitch M. An exponential formula for heart rate dependence of QT interval during exercise and cardiac pacing in humans: reevaluation of Bazett's formula. *Am J Cardiol* 1984; **54**: 103–8.
60. Baig MW, Boute W, Begemann M, *et al*. Nonlinear relationship between pacing and evoked QT intervals. *PACE* 1988; **11**: 753–9.
61. Baig MW, Wilson K, Boute W, *et al*. Improved pattern of rate responsiveness with dynamic slope setting for the QT sensing pacemaker. *PACE* 1989; **12**: 311–20.
62. Boute W, Gebhardt U, Begemann MJS. Introduction of an automatic QT interval drive rate responsive pacemaker. *PACE* 1988; **11**: 1804–14.
63. Mehta D, Lau CP, Ward DE, *et al*. Comparative evaluation of chronotropic response of activity sensing and QT sensing rate responsive pacemakers to different activities. *PACE* 1988; **11**: 1426–31.
64. Donaldson RM, Fox K, Rickards AF. Initial experience with a physiological, rate responsive pacemaker. *Br Med J* 1983; **286**: 667–71.
65. Fananapazir L, Rodemaker M, Bennet DH. Reliability of the evoked response in determining the paced ventricular rate and performance of the QT or rate responsive (TX) pacemaker. *PACE* 1985; **8**: 701–14.
66. Hedman A, Norlander R. Changes in QT and QTa intervals induced by mental and physical stress with fixed rate and atrial triggered ventricular inhibited cardiac pacing. *PACE* 1988; **11**: 1426–31.
67. Brown KR, Prystowsky E, Heger JJ, *et al*. Modulation of the QT interval by the autonomic nervous system. *PACE* 1983; **6**: 1050–6.
68. Bexton RS, Vallin HO, Camm AJ. Diurnal variation of the QT interval: influence of the autonomic nervous system. *Br Heart J* 1985; **55**: 253–8.
69. Djorddjevic M, Kocovic D, Pavlovic S, *et al*. Circadian variations in heart rate and STIM-T interval; adaptation for night time pacing. *PACE* 1989; **12**: 1757–62.
70. Jordaens L, Backers J, Moerman E, *et al*. Catecholamine levels and pacing behavior of QT-driven pacemaker during exercise. *PACE* 1990; **13**: 603–7.
71. Fyfe T, Robinson JF. Failure of Quintech TX pacemaker caused by loss of stimulus: T interval shortening during exercise. *Br Heart J* 1986; **56**: 391–3.

72. Travill C, Ingram A, Vardas P, et al. Inadequate rate response of a stimulus: T sensing pacemaker (abstract). PACE 1987; **10**: 1231.
73. Robbens EJ, Clement DL, Jordaeus LJ. QT related rate responsive pacing during acute myocardial infarction. PACE 1988; **11**: 339–42.
74. Edelstam C, Hedman A, Nordlander R, et al. QT sensing rate responsive pacing and myocardial infarction. PACE 1989; **12**: 502–4.
75. Maisch B, Langenfeld H. Rate adaptive pacing: clinical experience with three different pacing systems. PACE 1986; **9**: 997–1004.
76. Boute W, Derrien Y, Wittkampf FHM. Reliability of evoked endocardial T-wave sensing in 1500 pacemaker patients. PACE 1986; **9**: 948–53.
77. Wirtzfeld A, Goedl-Meinen L, Bock T, et al. Central venous oxygen saturation for the control of automatic rate-responsive pacing. PACE 1982; **5**: 829–35.
78. Wirtzfeld A, Heinze R, Liess HD, et al. An active optical sensor for monitoring mixed venous oxygen-saturation for an implantable rate-regulating pacing system. PACE 1983; **6**: 494–7.
79. Casaburi R, Daly J, Hansen JE, et al. Abrupt changes in mixed venous blood gas composition after the onset of exercise. J Appl Physiol 1989; **67**: 1106–12.
80. Stangl K, Wirtzfeld A, Heinze R, et al. First clinical experience with an oxygen saturation controlled pacemaker in man. PACE 1988; **11**: 1882–7.
81. Farerestrand S, Ohm OJ, Stangeland L, et al. Long-term clinical performance of a central venous oxygen saturation sensor for rate adaptive cardiac pacing. PACE 1994; **17**: 1355–72.
82. Lau CP, Tai YT, Leung WH, et al. Rate adaptive cardiac pacing using right ventricular venous oxygen saturation: quantification of chronotropic behavior during daily activities and maximal exercise. PACE 1994; **17**: 2236–46.
83. Lau CP, Tai YT, Leung WH, et al. Rate adaptive cardiac pacing using right ventricular venous oxygen saturation: quantification of chronotropic behavior during daily activities and maximal exercise. PACE 1994; **17**: 2236–46.
84. Stangl K, Wirtzfeld A, Heinze R, et al. A new multisensor pacing system using stroke volume, respiratory rate, mixed venous oxygen saturation and temperature, right atrial pressure, right ventricular pressure, and dP/dt. PACE 1988; **11**: 712–24.
85. Mason DT. Usefulness and limitations of the rate of rise of intraventricular pressure (dp/dt) in the evaluation of myocardial contractility in man. Am J Cardiol 1969; **23**: 516–27.
86. Gleason WL, Braunwald E. Studies of the first derivative of the ventricular pressure pulse in man. J Clin Invest 1962; **41**: 80–91.
87. Bennett T, Sharma A, Sutton R, et al. Development of a rate adaptive pacemaker based on the maximum rate of rise of right ventricular pressure (RV dp/dt max). PACE 1992; **15**: 219–34.
88. Ovsyshcher I, Guetta V, Bonday C, et al. First derivative of right ventricular pressure, dp/dt, as a sensor for a rate adaptive VVI pacemaker: initial experience. PACE 1992; **15**: 211–18.
89. Kay GN, Philippon F, Bubien RS, et al. Rate modulated pacing based on right ventricular dP/dt: quantitative analysis of chronotropic response. PACE 1994; **17**: 1344–54.
90. Lau CP, Camm AJ, Rate-responsive pacing: technical and clinical aspects: In: El-Sherif N, Samet P (eds), Cardiac Pacing and Electrophysiology. Philadelphia: W.B. Saunders, 1991: 524–44.
91. Candinas R, Mayer IV, Heywood T, et al. Influence of exercise induced myocardial ischemia on right ventricular dP/dt: potential implications for rate responsive pacing. PACE 1995; **18**: 2121–7.
92. Alt E, Hirgstetter C, Heinz M, et al. Rate control of physiological pacemakers by central venous blood temperature. Circulation 1986; **73**: 1206–12.
93. Fearnot NE, Smith HJ, Sellers D, et al. Evaluation of the temperature response to exercise testing in patients with single chamber, rate adaptive pacemakers: a multicenter study. PACE 1989; **12**: 1806–15.
94. Arakawa M, Kambara K, Hiroyasu I, et al. Intermittent oversensing due to internal

insulation damage of temperature sensing rate responsive pacemaker lead in subclavian venipuncture method. *PACE* 1989; **12**: 1312–16.

95. Shellock FG, Rubin SA, Ellrodt AG, *et al*. Unusual core temperature decrease in exercising heart failure patients. *J Appl Physiol* 1983; **52**: 544–50.

96. Zegelman M, Winter UJ, Alt E, *et al*. Effect of different body-exercise modes on the rate response of the temperature-control pacemaker Nova MR. *Thorac Cardiovasc Surg* 1990; **38**: 181–5.

97. Cammilli L, Alcidi L, Papeschi G. A new pacemaker autoregulating the rate of pacing in relation to metabolic needs. In: Watanabe Y (eds), *Proceedings of the Fifth International Symposium, Tokyo*. Amsterdam: Excerpta Medica, 1976; 414–19.

98. Cammilli L, Alcidi L, Papeschi G. Blood pH as a signal for rate responsive pacemaker. *PACE* 1987; **10**: 1209–14.

99. Salo RW, Pederson BD, Olive AL, *et al*. Continuous ventricular volume assessment for diagnosis and pacemaker control. *PACE* 1984; **7**: 1267–72.

100. McGoon MD, Shapland JE, Salo R, *et al*. The feasibility of utilizing the systolic pre-ejection interval as a determinant of pacing rate. *JACC* 1989; **14**: 1753–8.

101. Mckay RG, Spears JR, Aroesty JM, *et al*. Instantaneous measurement of left and right ventricular stroke volume and pressure volume relationship with an impedance catheter. *Circulation* 1984; **69**: 703–10.

102. Lau CP, Wong CK, Cheng CH, *et al*. Importance of heart rate modulation on cardiac hemodynamics during post-exercise recovery. *PACE* 1990; **13**: 1277–85.

103. Spodick DH, Quarry-Pigoh VM. Effect of posture on exercise performance: measurement by systolic time intervals. *Circulation* 1973; **48**: 74–8.

104. Whitsett TL, Naughton J. The effect of exercise on systolic time intervals in sedentary and active individuals and rehabilitated patients with heart disease. *Am J Cardiol* 1971; **27**: 352–8.

105. Ponget JM, Harris WS, Mayron BR, *et al*. Abnormal responses of systolic time intervals to exercise in patients with angina pectoris. *Circulation* 1971; **43**: 289–98.

106. Occhetta E, Perucca A, Magnani A, *et al*. Reliability of right ventricular impedance as a biological sensor in dual-chamber rate-responsive pacing. *Eur J CPE* 1993; **3**: 245–51.

107. Ruiter JH, Heemels JP, Kee D, *et al*. Adaptive rate pacing controlled by the right ventricular preejection interval: clinical experience with a physiological pacing system. *PACE* 1992; **15**: 886–94.

108. Schaldach M, Hutten H. Intracardiac impedance to determine sympathetic activity in rate responsive pacing. *PACE* 1992; **15**: 1778–86.

109. Pichlmaier AM, Braile D, Ebner E, *et al*. Autonomic nervous system controlled closed loop cardiac pacing. *PACE* 1992; **15**: 1787–91.

110. Callaghan F, Vollmann W, Livingston A, *et al*. The ventricular depolarization gradient: effects of exercise, pacing rate, epinephrine, and intrinsic heart rate control on the right ventricular evoked response. *PACE* 1990; **12**: 1115–30.

111. Paul V, Garrett C, Ward DE, *et al*. Closed loop control of rate adaptive pacing: clinical assessment of a system analyzing the ventricular depolarization gradient. *PACE* 1989; **12**: 1896–920.

112. Singer I, Olesh J, Brennan F, *et al*. Initial clinical experience with a rate responsive pacemaker. *PACE* 1989; **12**: 1458–64.

113. Lasaridis K, Paul VE, Katritsis D, *et al*. Influence of propranolol on the ventricular depolarization gradient. *PACE* 1991; **14**: 787–92.

114. Singer I, Brennan AF, Steinhaus B, *et al*. Effects of stress and beta-1 blockade on the ventricular depolarization gradient of the rate modulating pacemaker. *PACE* 1991; **14**: 460–9.

115. Occhetta E, Perucca A, Rognoni G, *et al*. Experience with a new myocardial acceleration sensor during dobutamine infusion and exercise test. *Eur J CPE* 1995; **5**: 204–9.

116. Rickards AF, Bombardini T, Corbucci G, *et al*. An implantable intracardiac accelerometer for monitoring myocardial contractility. *PACE* 1996; **19**: 2066–71.

117. Wood JC, Fensten MP, Lim MJ, *et al.* Regional effects of myocardial ischemia on epicardially recorded canine first heart sound. *J Appl Physiol* 1994; **76**: 291–302.
118. Provenier F, van Acker R, Backers J, *et al.* Clinical observations with a dual sensor rate adaptive single chamber pacemaker. *PACE* 1992; **15**: 1821–5.
119. Connell DT and the Topaz Study Group. Initial experience with a new single chamber dual sensor rate responsive pacemaker. *PACE* 1993; **16**: 1833–41.
120. Leung SK, Lau CP, Wu CW, *et al.* Quantitative comparison of rate response and oxygen uptake kinetics between different sensor modes in multisensor rate adaptive pacing. *PACE* 1994; **17**: 1920–7.
121. Lau CP, Leung SK, Guerola, *et al.* Efficacy of automatically optimized rate adaptive dual sensor to simulate sinus rhythm: evaluation by continuous recording of sinus and sensor rates during exercise testing and daily activities. *PACE* 1996; **19**: 1672–7.
122. Cowell R, Morris-Thurgood J, Paul V, *et al.* Are we being driven to two sensors? Clinical benefits of sensor cross-checking. *PACE* 1993; **16**: 1441–4.
123. van Krieken FM, Perrins JP, Sigmund M. Clinical results of automatic slope adaptation in a dual sensor VVIR pacemaker. *PACE* 1992; **15**: 1815–20.
124. Lau CP, Leung SK, Lee SFI. Delayed exercise rate response kinetics due to sensor cross-checking in a dual sensor rate adaptive pacing system: the importance of individual sensor programming. *PACE* 1996; **19**: 1021–5.
125. Kay GN, Ashar MS, Bubien R, *et al.* Relationship between heart rate and oxygen kinetics during constant workload exercise. *PACE* 1995; **18**: 1853–60.
126. Leung SK, Lau CP, Tang MO, *et al.* New integrated sensor pacemaker: comparison of rate responses between an integrated minute ventilation and activity sensor and single sensor modes during exercise and daily activities and nonphysiological interference. *PACE* 1996; **19**: 1664–71.
127. Ovsyshcher I, Guldal M, Karazguz R, *et al.* Evaluation of a new rate adaptive ventricular pacemaker controlled by double sensors. *PACE* 1995; **18**: 386–90.
128. Alt E, Combs W, Fotuhi P, *et al.* Initial clinical experience with a new dual sensor SSIR pacemaker controlled by body activity and minute ventilation. *PACE* 1995; **18**: 1487–95.
129. Mitsui T, Hori M, Suma K, *et al.* Optimal heart rate in cardiac pacing in coronary sclerosis and non-sclerosis. *Ann NY Acad Sci* 1988; **16**: 745.
130. Bornzin GA, Arambula ER, Florio J, *et al.* Adjusting heart rate during sleep using activity variance. *PACE* 1994; **17**: 1933–8.
131. Mianulli M, Birchfield D, Yakimow K, *et al.* The relationship between fitness level and daily heart rate behavior in normal adults: implication for rate-adaptive pacing (abstract). *PACE* 1995; **18**: 870.
132. Mianulli M, Birchfield D, Yakimow K, *et al.* Daily heart rate behavior in normal adults: implication for rate-adaptive pacing (abstract). *PACE* 1995; **18**: 1160.
133. Norlander R, Hedman A, Pehrsson JK. Rate-responsive pacing and exercise capacity (editorial). *PACE* 1989; **12**: 749–51.
134. Gentzler RD, Lucus E, and the North American Trilogy™ DR+ Phase-I Clinical Investigators. Automatic sensor adjustment in a rate modulated pacemaker. *PACE* 1996; **19**: 1809–12.
135. Kristensson BE, Karlsson O, Ryden L. Holter-monitored heart rhythm during atrioventricular synchronous and fixed-rate ventricular pacing. *PACE* 1986; **9**: 511–18.
136. Lau CP, Leung WH, Wong CK, *et al.* Adaptive rate pacing at submaximal exercise: the importance of the programmed upper rate. *J Electrophysiol* 1989; **3**: 283.
137. Leung SK, Lau CP, Choi YC, *et al.* Does the programmed lower rate affect the rate response in rate adaptive pacemakers? (abstract). *PACE* 1992; **15**: 579.
138. Lau CP, Tse WS, Camm AJ. Clinical experience with Sensolog 703: a new activity-sensing, rate-responsive pacemaker. *PACE* 1988; **11**: 1444–55.
139. Hayds DL, Higano ST. Utility of rate histograms in programming and follow up of a DDDR pacemaker. *Mayo Clin Proc* 1989; **64**: 495–502.
140. Mahaux V, Waleffe A, Kulbertus HE. Clinical experience with a new activity-sensing, rate-modulated pacemaker using autoprogrammability. *PACE* 1989; **12**: 1362–8.

141. Leung SK, Lau CP, Tang MO. Appropriateness of automatic versus manual optimization in a dual sensor rate response pacemaker (abstract). *Eur J CPE* 1996; **6**(1): 168.
142. Mianulli M, Birchfield D, Yakimow K, *et al.* Do elderly pacemaker patients need rate adaptation: implications of daily heart rate behavior in normal adults (abstract). *Eur J CPE* 1996; **6**(1): 182.
143. Lau CP, Pietersen A, Ohm O, *et al.* Automatic implant detection for initiating lead polarity programming and rate adaptive sensors: multicentre study (abstract). *PACE* 1996; **19**: 592.
144. Leung SK, Leung Z, Lau CP. Is subthreshold determination of lead impedance during daily activities possible? *Eur J CPE* 1996; **6**(1): 218.
145. Leung SK, Lau CP, Leung Z, *et al.* Is automatic sensor programming possible for combined activity and minute ventilation sensors (abstract). *Eur J CPE* 1996; **6**(1): 199.
146. Lau CP, Leung SK. Clinical usefulness of rate adaptive pacing systems: what should we assess? *PACE* 1994; **17**: 2233–5.
147. Leung SK, Lau CP, Tang MO, *et al.* Cardiac output is a sensitive indicator of difference in exercise performance between single and dual sensor pacemakers. *PACE* 1997; (in press).
148. Jutzy RV, Florio J, Isaeff DM, *et al.* Comparative evaluation of rate modulated dual chamber and VVIR pacing. *PACE* 1990; **13**: 1838–46.
149. Sulke N, Tan K, Kamalvand K, *et al.* Dual sensor VVIR mode pacing: is it worth it? *PACE* 1996; **19**: 1560–7.
150. Lukl J, Doupal V, Heinc P. Quality of life during DDD and dual sensor VVIR pacing. *PACE* 1994; **17**: 1844–8.
151. Leung SK, Lau CP, Tang MO, *et al.* An integrated dual sensor system automatically optimized by target rate histogram. *PACE* 1997; in press.
152. Lau CP. *Rate Adaptive Cardiac Pacing, Single and Dual Chamber.* Mount Kisco, NY: Futura, 1993.

15

Minimizing Complications in Pacemaker Surgery

J. Brandt and H. Schüller

The objectives of a pacemaker implantation procedure are evident: placement of a pacing system optimal for the individual patient, with a minimum of immediate and long-term complications. Controversies remain regarding how to reach this goal. Like all surgical procedures, a pacemaker implantation consists of various manoeuvres, which can all be performed in several different ways. Critical evaluation of different techniques of implantation is difficult: the experience and skill of implanters differ, and a method which is safe in some hands may be less successful in others. Comparative studies providing guidance are consequently few. Nevertheless, the literature on complications in pacemaker surgery provides a basis for an analysis of different technical considerations of pacemaker implantation, the aim being to recommend a step-by-step implantation procedure with a minimal risk of short- and long-term problems (see Table 15.1).

Table 15.1 Potential complications in pacemaker surgery

Pneumothorax
Arterial puncture
'Subclavian crush' lead damage
Lead entrapment
Myocardial perforation
Lead misplacement
Lead dislodgement
Undersensing
Oversensing (myopotentials, far-field QRS complexes)
Exit block
Pectoral muscle or phrenic nerve stimulation
Pulse generator pocket haematoma
Infection
Pulse generator or lead erosion

Left-Sided or Right-Sided Implantation?

If a unipolar pacemaker system is used – or unipolar sensing is programmed – myopotentials may cause inhibition and/or triggering of the pulse generator. In a right-handed patient, this risk is theoretically greater if the pulse generator is placed in the right pectoral region, and vice versa. As a rule, pacemaker implantation on the left side can be recommended for the majority of patients.

Skin Preparation and Antibiotics

As foreign bodies are inserted during pacemaker implantation, careful skin preparation and a sterile technique are mandatory to minimize the risk of infection. Regarding the use of prophylactic antibiotics, studies have shown conflicting results. Some have found no differences between treated and untreated patients, whereas others have demonstrated a protective effect of antibiotic prophylaxis.[1] A recent randomized study has shown a significantly lower risk of infections with systemic antibiotic administration, which can therefore currently be recommended.[2] The bacterial spectrum of pacemaker infections indicates that an antistaphylococcal agent should be used,[1] but the optimal drug and the ideal duration of treatment remain controversial. The microbiological environment at the implanting centre will also influence these factors. Possibly, local deposition of an antibiotic in the pacemaker pocket during implantation may be sufficient.[1,3]

Supraclavicular or Infraclavicular Venous Access?

From a cosmetic point of view, access to the heart through infraclavicular blood vessels (subclavian or cephalic veins) is preferable to supraclavicular lead introduction (internal or external jugular veins). A supraclavicular approach necessitates the forming of a sharp bend of the pacemaker lead in a region where the overlying skin is thin; furthermore, tunnelling of the lead to the pulse generator pocket in the infraclavicular region will then be necessary.

Subclavian Venepuncture or Cephalic Vein Cutdown?

Puncture of the subclavian vein is associated with a small but significant risk of pneumothorax and arterial puncture, even in trained hands. In a recent large study, these complications occurred in 1.9% and 2.7% respectively.[4] Another consideration is the 'subclavian crush' phenomenon, where mechanical interference with structures below the clavicle results in subsequent damage to the lead.[5-7] There is evidence that the risk of this complication is highest if the lead is inserted through a medial puncture of the subclavian vein and the risk lower if the puncture is more lateral.[5,8] 'Subclavian crush' is not seen if the cephalic vein is used. There are no randomized studies of different routes of lead implantation and one recent long-term investigation failed to show differences in the incidence of lead complications following subclavian venepuncture versus cephalic vein cutdown.[9] Nevertheless, lead introduction using the cephalic vein must currently be recommended. Even a very small cephalic vein may be used, if it is entered under direct vision with a cannula through which a guide-wire is then passed (the Seldinger technique), allowing subsequent placement of a standard introducer set. Once the introducer is in the venous system, the technique of retaining the guide-wire and using it for a subsequent lead introduction obviates the need for repeated cutdowns or venepunctures.[10]

If the cephalic vein cannot be used, the subclavian venepuncture should not be done too medially, to lessen the risk of 'subclavian crush'. Several different techniques for a safe subclavian cannulation have been advocated,[11–13] but no prospective comparative studies have been published. When the guide-wire has entered the vessel, passing of the wire tip below the diaphragm confirms that the guide-wire is in the venous system, and not accidentally placed in the subclavian artery. If the implanter is in doubt, this should be done before an introducer is inserted.

Choice of Lead: Unipolar or Bipolar?

Bipolar leads have the advantages of lack of myopotential oversensing, pectoral muscle stimulation and a very small risk of far-field QRS complex sensing in the atrium.[14,15] Furthermore, automatic implantable defibrillators currently used have a propensity to sense unipolar pacing impulses and interpret them as QRS complexes, which may interfere with the function of such systems. In patients where implantation of a defibrillator is indicated – or can be anticipated – bipolar pacing systems should therefore be used. However, bipolar leads are necessarily of a more complicated design than unipolar leads, and thus more prone to long-term lead failure. In most pacemaker patients, the choice of a unipolar or bipolar system therefore remains controversial, with valid arguments existing for both principles.

Lead Advancement

Advancement of a pacing lead through the venous system is facilitated if the lead stylet is not inserted fully, and the distal part of the lead is therefore more flexible. This also reduces the small risk of perforation of the right ventricle when the tricuspid valve is passed. If a nonretractable screw-in lead without a tip cover is used, it should be advanced with counterclockwise rotation so that it does not get stuck in the vessel wall or in unintended positions in the heart.

Sometimes the lead inadvertently enters the coronary sinus. With anterioposterior fluoroscopy, the lead will then curve in a somewhat more cranial direction than if it passes into the right ventricle. If doubt remains regarding the lead position, it can be gently advanced further. If the lead is in the right ventricle, the tip will then proceed through the pulmonary valve and into the right or left pulmonary artery. The lead may then be withdrawn and the tip finally placed in the right ventricle. Recording of the intracardiac electrogram also indicates whether the lead is in the coronary sinus, as a QRS complex with no injury current (ST-elevation) will then be seen. Alternatively, lateral fluoroscopy will show if the lead is in a coronary sinus position, as it will then follow the posterior border of the heart shadow.

Lead Positioning

Adequate positioning implies lead tip stability, satisfactory intracardiac signal configuration and amplitude and an acceptable stimulation threshold.

Stability of the fixation of a ventricular lead can be evaluated by withdrawing the stylet about 10 cm and then advancing the lead body, making it form a loop in the right ventricle with the bloodstream exerting a pull on the lead. The same dislodgement test may be used with an atrial lead, if it is not preshaped; if so, evaluation of lead tip fixation is more difficult. Generally, the risk of postoperative dislodgement is lower with screw-in leads than with passive-fixation electrodes, but thresholds tend to be somewhat higher with active-fixation leads. Most series using modern atrial pacing leads report a dislodgement rate of 2–5%.[4,16]

Atrial and ventricular *intracardiac signals* should preferably be evaluated both by direct recording of the intracardiac electrogram and by measuring the signals by means of a pacing systems analyser. In addition to the signal amplitude and slew rate data, intracardiac electrogram recording can provide information on retrograde (ventriculo-atrial) conduction.

The *stimulation threshold* should be measured in volts, with the impulse duration specified.[18] Generally, stimulation thresholds should not exceed 1.0 volt at 0.5 ms impulse duration; however, it must be recognized that active fixation leads with an electrically active screw frequently show higher thresholds immediately after the placement, which will decline within minutes. Substantial variations in the pacing threshold and/or the signal amplitude during the measurement may indicate instability of the lead tip, requiring adjustment of the position. Phrenic nerve stimulation should also be ruled out, especially when a lead is placed laterally in the right atrium.

Localization of the Pacemaker Pocket

The gradual reduction of the size of cardiac pulse generators has permitted the placement of a subcutaneous pacemaker pocket in the pectoral region even in very small adults and in most children, obviating the need for tunnelling of the pacemaker lead. In very lean patients, the pulse generator may be placed under the fascia of the pectoral muscle, or under the muscle itself. In these cases, unipolar pacing carries the risk of pectoral muscle stimulation, and a bipolar system should therefore be used.

Haemostasis

In recent years the number of patients treated with anticoagulants (warfarin or coumadine) or antiplatelet drugs has increased, owing to the benefits of these medications in conditions such as atrial fibrillation, stroke, thrombosis, valvular heart disease and coronary heart disease.

Anticoagulants are best discontinued a few days prior to pacemaker implantation, but the risk of peroperative bleeding must be weighed against the perils of treatment interruption in the individual case. The effect of *antiplatelet drugs* is long-lasting, but the risk of bleeding is less than with anticoagulants; consequently, pacemaker surgery may be performed without discontinuing these drugs.

Pacemaker Pocket Drainage?

The argument in favour of a closed pacemaker pocket drainage in the immediate postoperative period is a reduced risk of haematoma and seroma, conditions which may increase the need for surgical reintervention and predispose to postoperative pocket infection. However, the drainage itself may theoretically increase the risk of bacterial invasion of the pocket. Presently, the value of pocket drainage is debatable; it may be warranted in patients with an increased risk of peroperative bleeding (e.g. coagulation disorders or anticoagulant treatment).

Who Should Implant Cardiac Pacemakers?

The procedure likely to result in a minimal complication rate is summarized in Table 15.2. An implanter should master these surgical techniques and be able to obtain and interpret the recordings described, with both single- and dual-chamber systems. Furthermore, data have indicated that 'infrequent implanters' – defined as performing

Table 15.2 Recommendations for pacemaker implantation with a minimum of complications

---

Left-sided implantation (if the patient is right-handed)
Antibiotic prophylaxis
Sterile implantation technique
Infraclavicular venous access:
    Cephalic vein cutdown (first choice)
    Subclavian venepuncture (second choice)
Retained guide-wire technique
Retraction of the stylet when the lead enters the right ventricle
Screw-in atrial leads
Routine lead-tip stability testing
Recording of the intracardiac electrogram
Pacing systems analyser measurement of signals and thresholds
Pectoral pulse generator placement: subfascial or submuscular if needed
Experienced and active implanter

---

fewer than 12 operations per year – have considerably higher complication rates.[19] A final – and hardly controversial – conclusion is that operations are best made by an experienced implanter, who performs procedures frequently enough to keep up the skills required.

Complications requiring reoperation are in modern patient series reported to be around 5%.[4,16] In order to assure acceptable complication rates, continuous monitoring and reporting of complications related to pacemaker surgery are important.

References

1. Bluhm G. Pacemaker infections. *Acta Med Scand* 1985; suppl. **699**: 1–62.
2. Mounsey JP, Griffith MJ, Tynan M, *et al*. Antibiotic prophylaxis in permanent pacemaker implantation: a prospective randomised trial. *Br Heart J* 1994; **72**: 339–43.
3. Ramsdale DR, Charles RG, Rowlands DB, *et al*. Antibiotic prophylaxis for pacemaker implantation: a prospective randomized trial. *PACE* 1984; **7**: 844–9.
4. Aggarwal RK, Connelly DT, Ray SG, *et al*. Early complications of permanent pacemaker implantation: no difference between dual and single chamber systems. *Br Heart J* 1995; **73**: 571–5.
5. Magney JE, Flynn DM, Parsons JA, *et al*. Anatomical mechanisms explaining damage to pacemaker leads, defibrillator leads, and failure of central venous catheters adjacent to the sternoclavicular joint. *PACE* 1993; **16**: 445–57.
6. Magney JE, Parsons JA, Flynn DM, *et al*. Pacemaker and defibrillator lead entrapment: case studies. *PACE* 1995; **18**: 1509–17.
7. Roelke M, O'Nunain SS, Osswald S, *et al*. Subclavian crush syndrome complicating transvenous cardioverter defibrillator systems. *PACE* 1995; **18**: 973–9.
8. Jacobs DM, Finks AS, Miller RP, *et al*. Anatomical and morphological evaluation of pacemaker lead compression. *PACE* 1993; **16**: 434–44.
9. Helguera ME, Maloney JD, Pinski SL, *et al*. Long-term performance of endocardial pacing leads. *PACE* 1994; **17**: 56–64.
10. Belott PH. A variation on the introducer technique for unlimited access to the subclavian vein. *PACE* 1981; **4**: 43–8.
11. Fyke FE. Doppler-guided extrathoracic introducer insertion. *PACE* 1995; **18**: 1017–21.
12. Lamas GA, Fish RD, Braunwald NS. Fluoroscopic technique of subclavian venous puncture for permanent pacing: a safer and easier approach. *PACE* 1988; **11**: 1398–401.
13. Magney JE, Staplin DH, Flynn DM, *et al*. A new approach to percutaneous subclavian venipuncture to avoid lead fracture or central venous catheter occlusion. *PACE* 1993; **16**: 2133–42.
14. Brandt J, Fåhraeus T, Schüller H. Far-field QRS complex sensing via the atrial pacemaker lead. I: Mechanism, consequences, differential diagnosis and countermeasures in AAI and VDD/DDD pacing. *PACE* 1988; **11**: 1432–8.
15. Brandt J, Fåhraeus T, Schüller H. Far-field QRS complex sensing via the atrial pacemaker lead. II: Prevalence, clinical significance and possibility of intraoperative prediction in DDD pacing. *PACE* 1988; **11**: 1540–4.
16. Chauhan A, Grace AA, Newell SA *et al*. Early complications after dual-chamber versus single-chamber pacemaker implantation. *PACE* 1994; **17**(II): 2012–15.
17. Preston TA, Barold SS. Problems in measuring threshold for cardiac pacing: recommendations for routine clinical measurement. *Am J Cardiol* 1977; **40**: 658–60.
18. Parsonnet V, Bernstein AD, Lindsay B. Pacemaker-implantation complication rates: an analysis of some contributing factors. *JACC* 1989; **13**: 917–21.

Is There an Optimal Method of Lead Extraction?

C. L. Byrd

Management of biological complications and/or device failures may necessitate the revision or removal of implanted pacing and defibrillator hardware. However, the removal of transvenous leads from their encapsulating binding tissue has proved to be both technically challenging and potentially dangerous. Until recently, procedures did not exist to consistently and successfully manage these device-related complications without major surgery. Transvenous leads were initially removed by pulling (direct traction), tearing the leads free from the binding tissue. This uncontrolled application of force was replaced by tools for the mechanical ablation of binding tissue as intravascular lead extraction procedures were developed.[1-4] These procedures were based upon the use of telescoping sheaths to focus the application of force to the binding tissue. Advancing the sheaths through the vasculature to the myocardial wall is the more dangerous portion of these procedures. Once the sheaths are near the heart wall, the electrodes can generally be safely removed.

A new device, an excimer laser sheath, has recently been developed as an alternative to the inner telescoping sheath used in mechanical ablation. With the new technique, known as laser or photo ablation, the excimer laser sheath is used to vaporize the encapsulating binding tissue. This allows a more gentle and efficient separation of the lead from binding tissue. The device is currently in the final stages of its FDA IDE study and should be commercially available in the near future.

An electrosurgical ablation device is also under development. The results of initial animal testing are promising, though clinical studies have yet to be done to explore its efficacy for lead extraction and safety, especially the margin of safety with respect to fibrillation.

The following sections of this chapter will more fully describe why leads are difficult to remove, contemporary views regarding the indications for lead removal and techniques and results for removing leads using the conventional mechanical ablation or the new laser ablation.

Why Leads are Difficult to Remove

The pathophysiology associated with implanted leads explains the difficulties in lead removal. Knowing the factors that influence the formation of clot and the tensile strength of the binding encapsulating fibrous tissue is necessary to ensure safe extraction of an intact lead. Failure to understand the characteristics of the environment from which the lead is being removed can contribute to a poor result or an unnecessarily dangerous procedure.

Tissue is injured when a lead is inserted into a vein, advanced into the heart chamber and implanted on the endocardial surface of the heart wall, using either a passive or an active fixation device.[5] The tissue injury ranges from tissue disruption to transient or chronic pressure-induced injury of the vein and heart wall. Injury to the vein and heart wall activates the coagulation mechanism and predisposes the tissue to clot formation. Stasis of flow and turbulence of flow along the lead also cause clot formation. The resultant clot formation and maturation into encapsulating fibrous tissue occurs, binding the leads to the vein, to the heart wall and one to another.[6-8]

Some clinical issues related to clot formation and maturation into fibrous tissue are listed in Table 16.1. The size of the initial clot is related to the magnitude of the tissue injury and to contributing factors such as stasis and turbulence of flow. For example, implantation in the trabeculated right ventricle causes injury, stasis and turbulence. Significant clot formation is usually present in the ventricle. Much of the clot is likely to undergo lysis prior to maturation into fibrous tissue, but quantitative experimental and clinical data are not available regarding the degree of lysis. Lead characteristics are another factor in tissue injury.[9,10] Large, stiff leads cause more injury than small, supple leads. A present-day example is the contrast between 3–4Fr pacing leads and 10–11Fr defibrillator leads.

Table 16.1   Clot formation and maturation into encapsulating fibrous tissue

Clinical characteristics[a]	Variables
Initial clot size	Tissue injury
	Stasis of flow
	Turbulence
Clot lysis	Unknown (0–100%)
Clot maturation	Inflammatory reaction resulting in fibrous tissue
Continued clot formation	Unknown factors
	Anticoagulation
Tensile strength of fibrous tissue	Age of patient
	Implant duration
	Thickness and length of fibrous tissue
	Number of leads implanted
	Initial implant *vs* acute on chronic implant
	Steroids

[a] First is the size of the initial clot, and second is the amount of this clot involved in the maturation process. The clot can undergo lysis ranging from zero to 100%. Third, clots may continue to form during maturation. The fourth property is the increase in tensile strength of the fibrous tissue with time; this involves the deposition of calcium phosphate and carbonate. Circumferential calcium deposition is stronger than bone.

Continued clot formation is known to occur during the maturation process. Chronic animal studies show acute clot formation in areas of encapsulating fibrous tissue. The clinical significance of these findings is not clear. Although not all mechanisms for new clot formation are known, examples include stasis and sepsis. Sepsis can cause a large infected peduncular clot attached to the lead and/or heart wall. Their potential for embolization to the lungs, occlusion of the tricuspid valve and septicaemia makes them dangerous.

Another special case is propagation of a thrombus in a thrombosed vein. Large clot formation can cause thrombosis of the vein. Subclavian and/or brachiocephalic vein thrombosis is common. It occurs both acutely and chronically, and may be associated with transient swelling of the arm. Propagation of a thrombus back near the brachial vein is rare; but if it occurs, and if the collateral drainage is poor, this can cause permanent swelling of the arm.[11–14]

Maturation of a clot into encapsulating fibrous tissue is an inflammatory reaction. The clot is gradually replaced with fibrous tissue. Fibrous tissue forms a protective barrier between the foreign body and normal tissue and has substantial tensile strength (the maximum tension the tissue can take without breaking).

The tensile strength of clot and early thrombosis is weak; leads can easily be torn free without damaging the vein or heart wall. Once replaced by encapsulating fibrous tissue, however, the tensile strength is significant, even when new. Trying to free the lead using traction can tear the vein or heart wall. Factors influencing the tensile strength include the age of the patient, duration of the implant, the thickness of the tissue, the length of the tissue along the lead body, the number of leads implanted and whether a lead was an initial implant or a replacement lead.

The age of the patient is important. Young, active patients have fibrous tissue with greater tensile strength than the old and sedentary. Leads which are easy to remove from a 90-year-old may be extremely difficult to remove from someone less than 40. Also, the deposition of calcium salts occurs much faster in young patients. A lead implant for 8 years in a young patient is more likely to have calcified binding tissue than a lead implanted for 8 years in an elderly patient.

The effects of implant duration, and the thickness and length of the binding encapsulating tissue, on the tensile strength are intuitively obvious. Quantification of these factors is not possible because of the influence of age and number of leads. The effect of the number of leads implanted on the tensile strength is less intuitive. Leads are bound not only to the tissue but to each other. In some cases, the binding tissue mass is large, encompassing all leads passing through the region and the wall. Removing leads from these masses can be dangerous, especially at the junction of the SVC and atrium.

The maturation characteristics of fibrous tissue associated with an initial implant, in comparison with a replacement implant through the same site, are not intuitively obvious. A new replacement lead inserted through a chronic implant site is likely to have fibrous tissue properties of the old fibrous tissue soon after implanting. As an example, suppose a 12-year-old lead is removed, and a new lead reimplanted through the same conduit. Within weeks, the old encapsulating fibrous tissue will have contracted around the new lead. The new lead now has many of the encapsulation properties of the old lead. In some cases, after many months it can be more difficult to remove than the original lead. Therefore, duration of implant must be qualified as an initial process or as a reimplant process.

Should Leads be Removed?

Because of the difficulty and risks of lead removal, the traditional viewpoint has been that once a lead is implanted, it should remain implanted even if it fails to function, unless there is a compelling reason to remove it.[15] As indications have expanded in recent years, some physicians now hold a viewpoint that a superfluous lead should be removed unless there is a compelling reason to leave it in place. The indications for lead removal will be discussed from both viewpoints.

Premise: In General, Leads Should Not Be Removed

The indications for lead removal were initially classified as 'mandatory', 'necessary' or 'discretionary' conditions (Table 16.2). These categories were based on clinical situations in which leaving the lead in place would be life-threatening, would cause significant morbidity or might cause significant morbidity. This reasoning is based on clinical observations of the natural history of lead complications. Fundamental to this approach is the view that leads generally should not be removed. The decision to remove a lead was made by comparing the perceived risk of mortality and morbidity thought to be inherent in an extraction procedure to the risk of mortality and morbidity from leaving the lead implanted.

Mandatory conditions are the only indications everyone agrees upon for lead extraction. All such leads must be removed. If the extractor does not have experience using a transvenous procedure, an open heart procedure is used instead. The same situation does not exist for leads with necessary and discretionary conditions, which include all superfluous leads (except those that are migrating or causing electrical interference). The incidence of lead removal for necessary and discretionary conditions is dependent on the experience of the extracting physician. An experienced extractor removes most of these leads. Exceptions include patients whose physical condition precludes a safe procedure, or whose life expectancy is such that the lead-related risk does not present a significant threat.

Indications for lead removal can also be based on the pathophysiology of implanted leads. One example is to consider both the lead's biological interface with the body and the lead's clinical utility (Figure 16.1). This approach emphasizes the underlying

Table 16.2   Indications for lead extraction based on the clinical condition of the patient

Graded clinical indications (conditions)	Clinical situations in which *not* removing the lead:
Mandatory	would be life threatening
Necessary	would cause significant morbidity
Discretionary	may cause significant morbidity

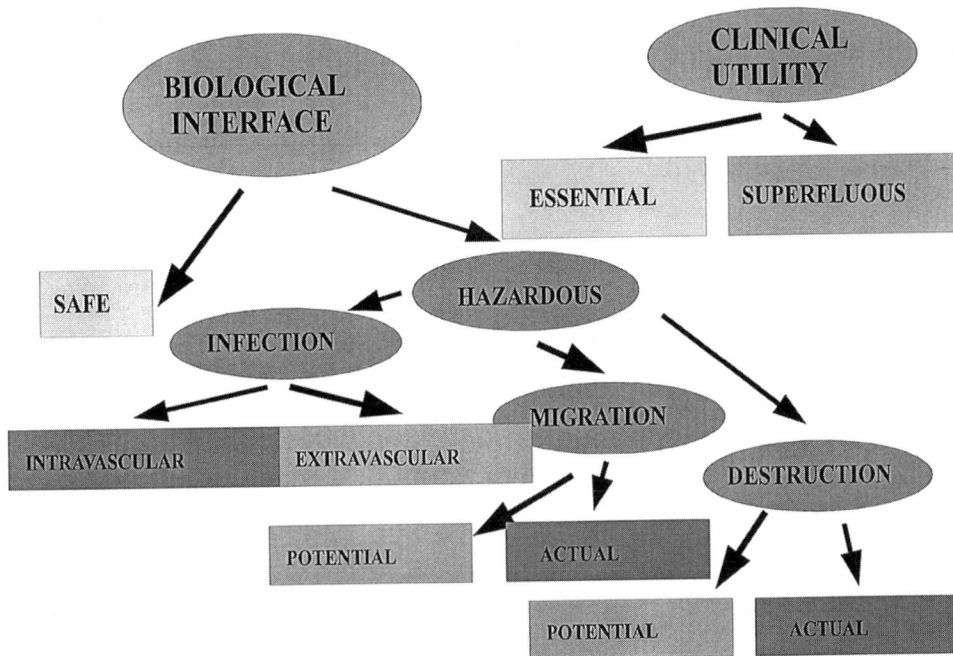

Figure 16.1 Lead status.

lead and/or biological problem, but does not grade the clinical magnitude of the problem. Combining this approach with the clinical conditions (Table 16.3) for lead extraction results in a presentation of the currently accepted indications for lead removal.

Complications associated with the biological interface include infection, lead migration and tissue destruction, and may potentially include calcification of the encapsulating tissue. Infections are separated into intravascular and extravascular

Table 16.3 Summary of combined indications

Lead-related indications	Lead status	Clinical condition	Action
Abandoned	Superfluous	Necessary or discretionary	?
Infected	Extravascular	Necessary	Removal[a]
Infected	Intravascular	Mandatory	Removal
Migrating	Potential	Necessary or discretionary	?
Migrating	Actual	Mandatory	Removal
Disruption	Potential	Necessary or discretionary	Removal[a]
Disruption	Actual	Mandatory	Removal

[a] Most leads are treated this way, but not all.
? There is no agreement on how to manage these conditions. Experienced physicians generally remove these leads if the patient's physical condition is satisfactory.

infections. Intravascular infections are life-threatening and are a mandatory condition for lead removal. Extravascular infections cause significant morbidity and are a necessary condition for lead removal.

'Destructive leads' are a new group. The example seen thus far is that of leads with J-shaped retention wires that may fracture and protrude from the lead (Telectronics Accufix™ or Encor™ leads). A protruding retention wire has potential to puncture or tear the wall of the heart and/or great vessels or to migrate. Indications for removal of destructive leads and migrating leads are subdivided by whether the event has actually occurred or has the potential to occur. Actual events are mandatory conditions, whereas potential events are necessary conditions.

Calcification of the encapsulating tissue represents a different type of problem. Complications associated with its presence have to date been related to the difficulty of removing leads. Calcified tissue cannot be dilated or torn free. The only way to remove this tissue is to pass a sheath over the calcified region, peel it from the vein or heart wall and include it with the extracted lead body. The risk associated with this approach is the risk of tearing vascular tissue and/or creating a false passage following a misadventure while applying excessive force.

Primary complications from calcified encapsulating tissue have not been reported in the literature, probably because tissue calcification is a progression of the natural encapsulation process from a supple to a rigid structure, occurring over a long period. This allows surrounding tissues time to compensate. However, multiple rigid leads in the right ventricle could compromise the compliance of the right heart wall and reduce the contractile motion (diastolic and systolic dysfunction). Although a theoretical possibility, this condition has not been documented to the author's knowledge.

The utility of an implanted lead is based on its function. A lead is either essential to the electrical performance of the pulse generator or it is superfluous. All abandoned leads are superfluous. The removal of superfluous leads is classified as either a necessary or discretionary condition. Superfluous leads present the same risk as any functional implanted lead for developing a time-dependent biological interface complication. In addition, these leads may interfere with the electrical performance of essential leads. For example, a retained ICD lead may interfere electrically with the function of an essential lead.

Removal of superfluous leads, in the absence of a biological interface complication, is currently controversial. One reason is the perception that leads were designed to be implanted for the lifetime of a patient, and consequently should do no harm. This misconception has been perpetuated by lack of data on the natural history of long lead implants. Some physicians prefer to set qualifying conditions for removal of super-fluous leads. These include setting a limit on implant duration or on the maximum number of leads considered safe to abandon in the superior veins, to pass through the tricuspid valve and/or to reside in the right ventricle. These quantifying conditions are largely intuitive. Data concerning these qualifying conditions do not exist and would be extremely difficult to collect.

A positive argument for removing superfluous leads is to relate the dangers of lead extraction to the duration of implantation, to the number of chronic leads implanted and to the experience of the extractor. For example, it is less dangerous to remove leads implanted for less than 4–6 years than to remove leads implanted for greater than 8–10 years. It is more dangerous to remove multiple leads implanted for varying lengths of time. The implication of this argument is to remove leads when it is safer. The risk and morbidity are related to physician experience and are low for most experienced extractors.

Premise: All Leads Should Be Removed

The initial indications grading the clinical condition (mandatory, necessary and discretionary) were based on the need to justify extracting a lead. The logic for this approach is that leads are generally well tolerated by the body and should not be removed unless one is forced to do so. What happens if the argument is reversed and a justification for not removing a lead must be made? The supposition for this approach is that leads are not tolerated well by the body over long periods of time; i.e. the presence of a lead has the potential of being a progressive detrimental process to the veins and heart.

For this supposition to be true, the risk associated with the removal of leads must be minimal, and it must be detrimental to leave superfluous leads implanted. If this hypothesis is correct, then contraindications should be related to the patient's physical condition and ability to safely undergo the lead extraction procedure. If a standard procedure is assumed to include general anaesthesia and a worst-case scenario is a median sternotomy for a complication, the patient must be able to tolerate these procedures. (In the author's experience, procedures performed under general anaesthesia are easier and probably safer than those performed using conscious sedation.)

One method of grading a patient's physical condition is to use Classes I–V as proposed by the American Society of Anesthesiologists[16] (Table 16.4). It essentially

Table 16.4 Relationships between the American Society of Anesthesiologists' classes of physical status and contraindications for lead removal

Class	System disease[a]	Excluded from lead removal
I	None	No contraindication
II	Mild to moderate	No contraindication
III	Significant	No contraindication
IV	Severe	'Necessary' may be contraindicated 'Discretionary' is contraindicated
V	Moribund	Contraindicated

[a] Moribund means the patient pathology is lethal regardless of whether it is corrected or not. Lead extraction is contraindicated in all Class V patients. Class IV patients have severe systemic disease such as end-stage heart and/or respiratory disease; these patients can survive an extraction procedure, but the hospitalization will probably involve intensive care and be prolonged. All 'mandatory' and many 'necessary' conditions for lead extractions qualify in this group. There are no restrictions for Classes I–III.

Table 16.5 Summary of indications for lead extraction

Biological interface		ASA physical status class					Social[a]
Event	Modifier	I	II	III	IV	V	
Infection	Intravascular	E	E	E	E	N	E
Infection	Extravascular	E	E	E	C	N	N
Migration	Actual	E	E	E	E	N	E
Migration	Potential	E	E	E	N	N	N
Destruction	Actual	E	E	E	E	N	E
Destruction	Potential	E	E	E	C	N	N
Superfluous	Noncalcified	E	E	E	C	N	N
Superfluous	Calcified	C	C	C	N	N	N

[a] Social = dementia and/or terminal illness (short time to live).
E = extraction; C = conditional extraction (extract in most situations); N = no extraction.

shows that the only patients who are *not* candidates for general anaesthesia are Class V moribund patients. This would therefore be the only absolute contraindication to lead extraction. Consequently, patients in Classes I–IV would be candidates for all 'mandatory' and most 'necessary' procedures.

Relative contraindications include calcified encapsulating tissue and social constraints. Leads encapsulated with calcified tissue, usually implanted for 10–15 years or more, are difficult to remove. Since an extensive procedure may be required, superfluous calcified leads would probably not be removed from elderly patients, but would generally be removed from young patients. Social factors such as decreased life expectancy, dementia and economic considerations are based on the standard of care in the community and judgement issues. Table 16.5 is a summary of the current indications for lead extraction. Many physicians experienced in lead extraction are currently using this rationale for extracting leads.

Regardless of the rationale used for removing leads, there has been a marked expansion of indications in recent years. Some of the reasons for this expansion are given in Table 16.6. They are interrelated. A decrease in the risk and morbidity of the procedure, increased experience of the extractor and availability of more sophisticated equipment are all related. The increase in the number of leads extracted provides more experience, allowing procedures to be done in a safer and more expeditious manner. As the number of procedures increases, more extractors will be trained and the procedure ought to become more economic.

Table 16.6 Generalizations regarding increase in lead removal

Risk and morbidity of procedure decreases
Experience of extractors increases
Extraction equipment more sophisticated
The number of leads under recall increases
Superfluous leads are being removed

How are Leads Removed?

This section discusses techniques for lead extraction, either by simply pulling on the lead or by the use of devices for mechanical and laser ablation of binding fibrous tissue. This discussion will not cover cardiopulmonary bypass, techniques for partial lead extraction or anecdotal techniques not qualifying as an extraction procedure. An extraction procedure is defined as a technique which can be applied to a consecutive series of patients using a planned series of manoeuvres to perform a task with predictable results. That is, the technique can be applied in a prescribed manner and obtain the predetermined result. Cardiopulmonary bypass is a procedure, but it is not competitive with the mechanical ablation approach. Cardiopulmonary bypass is not applicable to all patients, and the morbidity and mortality rates are prohibitive.[17] In contrast, procedures for mechanical ablation and laser ablation of encapsulating tissue are well-developed.

Lead Extraction Prior to Lead Extraction Devices

Initially leads were removed by pulling (traction) on the exposed extravascular portion of the lead. The object was to tear the lead free from the scar tissue at the binding sites, including the tissue binding the electrode to the heart wall. This traction force was applied not only to the binding sites, but also to those tissues surrounding the binding sites. If the weakest tissue was the binding site, the lead was successfully removed. Otherwise, an avulsion of the surrounding tissue and/or a tearing of the vein or heart wall would occur. A resultant haemorrhage into the thorax or pericardium caused a life-threatening cardiovascular emergency (haemothorax or cardiac tamponade).

In some cases, the lead started to stretch, unwind or break. Some physicians cut such leads and let them retract into the implant vein. Leaving a damaged lead or lead segment behind had the potential of causing a later complication such as vein thrombosis, lead migration or septicaemia if infected. Failure to remove an infected lead by traction resulted in lead removal by a cardiac surgical procedure, with or without bypass.

In the 1960s and early 1970s, most leads could be removed by traction, since the implant duration was short and the fixation mechanisms (flanges) were not very effective. Traction techniques included manually pulling on a surgically exposed lead or using some sort of chronic traction device, such as weights or elastic bands. Transfemoral snares were used to grasp the lead body and pull it out of both the superior veins and heart wall. The transfemoral traction approach was more successful than applying traction at the vein entry site. Consequently, it became a popular approach.

When tined passive fixation devices were added to pacing leads, the difficulty of separating the leads from the heart wall increased. In addition, the increased duration of lead implants (related to increased longevity of pulse generators) resulted in greater tensile strength at the binding site. With the advent of dual-chamber pacing, the presence of multiple leads became commonplace. These three factors significantly increased the difficulty of removing transvenous leads and caused higher extraction-related complication rates. The poor results with traction techniques were responsible for the development of lead extraction devices.

Mechanical Ablation Devices for Lead Extraction

The first attempts at lead extraction devices involved a locking stylet and telescoping plastic sheaths (Cook Vascular Inc., Leechburg, PA, USA).[18,19] The locking stylet was advanced inside the coil lumen and locked at the tip of the lead, to reinforce the lead and deliver extraction force to the tip. The stylet also provided a 'handle' to maintain adequate tension on the lead while advancing telescoping sheaths. The telescoping sheaths were used to focus the traction forces to a specific binding site, while the binding tissue was mechanically ablated. The goal was to eliminate the avulsion and/or tearing of the tissue surrounding the binding sites in the vasculature and at the myocardium. 'Counterpressure' and 'countertraction' are the two words used to describe these procedures.

Counterpressure is a 'pushing' by the sheaths against the binding sites, causing pressure against the binding tissue (Figures 16.2–16.4). This pressure is countered by the tissue surrounding the binding site, so that a shearing force is applied to the vein wall. *Countertraction* is the opposite. With countertraction, traction is applied to the lead while the sheaths are held stationary, so that the binding site is pulled against the sheaths (Figure 16.5). The traction forces are countered by the sheaths. Counter-traction applies force only to the binding tissue (with no shearing force on the wall).

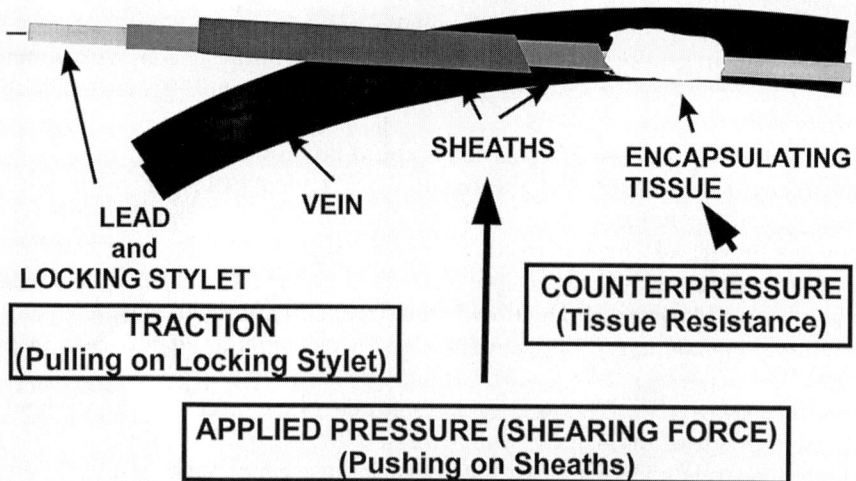

Figure 16.2 The principle of counterpressure.

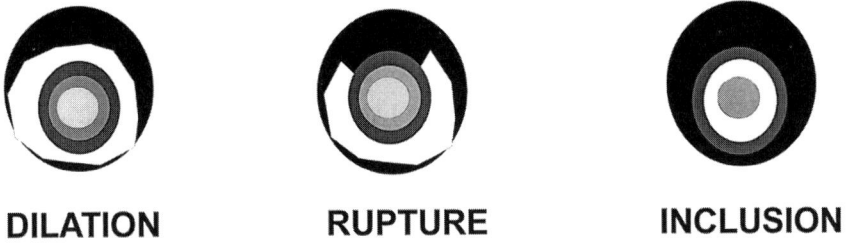

DILATION   **RUPTURE**   **INCLUSION**

Figure 16.3 Dilation, rupture and inclusion in the counterpressure technique.

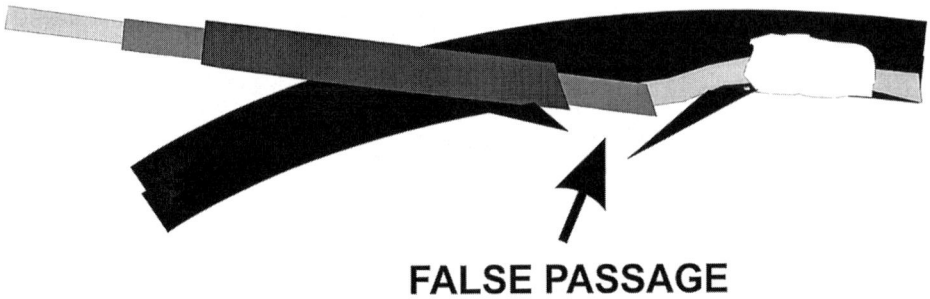

FALSE PASSAGE

Figure 16.4 An example of false passage during the counterpressure technique. A complication may be associated with a tear outside the vein or heart wall with haemorrhaging. Bleeding into the thoracic cavity causes loss of blood volume, while bleeding into the pericardium can result in tamponade.

Counterpressure and countertraction are applied by the sheaths in the superior veins; countertraction is also applied at the myocardium.

Passage of the telescoping sheaths through the superior veins and to the heart involves both counterpressure and countertraction. When the sheaths are against only the binding tissue within the veins and heart, countertraction is applied. Countertraction will dilate and/or tear the binding tissue. This is usually a safe procedure. In contrast, when the sheaths are only partially against the binding tissue, counter-

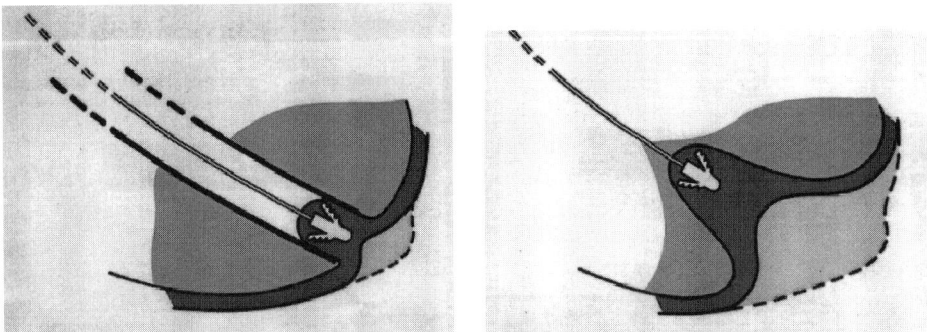

Figure 16.5 The principle of countertraction. Left: countertraction. Right: manual traction.

pressure is applied. Counterpressure will tear the binding tissue and/or peel it off the wall.

Passage of the sheaths through the veins and heart requires experience and judgement to avoid tearing the wall and creating a false passage. This is the dangerous part of a lead extraction. Although tearing the wall is theoretically possible for both countertraction and counterpressure, the shearing force caused by counter-pressure intuitively seems to pose the greater risk. The author has experienced two sheath-related tears of the distal superior vena cava resulting in pericardial tampo-nade. It could not be determined whether countertraction or counterpressure caused the longitudinal tear in the vein wall.

Removal of the lead from the implantation site on the heart wall involves only countertraction, and is generally safe when judiciously applied. The outer sheath is placed 1–2 cm from the heart wall and held stationary while traction is carefully applied. The heart wall is pulled against the sheaths with only the fibrous tissue between the sheath and the heart wall. When the electrode is torn free from this tissue, it is pulled into the sheath and the heart wall falls away. The author has not torn an atrial or ventricular wall using countertraction.

In some cases, the telescoping sheaths cannot be passed over the lead through the superior veins into the heart. Examples include a broken or cut lead that is completely intravascular, or a lead whose fibrous binding tissue has a tensile strength greater than that of the lead or greater than the forces that can be safely applied within the superior veins. Excessive force misdirected in the superior veins can result in a tear of the contiguous artery or rupture into the thoracic cavity; either causes massive haemorrhage. Consequently, alternative approaches were developed to remove these leads.

The transfemoral approach, transatrial approach and ventriculotomy are altern-atives to lead extraction using a superior approach. The transfemoral approach uses sheaths and snares passed through a percutaneous puncture into a femoral vein. It eliminates the need to advance sheaths through the binding sites in the superior veins. With the transfemoral approach, a portion of free lead body in the atrium is surrounded by a reversible loop made by the snares (Figure 16.6). (The loop should not be passed in the superior veins unless the lead is free of binding tissue.) In most cases, if a lead can be snared using a reversible loop in the atrium, the lead or lead remnant can be pulled down from the superior veins into the atrium by pulling on the lead body. The sheath is pushed against the lead body, binding the lead. As the lead is pulled into the atrium, the reversible loop is loosened, and the loop is manoeuvred more proximal on the lead body (toward the superior veins). The lead body is again bound by the sheath, and the lead is pulled further down. This sequence is repeated until the lead is freed from the superior veins and pulled into the atrium or inferior vena cava (IVC). It is important during such manoeuvres to apply traction only to the lead body in the superior veins; traction on the electrode at the heart wall is to be avoided.

When the proximal end of the lead has been freed and pulled into the atrium or IVC, the lead body is re-grasped by a stronger snare, such as the Dotter. Counter-pressure and countertraction are used to manoeuvre the sheaths to a site near the electrode and the electrode is removed by countertraction. This approach bypasses the

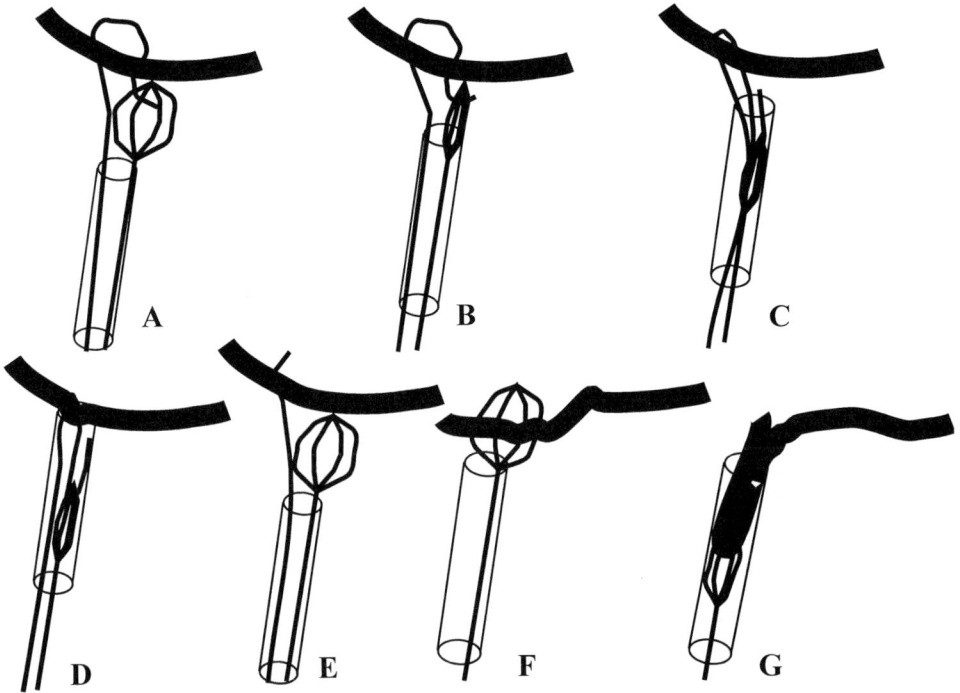

Figure 16.6 The snare technique. One way to construct a reversible loop is to use a Cook deflection catheter, a Cook Dotter basket snare and plastic sheaths. The snares make a reversible loop around the lead body, binding it against the plastic sheaths. The loosened loop is advanced proximally on the lead and pulled out of the superior veins. Although the reversible loop was originally used as an adjunct to the transfemoral approach, it is also used to snare and remove intravascular leads through the superior veins (vein entry site). The procedures include (A) curving the deflection sheath around the lead body, (B) entangling the deflection catheter in the Dotter basket snare, (C) pulling the Dotter snare into the plastic sheaths, closing the basket and tightly gripping the tip of the deflection catheter and (D) binding the lead body against the entrance to the plastic sheaths. Traction is then applied pulling the lead out of the superior veins. Care is taken not to pull on the electrode at the heart wall. The loop is loosened as needed to manoeuvre up the lead body. Once the lead is out of the superior veins (E), the loop is reversed and the deflection catheter removed (F). The proximal lead tip is entangled in the Dotter snare and (G) the Dotter basket is pulled into the plastic sheaths by gripping the lead and dragging it into the plastic sheaths for removal by mechanical and/or laser ablation.

superior veins. It is preferred by many extractors, since it avoids the danger of a misadventure in the superior veins. The transfemoral approach is more complicated and can take considerable time to manipulate the snares.

The transatrial approach (Figure 16.7) combines cardiac surgery with counter-pressure and countertraction techniques. Through a small incision (<6 cm), the third or fourth costal cartilage is removed, the pericardium opened and the atrium exposed. Through a purse-string suture, the leads are grasped by an instrument and pulled out of the superior veins and out the atriotomy. Telescoping sheaths are then passed over the leads to remove them from the heart wall.

The transatrial approach is used both as a primary and a secondary approach.[20] For example, patients with an occluded superior vena cava would have removal of old

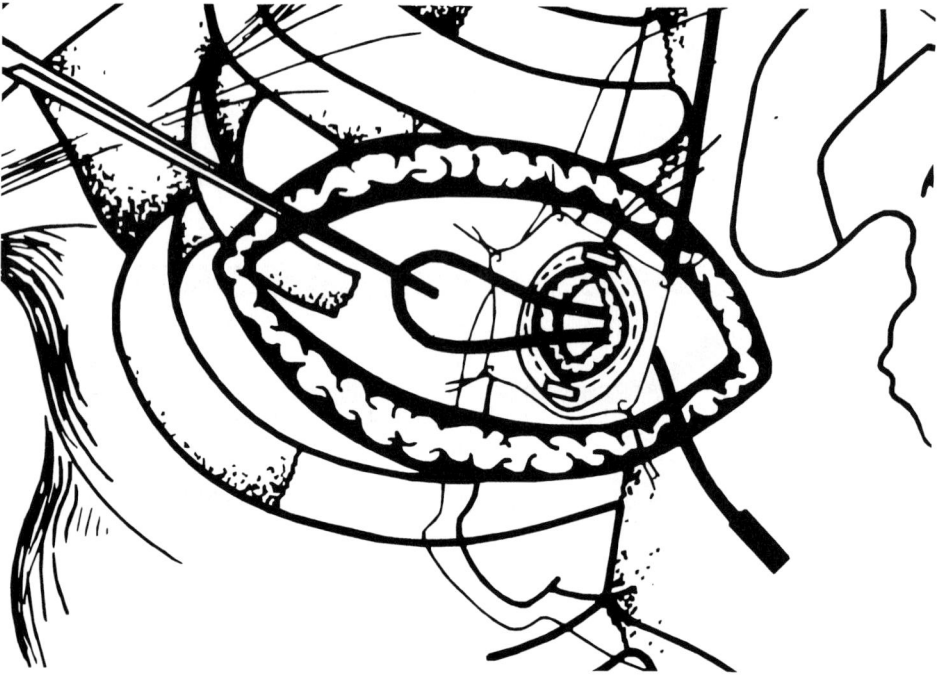

Figure 16.7   The transatrial approach.

leads and insertion of new leads through the transatrial approach. It is a way of implanting state-of-the-art bipolar transvenous pacing leads into the heart without using the superior veins.

A ventriculotomy is used only as a last resort. For example, when an infected lead breaks within the heart and septicaemia persists, a ventriculotomy is used to remove that lead segment. Through a median sternotomy, the right ventricle is exposed. A stab wound is made over the electrode, which is grasped and the lead remnant pulled out of the heart. Cardiopulmonary bypass is not required for this procedure.

Laser Ablation Device for Lead Extraction

Recently, laser ablation has become a viable method for lead removal, using an excimer laser sheath developed by Spectranetics Inc. (Colorado Springs, CO, USA). After locking a stylet inside the coil lumen of the lead, the excimer laser sheath, in conjunction with an outer sheath, is manoeuvred over the lead to a binding site (Figure 16.8). The encapsulating fibrous tissue at the binding site is ablated (vaporized). The xenon-chloride laser emits electromagnetic radiation at 308 nm. This radiation causes photochemical disruption of many protein bonds and vaporizes water molecules. The photochemical action and vaporization of water is so rapid that tissue is fragmented into microscopic particulate matter and carried away by the

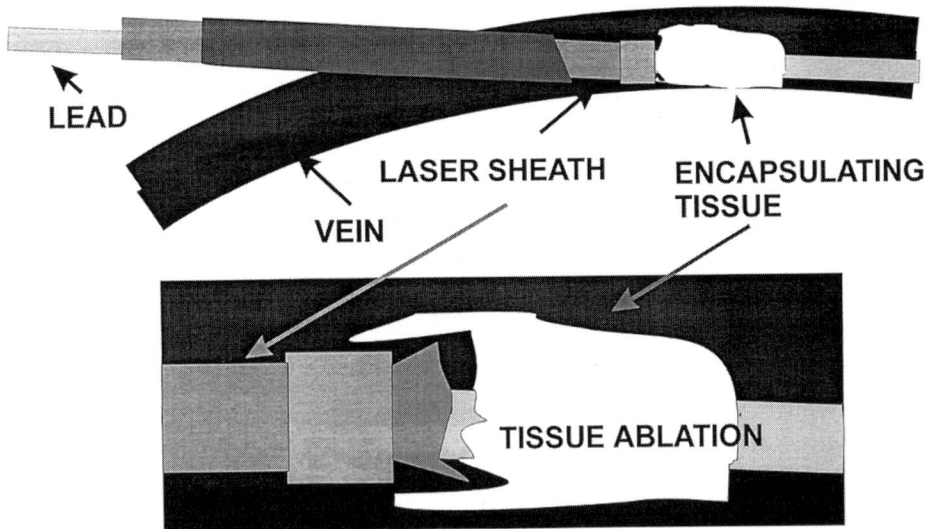

Figure 16.8   Principle of the Spectranetics excimer laser.

bloodstream (ablated). The excimer laser is capable of ablating all encapsulating tissues except deposits of calcium phosphate or carbonate.

The purpose of the excimer laser sheath is to replace those counterpressure and countertraction techniques used to pass sheaths to the heart wall. Mechanical force is replaced by laser ablation. All accessible leads not encapsulated in calcium salts can theoretically be removed from the superior veins. The electrode is still removed from the heart wall using countertraction (mechanical ablation). Most leads can be removed intact using laser ablation, since the tensile strength of the lead need only be sufficient to allow manoeuvring of the laser sheath.

Sheaths are not currently available for a transfemoral approach. Alternative approaches are rarely needed when the excimer laser sheath is available. However, for those leads that break or for leads which were left within the vascular system, snares are passed through the sheaths at the vein entry site. The snares and sheaths are manoeuvred in the same manner as for a transfemoral approach. Once the lead body is entrapped in a snare, the laser sheath is passed over the snare and lead, ablating the encapsulating tissue.

Ten-Year Experience: The Byrd Database

About the Database

Over a 10-year period (June 1986 to June 1995), 842 procedures were performed by the author on 764 patients, removing 1369 leads (Figures 16.9–16.14). These results reflect a consecutive experience, first using mechanical ablation extraction devices, and later using laser ablation devices as well. The experience with mechanical ablation is not only more extensive, but is representative of an established extraction technique.[21] The mechanical devices were developed early in the series and underwent only minor modifications thereafter. The superior vena cava (via vein entry site), inferior vena cava (transfemoral) and transatrial approaches were also developed early in the experience. For the majority of patients in the mechanical ablation series, therefore, the procedures were performed in much the same fashion as they are today. In contrast, the laser ablation experience is less extensive and more variable; it consists of the developmental stages of the excimer laser sheath and the evolution of the procedures from the first human extractions up to the procedure as used today.

The results may be influenced by the order in which leads were removed. Easier leads were generally removed first (leads implanted for a short duration before older leads, and atrial leads before ventricular leads of similar implant duration). A short-duration lead that was reimplanted in a chronic site was considered to have the implant duration of the chronic site, as previously discussed. Since removing one lead sometimes helps to free the other leads, it is logical to start with the easier leads. If leads have equal size and tensile strength, it is generally harder to remove a ventricular lead than an atrial lead. This is because there are more binding sites associated with a ventricular lead.

A limit of this database is that it records removal of a maximum of three leads during a single procedure (an atrial lead, a ventricular lead and a 'third lead' that may be atrial or ventricular). If more than three leads were removed, the additional leads were not recorded. (If a complication occurred during the removal of a fourth, fifth or sixth lead, the complication-related lead was included in the database as the third lead.) It is anticipated that the errors incurred by this limitation do not significantly affect the analysis, since only 12% of the patients had three leads removed and much fewer had four or more leads.

During the 10-year period, 764 patients underwent 842 procedures, indicating that more than one procedure was performed on 10% of the patients (Figure 16.9). Most of the patients who underwent multiple procedures presented with another lead problem years after their first procedure. A few had multiple procedures during the same admission to remove their leads. For example, infected leads would be removed on one day, and noninfected leads removed on another day when new leads were implanted. The percentage of atrial and ventricular leads removed were about equal (Figure 16.9).

The number of leads removed annually has recently increased (Figure 16.10). This reflects both an increase in the recognition and treatment of device-related complications and an increase in the number of leads under recall. The number of leads under recall being removed prior to reimplantation of a new lead has increased. In addition, because the Accufix™ and Encor™ leads are potentially destructive, many of those leads were removed prophylactically.

Extraction Approach

Figure 16.11 shows the approaches used to remove the 1369 leads. The majority, 1104 leads (80.64%), were removed from the vein entry site (superior vena cava approach).

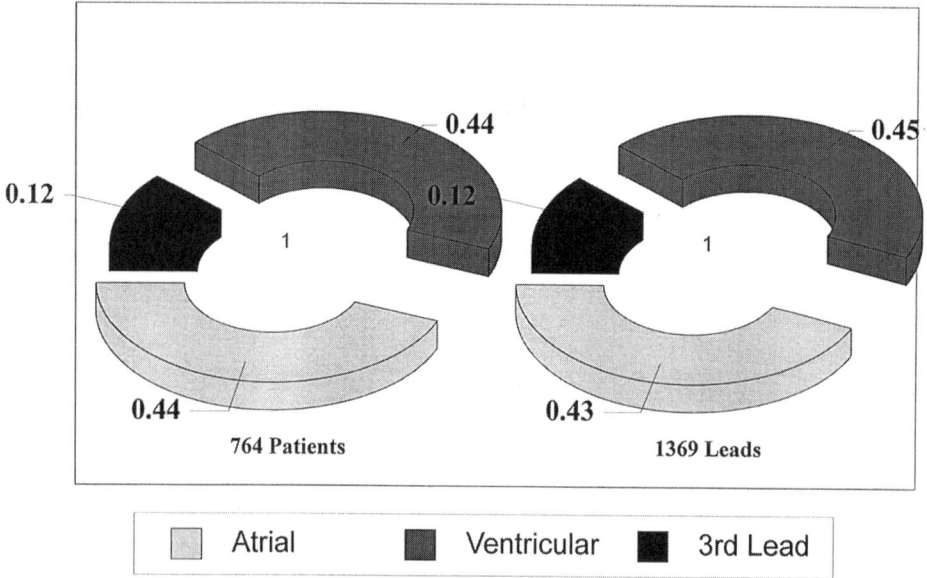

Figure 16.9 Byrd database: patients *vs* leads.

The transfemoral approach was used to remove 203 leads (14.83%). Only 62 leads (4.53%) were removed using the transatrial approach. These results reflect the author's personal preference to remove leads from the vein entry site when possible.

Utilization of the superior approach varied with respect to the type of lead removed. Use of the vein entry (SVC) approach decreased from 88.91% for 595 atrial

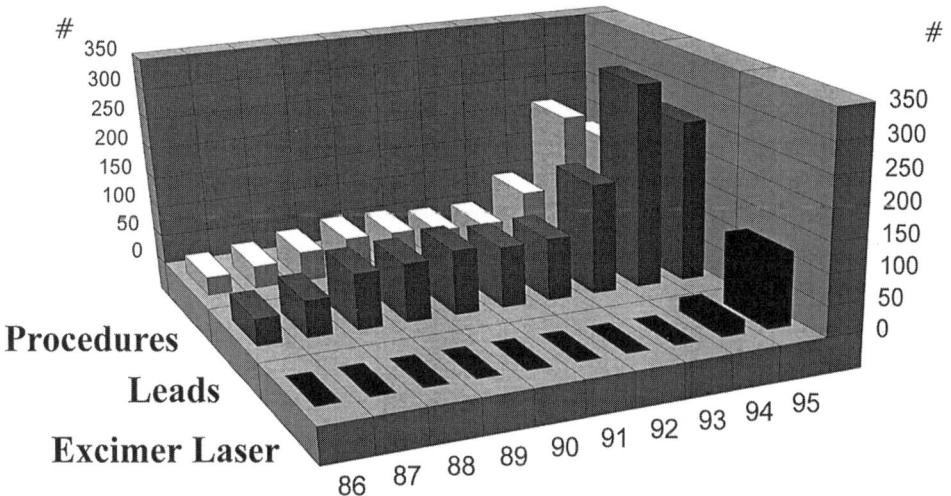

Figure 16.10 Byrd database: the course of the 10-year experience.

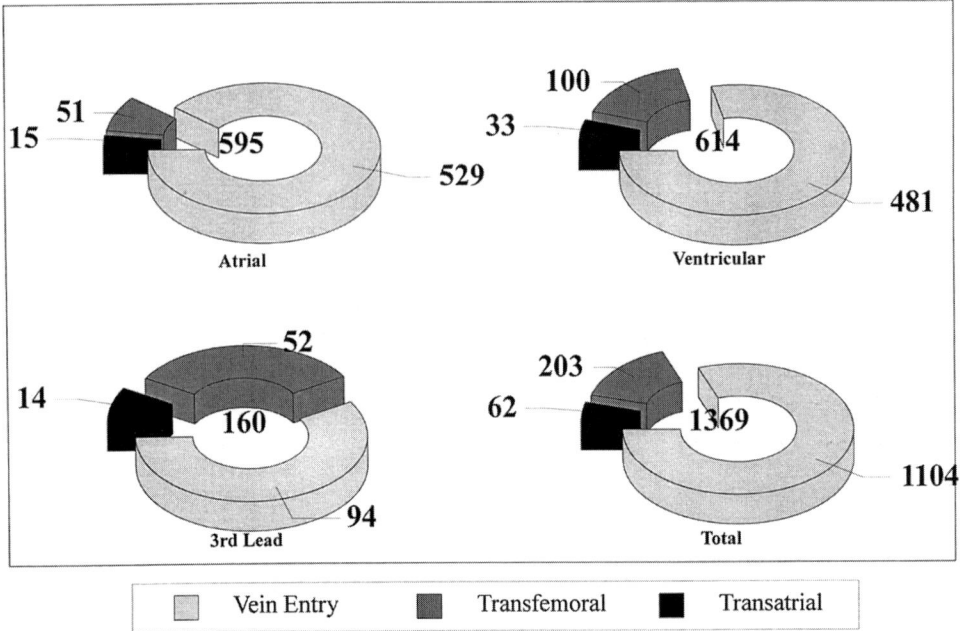

Figure 16.11   Byrd database: breakdown of lead extraction processes adopted.

leads, to 78.34% for 614 ventricular leads and to 58.75% for 160 third leads. Conversely, usage of the transfemoral (IVC) approach increased from 8.57% for atrial leads, to 16.29% for ventricular leads and to 32.50% for third leads. Usage of the transatrial approach showed a similar pattern: 2.52% for atrial leads, 5.37% for ventricular leads and 8.75% for third leads.

This change in the extraction approach with respect to lead group is related to three factors: binding sites, lead disruption and accessibility from the vein entry site. Duration of implant, number of leads implanted and lead size and stiffness are factors that increase the amount and tensile strength of the encapsulating binding tissue. Leads are bound to each other and to the heart wall. The inability to safely manoeuvre the telescoping sheaths past a binding site is intuitively obvious. However, the type of sheath used does influence the forces applied. Stainless steel sheaths were used at the vein entry site. An unlimited amount of force can be transmitted using these sheaths. The failure rate for actually entering the venous system is low. Also, this is a relatively safe region to apply force. No complications were encountered passing these sheaths into the subclavian vein. Before the vein path curved, the stainless steel sheaths were changed to the more malleable Teflon® sheaths. Within the subclavian vein, creation of a false passage following a misadventure with the sheaths is possible. The malleable Teflon® sheaths helped limit the applied force. Significant damage to the tips of these sheaths when trying to pass a binding site was generally considered a failure for the superior approach, and the transfemoral or transatrial approach was then tried.

Lead disruption is a relative factor in the extraction approach. Lead disruption is a function of lead fragility. In many early lead models, ventricular leads were more fragile than atrial leads. For most lead extractions, lead disruption was not a factor as long as traction could be applied. Lead disruption became an indication to change from mechanical ablation to laser ablation. In some situations, sheaths could not be passed over lead disruption sites because of the insulation being pushed forward. This is called a 'snow plow effect'. The insulation was pushed forward, forming a mass too large for the sheaths to pass. In this situation, an alternative was sometimes necessary.

The approach used depends on the availability of venous access. If the superior vein on the implant side cannot be accessed, an alternative approach is necessary. In many cases this vein was available either from a vena puncture using an introducer or from a sheath left in place. For example, if a lead had been removed via the vein entry site and a sheath was left in the vein, snares could be passed down that sheath and used to extract an intravascular lead. Intravascular leads could be extracted by entrapment in snares and the passage of sheaths over the snares to the lead. This technique was perfected for the transfemoral approach, but worked just as well when applied through the superior veins (cephalic, subclavian or jugular).

Leads were removed from the heart wall using countertraction, traction and, in some situations, a combination of both. Removal by countertraction is the preferred method. Only those leads implanted for 6 months or less were removed preferentially by manual traction (pulling on the lead). After 6 months, the telescoping Teflon® sheaths were used with the intention to remove the leads by countertraction. The leads were occasionally freed from the heart wall by the traction forces used in manoeuvring the telescoping Teflon® sheaths through the binding sites. When this occurred, the lead was said to have been removed using manual traction. Lead removal from the heart wall, using the traction forces required to manipulate the Teflon® sheaths, appears to be generally safe. In this series, there were no accidents attributed to manual traction when used in this fashion. The malleable Teflon® sheaths seem to act as a crude traction gauge, giving an indication of, and a limit to, the amount of force applied.

A combination of countertraction and manual traction was responsible for freeing some electrodes from the heart wall. For example, countertraction was applied to exuberant binding tissue close to the heart wall, yet during manipulation of the sheaths the electrode was freed by manual traction. In this situation, it is unclear which method was actually responsible for freeing the electrode. Electrodes freed in this fashion were classified as removed by 'combined' techniques.

Figure 16.12 shows the data for freeing leads from the heart wall. For 1369 leads, countertraction was used for 948 (69.25%), manual traction for 368 (26.88%) and a combination in only 53 (3.87%). The high incidence of manual traction is attributable to the atrial leads: 238 atrial leads (40% of the atrial leads) were freed from the myocardium by manual traction. This is due to the increased incidence of active fixation devices and to a large number of Telectronics Accufix™ leads being removed, most of which had been implanted for less than 4 years. The incidence of extractions using countertraction increased with the difficulty factor. In contrast to the atrial leads, countertraction was used for 76.87% of the ventricular leads removed, and 86.25% of the third leads removed.

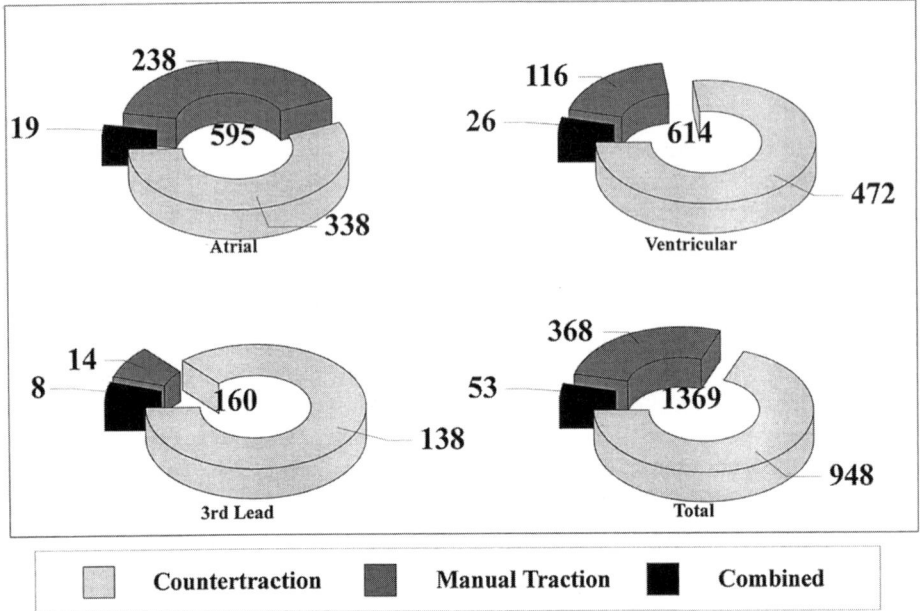

Figure 16.12   Byrd database: lead extraction from heart walls.

Excimer Laser Experience

Figure 16.13 shows the incidence of mechanical ablation, manual traction and excimer laser ablation extraction techniques. The Spectranetics excimer laser was used only during the last 2 years of this study to remove 142 leads (10.37% of the total 1369 leads). The excimer laser study population is shown in Figure 16.14. This study encompasses both the developmental phase and the author's experience during most of the formal FDA IDE multicentre study.

Throughout the entire study, the performance of the 12Fr excimer laser sheaths has been a positive adjunct to the telescoping sheaths. The inner Teflon® sheath is removed and the laser sheath inserted over the lead. The 16Fr outer Teflon® sheath is an integral part of the extraction procedure. It dilates ablated tissue, helps prevent binding of the laser sheath, is used to apply countertraction at the heart wall and is used as a conduit for reimplanting a new lead through the chronic explant site.

The transfemoral approach, used for 14.8% of the leads removed by mechanical ablation techniques, was not used in conjunction with the excimer laser. The implication is that laser ablation is more effective than mechanical ablation in passing through the superior vein binding sites with less force. The transatrial approach was used as a primary approach in conjunction with laser ablation in only two patients, removing three leads.

Because laser ablation has been more effective in removing leads intact, the author's expectations regarding complete removal of the lead have changed during the laser ablation study. Using mechanical ablation, the incidence of lead disruption at or near

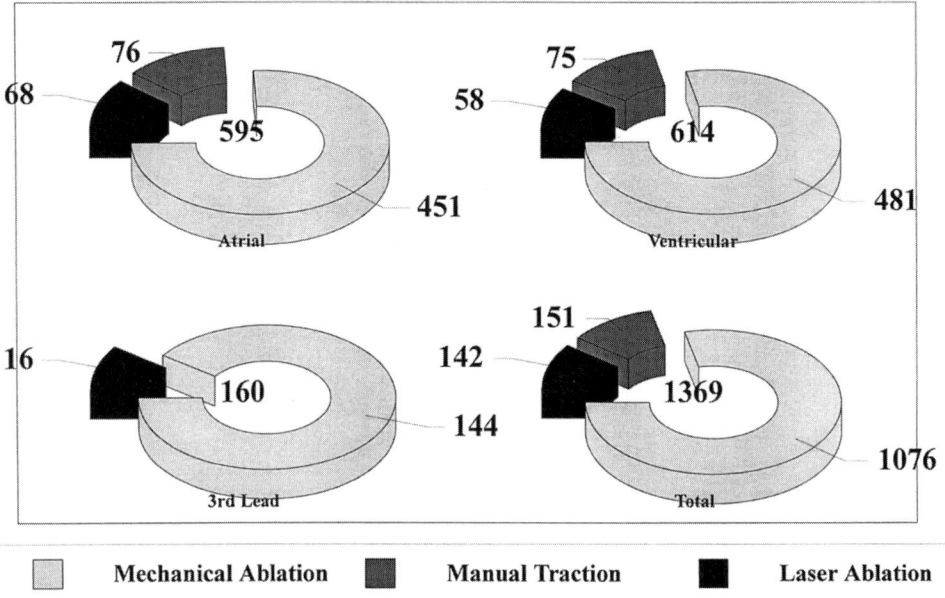

| | Mechanical Ablation | | Manual Traction | | Laser Ablation |

Figure 16.13 Byrd database: conventional *vs* excimer laser sheaths (summary of first- and second-generation devices).

the electrode was about 11%; lead fragments were snared using a transfemoral approach in some of these cases, but one or more electrodes was left implanted for 7%. Although only one patient with an infected lead, in whom a portion of insulation was also left behind, required later removal of the remaining fragment, the obvious preference is to remove the lead intact. For all but 1 of the 142 leads removed with laser ablation, intact removal of the lead was achieved. Using laser ablation, the author has come to expect complete removal of the lead in nearly all cases.

Experience with Complications

In the 10-year experience outlined above, there were no deaths attributed to the lead extraction procedure. Two patients had tears, one of the SVC and the other of the right atrium (Table 16.7). Both patients required an emergency median sternotomy and a surgical repair. Three patients developed pericardial effusion requiring drainage. Of these, one had a puncture of the right atrium sustained after the lead extraction, while reinserting a new lead. This complication may be unique to laser extraction procedures. One hypothesis is that the laser cores out a tunnel around the old lead. A replacement lead reinserted through this tunnel creates a false passage through the tunnel wall into the pericardium or into the right chest. To avoid this complication, the outer extraction sheath should be left in the right atrium and the replacement lead inserted through this conduit. The sheath can then be safely removed and split to free the lead.

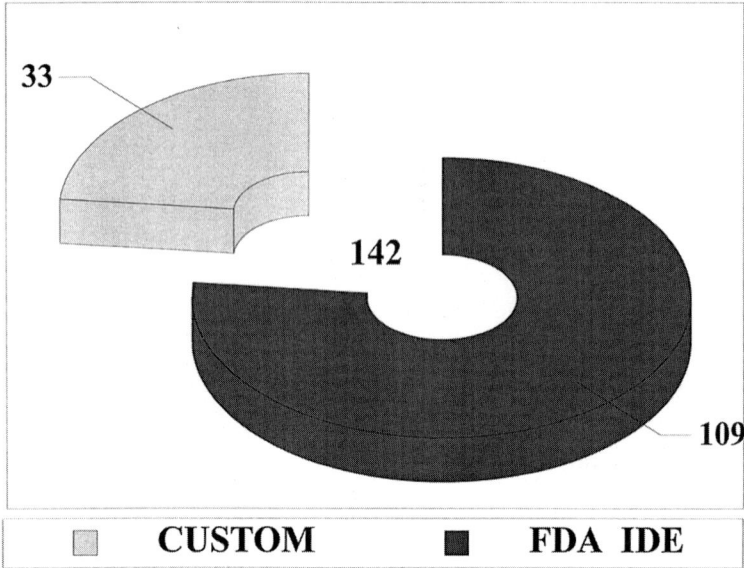

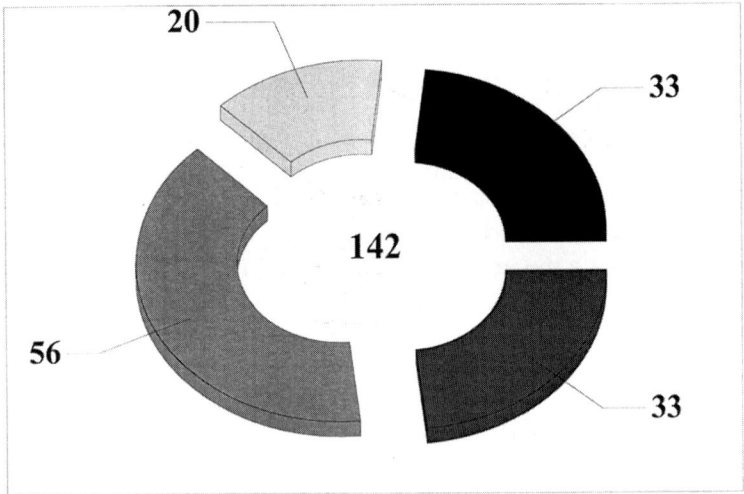

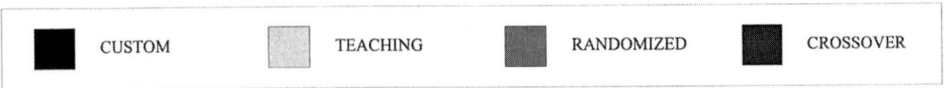

Figure 16.14 Byrd database of the Spectranetics excimer laser study on 84 patients.

In two patients pericardial effusions developed slowly, following uneventful lead extractions. In these patients, the leads were removed from the atrium by unscrewing the active fixation device and the leads fell free of the wall. These effusions were probably the result of bleeding from the fixation site. The incidence of this complication may be higher if the effusion is small and does not cause sufficient symptoms.

Table 16.7 Complications from haemorrhage

Number	Complication	Remarks
2	Tear of superior vena cava and tear of the right atrium	Median sternotomy and surgical repair
1	Puncture of SVC while reinserting a new pacing lead	Pericardial drainage
2	Patent active fixation device at implantation site	Pericardial drainage

Four deaths are known to have occurred within 4 weeks of the extraction procedure (Table 16.8). These deaths were considered related to underlying disease rather than to the extraction procedure. Pulmonary emboli (the cause of two deaths) was initially thought by the author to be a possible complication of extraction, especially when using the transfemoral approach. This worry was responsible for the transfemoral workstation concept and the emphasis upon avoiding retained debris at the femoral vein puncture site. However, both patients who died from pulmonary emboli had documented pulmonary emboli within weeks of the procedure. One patient was admitted in a coma secondary to a pulmonary embolus. Upon recovery from the coma, the patient was transferred with septicaemia (without vegetation) for lead removal. The lead removal was uneventful. However, immediately after extraction, the patient had massive pulmonary emboli from the inferior veins. The chest was opened, but the distal emboli in the pulmonary veins could not be removed and the patient died. This was confirmed at autopsy. The second patient has a pulmonary embolus associated with an attempted removal of infected leads about 7 days prior to a transfer for this procedure. The leads were removed, but the patient died 3 days postoperatively, prior to discharge. The rationale for excluding the lead extraction procedure as a cause of death for these two patients is that both had recent pulmonary emboli and there was nothing remarkable about the extraction procedure. The two other patients would probably have died of their concomitant disease processes. The lead extraction just corrected one of their pre-existing problems.

Table 16.8 Deaths from concomitant disease processes

Cause	Number	Remarks
Pulmonary embolus	2	Patients admitted from other institutions with diagnosis of acute pulmonary emboli from the inferior veins and septicaemia from an intravascular pacemaker lead infection; both patients died from recurrent pulmonary emboli (one died immediately and one died 3 days after surgery)
Congestive heart failure	1	Patient with severe COPD and CHF had an infected pacing system removed and a new pacemaker implanted 36 hours later; the initial recovery was uneventful and the patient was discharged on the second postoperative day; 2 weeks after discharge the patient developed heart failure and died
Unknown	1	28-year-old female with a corrected transposition of great vessels was rushed to a hospital emergency room 4 weeks after atrial lead removal and reimplantation; patient was pronounced dead without determining a cause; a post-mortem examination showed the cardiovascular system intact; a reason for the death was not determined

There are cardiovascular complications associated with lead extraction. These complications are caused by tearing of the veins and/or heart with bleeding into the chest and/or pericardial space. When they occur, it is imperative that emergency procedures be immediately instituted. Delays result in excessive blood loss into the chest cavity and/or cardiac tamponade. A prolonged period of poor perfusion will result in irreversible organ damage and death. It is recommended that leads only be removed in those environments where an emergency median sternotomy and/or thoracotomy can be performed in an expeditious fashion. Such an environment reduces the risk of the procedure to an acceptable level (with the risk of death approaching zero). This level of risk reduction must be approached if justification is to be found for removing superfluous leads.

Conclusions

The use of telescoping sheaths, the techniques for using those sheaths, the uses of snares in combination with the sheaths and, finally, the application of countertraction to separate the electrode from the heart wall, are all mechanical ablation techniques. Laser ablation is just a refinement of mechanical ablation techniques. Photoablation replaces the use of force at the binding sites. The author's database supports the contention that these techniques are efficacious and can be safe, although appropriate precautions must always be taken.

The best method of removing leads intact today seems to be laser ablation. Regarding the potential for complications, a larger patient experience with laser ablation must be accrued before it is possible to determine whether the complication rates vary with the technique used.

The best method for removing leads will continue to change as the technology improves. New technologies, such as electrosurgical ablation, await clinical evaluation. With each improvement, the goal of a consistently safe and efficacious transvenous lead extraction device comes closer to becoming a clinical reality.

References

1. Byrd CL. Management of implant complications. In: Ellenbogen KA, Kay GN, Wilkoff BL (eds), *Clinical Cardiac Pacing*. Philadelphia, PA: WB Saunders, 1995: 491–522.
2. Byrd CL, Schwartz SJ, Hedin NB. Lead extraction: techniques and indications. In: Barold SS, Mugica J (eds), *New Perspectives in Cardiac Pacing*. Mount Kisco, NY: Futura, 1993: 29–55.
3. Byrd CL, Schwartz SJ, Hedin N. Lead extraction: indications and techniques. *Cardiol Clin* 1992; **10**: 735–48.
4. Byrd CL, Schwartz SJ, Hedin N. Intravascular techniques for extraction of permanent pacemaker leads. *J Thorac Cardiovasc Surg* 1991; **101**: 989–97.
5. Anderson JM. Inflammatory response to implants. *ASAIO* 1988; **11**(2): 101–7.
6. Robboy SJ, Harthorne JW, Leinbach RC, *et al.* Autopsy findings with permanent pervenous pacemakers. *Circulation* 1969; **39**: 495–501.
7. Huang TY, Baba N. Cardiac pathology of transvenous pacemakers. *Am Heart J* 1972; **83**: 469–74.

8. Fishbein MC, Tan KS, Beazell JW, *et al.* Cardiac pathology of transvenous pacemakers in dogs. *Am Heart J* 1977; **93**: 73–81.
9. Schoen FJ, Harasaki J, Kim KM, Anderson C, *et al.* Biomaterial-associated calcification: pathology, mechanisms, and strategies for prevention. *J Biomed Mater Res: Appl Biomat* 1988; **22**(A1): 11–36.
10. Becker AE, Becker MJ, Caludon DG, *et al.* Surface thrombosis and fibrous encapsulation of intravenous pacemaker catheter electrode. *Circulation* 1972; **46**: 409–12.
11. Mazzetti H, Dussaut A, Tentori C, *et al.* Superior vena cava occlusion and/or syndrome related to pacemaker leads. *Am Heart J* 1993; **125**: 831–7.
12. Yakirevich V, Alagem D, Papo J, *et al.* Fibrotic stenosis of the superior vena cava with widespread thrombotic occlusion of its major tributaries: an unusual complication of transvenous cardiac pacing. *J Thorac Cardiovasc Surg* 1983; **85**: 632–4.
13. Doty DB, Doty JR, Jones KW. Bypass of superior vena cava: fifteen years' experience with spiral vein graft for obstruction of superior vena cava caused by benign disease. *J Thorac Cardiovasc Surg* 1990; **99**: 889–95.
14. Pauletti M, Di Ricco G, Solfanelli S, *et al.* Venous obstruction in permanent pacemaker patients: an isotopic study. *PACE* 1981; **4**: 36–42.
15. Byrd C. Rationale for the management of pacemaker and defibrillator complications. In: Oto MA (ed.), *Practice and Progress in Cardiac Pacing and Electrophysiology.* Dordrecht: Kluwer Academic, 1996; 239–48.
16. Goldstein A, Keats AS. The risk of anesthesia. *Anesthesiology* 1970; **33**: 125.
17. Furman S, Behrens M, Andrews C, *et al.* Retained pacemaker leads. *J Thorac Cardiovasc Surg* 1987; **94**: 770–2.
18. Fearnot NE, Smith HJ, Goode LB, *et al.* Intravascular lead extraction using locking stylets, sheaths, and other techniques. *PACE* 1990; **13**: 1864–70.
19. Byrd CL, Schwartz SJ, Hedin NB, *et al.* Intravascular lead extraction using locking stylets and sheaths. *PACE* 1990; **13**: 1871–2.
20. Byrd CL, Schwartz SJ, Sivina M, *et al.* Technique for the surgical extraction of permanent pacing leads and electrodes. *J Thorac Cardiovasc Surg* 1985; **89**: 142–4.
21. Sellers TD, Smith HJ, Fearnot NE, *et al.* Intravascular lead extraction: technique tips and US database results. *PACE* 1993; **16**: 1538.

17

Interaction Between a Pacemaker and an Implantable Cardioverter–Defibrillator

M. Fromer

Implantable cardioverter–defibrillators (ICDs) are designed to prevent sudden cardiac death. They do so by delivering an electrical discharge either via epicardial patches or via endocardial electrodes or both. Since the introduction of the third generation of ICDs in 1989,[1,2] the devices are also capable of ventricular stimulation with discrete pulses (Figure 17.1), either in the form of a rapid burst to break ventricular tachycardia or as ordinary pacemaker stimuli. The pacing function serves primarily to prevent shock-induced bradycardia or to prevent bradycardia or asystole. To focus a book chapter on ICDs and pacemakers implies that there is a potential harmful interaction between them.

Why is Pacing Therapy Needed in ICD Patients?

It is not the aim of this chapter to discuss antitachycardia pacing, but rather to address the issue of pacemaker therapy and pacemaker function in the global setting of ICD therapy.

The prevention of asystole is important in the prevention of sudden cardiac death (SCD). Holter recordings in victims of SCD have shown that asystole or brady-arrhythmias precede cardiac arrest in about 16% of the patients.[3] Severe bradycardia and electromechanical dissociation was seen in 62% of 21 cardiac-arrest patients suffering from advanced heart failure.[4] In addition, ageing of the population and ageing of the ICD patients increases the need of pacemaking therapy. The magnitude of the problem can also be estimated by the experience gained by Winkle et al.:[5] in their series 11% of the ICD patients also required pacemaker therapy against bradycardia, 17% in another group of 170 ICD patients[6] and fewer than 10% in a group of patients with nonthoracotomy leads.[7]

In the majority of ICD models actually available, simple programmable VVI pacing is on offer. Using 100% VVI pacing reduces ICD longevity considerably. Progress in

'219 CHART SPEED 25.0 mm/s

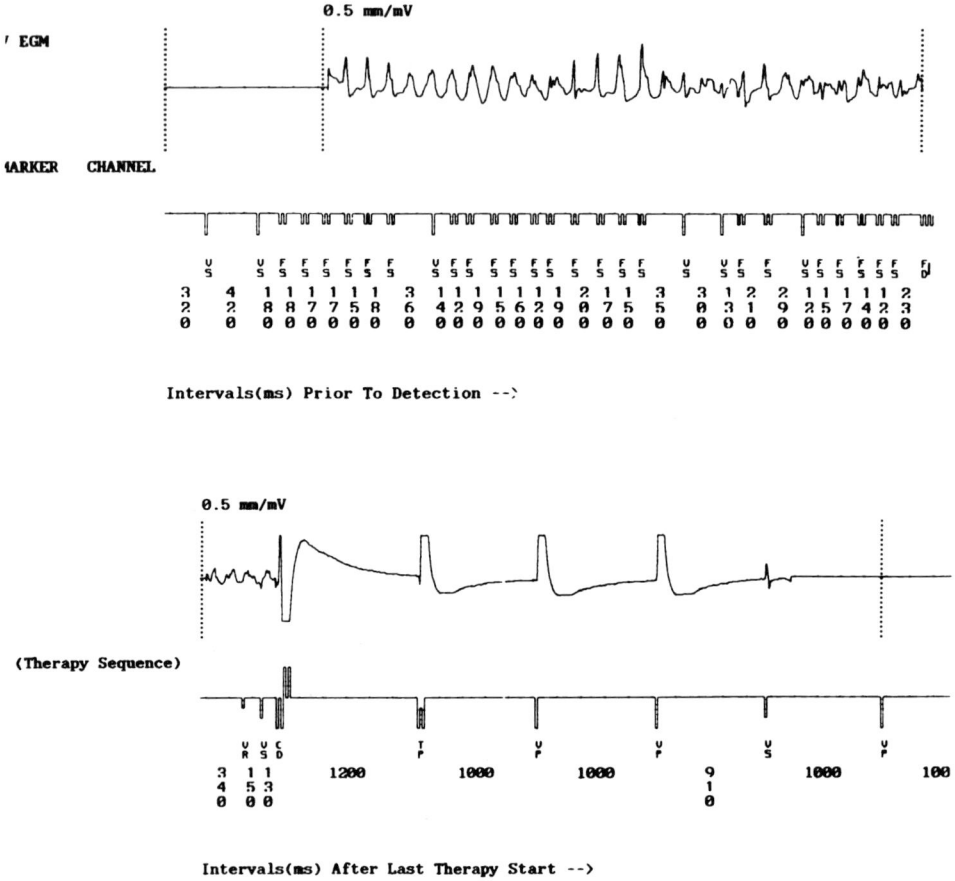

Figure 17.1 A spontaneous ventricular fibrillation episode, detected and terminated by an implantable defibrillator, a Medtronic PCD model 7219. After the high-voltage shock, there is a sinus bradycardia detected and VVI backup pacing is shown. The RR intervals are measured by the device in milliseconds.

device technology will allow us to incorporate rate-responsive VVI pacing and dual-chamber pacing, hopefully without compromising substantially ICD longevity. It can be anticipated that in 1997 various manufacturers will have such devices available. However, at time of indication for ICD therapy the need for additional dual-chamber pacing might not be obvious. This means that during the course of ICD therapy in some ICD patients, separate pacemakers will be implanted to treat sinus node dysfunction, bradycardic atrial fibrillation and AV conduction blocks. As soon as there are two separate units to be implanted the potential for complication increases. These complications would be mainly related to device function and surgical intervention.

Possible Harmful Device Interactions

Potentially harmful effects of the pacemaker on the ICD and of the ICD on the pacemaker have been observed. Whether these transient malfunctions are clinically important is difficult to assess. The malfunctions mainly consist of:

(a) loss of ventricular capture after ICD discharge;
(b) resetting of pacemaker function owing to ICD shock;
(c) ICD undersensing of ventricular fibrillation owing to continuous pacing during VF;
(d) oversensing of the pacemaker stimulus artefact leading to double counting and spurious VF detection;
(e) oversensing of the paced T-wave leading to double counting and device therapy;
(f) pacing at highest tracking rates during atrial arrhythmias.

Rate-responsive pacing may also lead to an overlap between pacing rate and programmed ventricular tachycardia detection rate.

The following are examples of ICD–pacemaker interactions. Figure 17.2 shows an interaction between a dual-chamber pacemaker and an induced ventricular fibrillation episode. The pacemaker is correctly inhibited during VF and after spontaneous cessation dual-chamber pacemaking reoccurs. Figure 17.3 demonstrates pacemaker dysfunction during ventricular fibrillation and after ICD discharge in a patient with a dual-chamber pacemaker.

Kelly *et al.*[8] reported oversensing during ventricular pacing in 3 out of 85 consecutive patients who were treated with a Ventitrex Cadence™ device and who required permanent antibradycardia pacing. It is important to know that the pacing was delivered by the Cadence™ device itself and not via a separate unit. This oversensing provoked ICD discharges. The authors concluded that this dysfunction was related to a specific feature in this device, whereby sensitivity during pacing is maximally increased to allow detection of low-amplitude arrhythmias. This can finally result in overdetection and overcounting. The implantation of a separate pacemaker solved the problem.

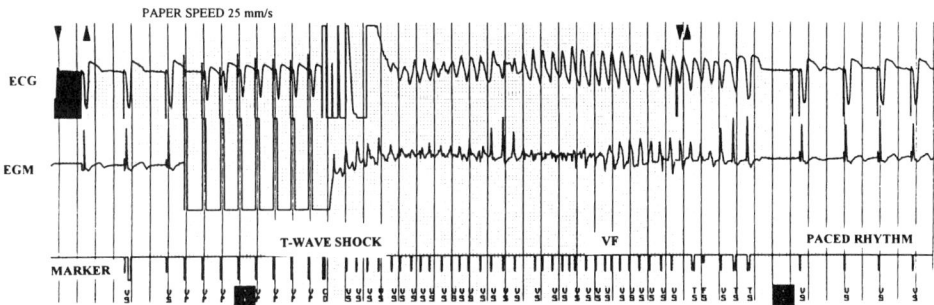

Figure 17.2 Function of a dual-chamber pacemaker and an induced ventricular fibrillation episode. The pacemaker is correctly inhibited during VF, and after spontaneous cessation of VF dual-chamber pacemaking reoccurs.

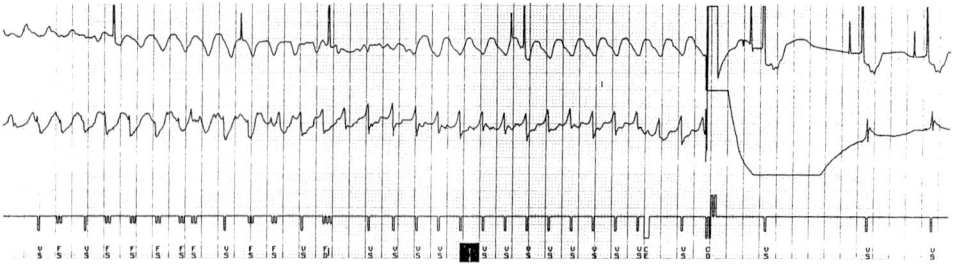

Figure 17.3 Interaction between a dual-chamber pacemaker and an ICD during VF and after a high-voltage discharge. During ventricular fibrillation, pacemaker artefacts are seen; they correspond to atrial and ventricular pacemaker artefacts in variable escape intervals. Assuming that the programmed pacemaker escape interval is 800 ms, there is pacemaker inhibition owing to oversensing after the first atrial and ventricular stimulus, perhaps due to oversensing of a T-wave.

Cohen et al.[9] reported on a small group of patients who had a permanent pacemaker and ICD implanted. The output of pacemaker stimuli during ventricular fibrillation was observed and this provoked delay of ICD discharge. Loss of capture after ICD shock was observed, as well as ICD discharge due to oversensing of pacemaker stimuli. As these series comprised patients with epicardial lead systems, there was no technical difficulty encountered by implanting the endovenous pacemaker leads.

Calkins et al.[6] reported on 30 patients who had an ICD and a pacemaker implanted. They noted: 'Despite a high incidence of transient pacemaker malfunction after defibrillator discharge and a demonstrated potential for double counting of pacemakers spikes and failure of AICD sensing during ventricular fibrillation, these interactions, for the most part, did not become clinically relevant.'

Callans et al.[10] pointed out that undersensing of a spontaneous sinus beat or of ventricular extrasystoles that trigger a pacemaker stimulus can lead to short–long–short coupling sequences with an important arrhythmic potential.

The above dysfunctions relate to the techniques available then. Today, sensing in ICDs is either true bipolar or integrated bipolar, and so is more accurate and less influenced by environmental signals. In pacemakers, bipolar sensing and pacing is available and more pacemakers today resist high-voltage discharges without resetting.

Surgical Aspects

The implantation of a transvenous ICD lead in patients who already have a pacemaker lead implanted at the right ventricular apex may cause some technical difficulties. Brooks et al.[7] reported on 11 of 177 patients with a nonthoracotomy lead system who also required pacemaker therapy. The authors remarked that pacemaker leads previously implanted at the apex interfered with the insertion of the endocavitary ICD lead, and vice versa. Indeed, placement of the ICD lead in these conditions is technically more difficult. It is preferable that the two leads be placed distant from one

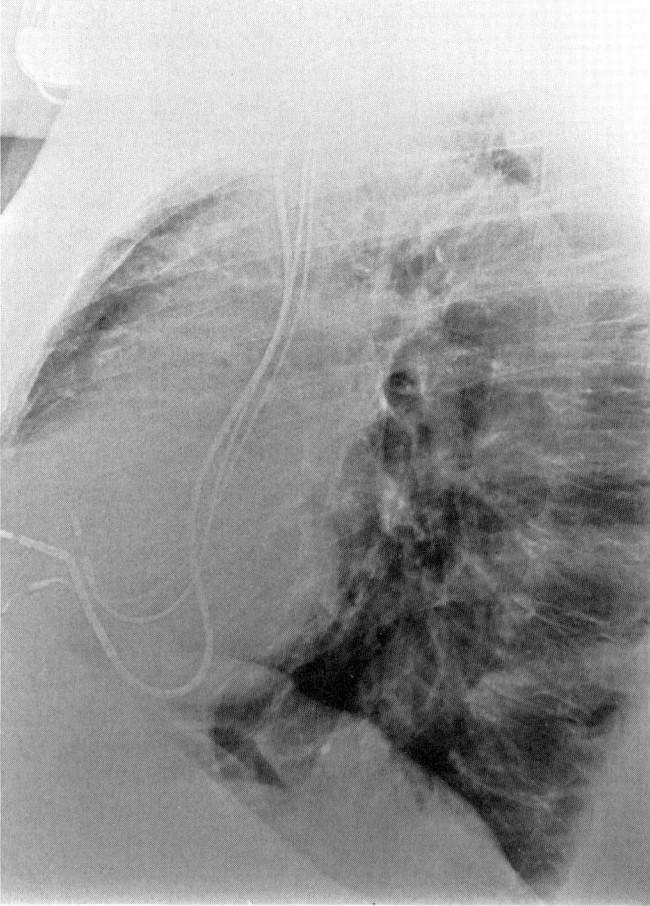

Figure 17.4 Lateral chest X-ray of a patient with a dual-chamber pacemaker lead system (right atrium and right ventricle) and a tripolar defibrillation lead. The active fixation defibrillation lead is implanted in the anterior septal area of the right ventricle. The ICD and pacemaker leads are separated from each other and both leads provide truly bipolar sensing.

another. One could direct either lead towards the high septum/outflow tract, as shown in Figure 17.4.

Some Practical Considerations

In some cases where there has been a pacemaker already positioned at the left subclavicular region, we have had to change the pacemaker position to the right side to allow implantation of the active can in the left pectoral area. However, it seems that placement of the ICD shell on the right side does not preclude effective defibrillation.

As the actual device technology offers mainly VVI or VVI(R) pacing, and since 100% pacing leads to reduction in device longevity, we prefer to implant a separate pacing unit, either a VVI(R) or a dual-chamber pacemaker.

Numerous interactions between the pacemaker and ICD may occur that have a potentially negative impact. Table 17.1 summarizes some of the interactions systematically.

If for sensing the ICD uses two widely spaced electrodes (as in integrated bipolar sensing), sensing of a pacemaker stimulus may occur more easily; in closely spaced, true bipolar electrodes this is less likely. Owing to sensing dysfunction during VF, the pacemaker may continue to deliver stimuli (Figure 17.3).

To prevent crosstalk between a pacemaker and an ICD, rigorous testing is mandatory. The principle is to programme the worst conditions for the crosstalk function to be tested. It might be best to start with testing of the ICD function, as the ICD must function correctly and VVI pacing is available in ICDs in any case. Interaction testing should start only when good sensing and pacing values have been obtained and after definitive placement of the ICD lead. To exclude double-counting by T-wave sensing during VVI pacing, the ICD detection sensitivity should be programmed to its most sensitive level and then categorization of the detected rhythm is noted. One has to keep in mind that the amplitude of the repolarization might fluctuate during follow-up. One has also to test whether the ICD detects the pacemaker spike or the ventricular response (evoked potential). If the pacemaker spike is detected, double-counting may occur and provoke a response by the ICD. If, for example, antitachycardia pacing is programmed as VT therapy, real ventricular tachycardia might result.

With the pacemaker sensitivity programmed to its least sensitive level, ventricular fibrillation should be induced to check whether the pacemaker is inhibited. If it is not, the sensitivity threshold for pacing inhibition should be assessed. A maximum output shock of the ICD should be delivered to make sure that the pacemaker is not reset by the high-voltage discharge. The post-shock pacing interval should be programmed to an escape interval that guarantees effective capture after the shock. Again VF should be induced to check that ventricular pacing during VF does not inhibit VF detection by the ICD and delay charging. This is done by programming the pacemaker to the V00 mode. An autothreshold amplifier feature in some ICDs decreases the sensitivity when signals of large amplitudes such as PM spikes are detected and leads to undersensing of VF.

Table 17.1 Some interactions between pacemakers and ICDs

Rhythm	PM activity	Potential ICD malfunction
Bradycardia	Pacing	T-wave sensing Rate double-counting
VT or VF	Undersensing → ventricular pacing continues	PM spike detection → VT or VF not detected
After high-energy discharge	Resetting of PM to asynchronous (V00) pacing loss of capture	PM spike detection → VT or VF not redetected

The final programming of the two units must be such that the pacemaker is inhibited during ventricular tachyarrhythmias and that there is no detection of pacemaking activity that could enter into a tachycardia detection window. This is of special importance in the case of DDD(R) or VVI(R) pacing.

ICDs having a DDD pacemaker function are now available, that use the atrial channel for detection of supraventricular arrhythmias.

References

1. Fromer M, Schläpfer J, Fischer A, Kappenberger L. Experience with a new implantable pacer-, cardioverter-, defibrillator for the therapy of recurrent sustained ventricular tachyarrhythmias: a step toward a universal tachyarrhythmia control device. *PACE* 1991; **14**: 1288–98.
2. Fromer M, Brachmann J, Block M, Siebels J, Hoffman E, Almendral J, Ohm O, den Dulk K, Coumel P, Camm AJ, *et al.* Efficacy of automatic multimodal device therapy for ventricular tachyarrhythmias as delivered by a new implantable pacing cardioverter–defibrillator: results of a European multicenter study incorporating 102 implants. *Circulation* 1992; **86**: 363–74.
3. Bayes de Luna A, Coumel P, Leclercq J. Ambulatory sudden cardiac death: mechanisms of production of fatal arrhythmia on the basis of data from 157 cases. *Am Heart J* 1989; **117**: 151–9.
4. Luu M, Stevenson WG, Stevenson LW, Baron K, Walden J. Diverse mechanisms of unexpected cardiac arrest in advanced heart failure. *Circulation* 1989; **80**: 1675–80.
5. Winkle RA, Mead RH, Ruder MA, Gaudiani VA, Smith NA, Buch WS, Schmidt P, Shipman T. Long-term outcome with the automatic implantable cardioverter–defibrillator. *JACC* 1989; **13**: 1353–61.
6. Calkins H, Brinker J, Veltri EP, Guarnieri T, Levine JH. Clinical interactions between pacemakers and automatic implantable cardioverter–defibrillators. *JACC* 1990; **16**: 666–73.
7. Brooks R, Garan H, McGovern BA, Ruskin JN. Implantation of transvenous nonthoracotomy cardioverter–defibrillator systems in patients with permanent endocardial pacemakers. *Am Heart J* 1995; **129**: 45–53.
8. Kelly PA, Mann DE, Damle RS, Reiter MJ. Oversensing during ventricular pacing in patients with a third-generation implantable cardioverter–defibrillator. *JACC* 1994; **23**: 1531–4.
9. Cohen AI, Wish MH, Fletcher RD, Miller FC, McCormick D, Shuck J, Shapira N, Delnegro A. The use and interaction of permanent pacemakers and the automatic implantable cardioverter defibrillator. *PACE* 1988; **11**: 704–11.
10. Callans DJ, Hook BG, Kleiman RB, Mitra RL, Flores BT, Marchlinski FE. Unique sensing errors in third-generation implantable cardioverter–defibrillators. *JACC* 1993; **22**: 1135–40.

Index

.